STATISTICAL METHODS FOR HEALTH CARE RESEARCH

Second Edition

Barbara Hazard Munro, PhD, FAAN

Dean and Professor
Boston College School of Nursing
Chestnut Hill, Massachusetts

Ellis Batten Page, EdD, MA

Professor
Educational Psychology and Research
Duke University
Durham, North Carolina

J. B. LIPPINCOTT COMPANY   Philadelphia

Sponsoring Editor: David P. Carroll
Coordinating Editorial Assistant: Patty L. Shear
Indexer: Ann Cassar
Design Coordinator: Melissa Olson
Interior Design: Susan Hess Blaker
Cover Designer: Lou Fuiano
Production Manager: Helen Ewan
Production Coordinator: Maura C. Murphy
Compositor: Circle Graphics
Printer/Binder: R.R. Donnelley & Sons Company, Crawfordsville
Cover Printer: R.R. Donnelley & Sons Company, Crawfordsville

Second Edition

The educational software that accompanies this text is MYSTAT, a registered trademark of SYSTAT, Inc., Evanston, Illinois. Copyright © 1988–1991, SYSTAT, Inc.

6 5 4 3 2

Library of Congress Cataloging in Publications Data

Munro, Barbara Hazard.
    Statistical methods for health care research / Barbara Hazard
Munro, Ellis Batten Page. — 2nd ed.
        p.   cm.
    Includes bibliographical references and index.
    ISBN 0-397-54982-2
        1. Nursing—Research—Statistical methods.   2. Medical care—
Research—Statistical methods.   I. Page, Ellis Batten.
        [DNLM: 1. Health Services Research—methods.   2. Statistics. WA
950 M968s]
    RT81.5.M86   1993
    610′ .72—dc20
    DNLM/DLC
    for Library of Congress   92-48308
                                                                        CIP

Any procedure or practice described in this book should be applied by the healthcare practitioner under appropriate supervision in accordance with professional standards of care used with regard to the unique circumstances that apply in each practice situation. Care has been taken to confirm the accuracy of information presented and to describe generally accepted practices. However, the authors, editors, and publisher cannot accept any responsibility for errors or omissions or for any consequences from application of the information in this book and make no warranty express or implied, with respect to the contents of the book.

Every effort has been made to ensure drug selections and dosages are in accordance with current recommendations and practice. Because of ongoing research, changes in government regulations and the constant flow of information on drug therapy, reactions and interactions, the reader is cautioned to check the package insert for each drug for indications, dosages, warnings and precautions, particularly if the drug is new or infrequently used.

Contributors

Leonard Braitman, PhD
Biostatistician
Office for Research Development
Albert Einstein Medical Center
Philadelphia, Pennsylvania

Jane Karpe Dixon, PhD
Associate Professor
Yale University School of Nursing
New Haven, Connecticut

Mairead L. Hickey, PhD, RN
Nurse Researcher and Manager
Nursing Research Program
Brigham and Women's Hospital
Boston, Massachusetts

Barbara S. Jacobsen, MS
Professor
University of Pennsylvania School of Nursing
Philadelphia, Pennsylvania

Acknowledgments

We would like to acknowledge the students who have heard our lectures and used our book for their input into the development of our ideas about how to teach statistical concepts. They include students from Schools of Nursing at Boston College, Yale University, and the University of Pennsylvania; and students at Duke University. Additionally, we would like to acknowledge the contributions of Madelon A. Visintainer to the first edition.

Preface

The purpose of the first edition of *Statistical Methods for Health Care Research* was to acquaint the reader with the statistical techniques most commonly reported in the research literature of the health professions. In that edition we attempted to keep mathematical calculations to a minimum and used computer printouts and examples from the literature to demonstrate specific techniques.

In this edition our purpose remains the same. We have added additional techniques, reduced even further the amount of calculations, and increased the emphasis on interpretation of computer printouts. All chapters have been revised and updated. New contributors have joined us. Professor Barbara S. Jacobsen from the University of Pennsylvania School of Nursing has written new chapters on organizing and displaying data, univariate descriptive statistics, and a section on probability. Her reputation as an outstanding teacher is evidenced in her work. Dr. Leonard E. Braitman, a biostatistician employed at the Office for Research Development, Albert Einstein Medical Center, Philadelphia, has contributed an in-depth look at confidence intervals and interpretation of the clinical and statistical significance of research results. Dr. Mairaid L. Hickey, Nurse Researcher at Brigham and Women's Hospital in Boston, has written a very clear description of structural equation models and latent variables. Her step-by-step description of the process with accompanying computer printouts makes these complex analyses understandable.

Dr. Jane K. Dixon, Associate Professor at Yale University School of Nursing and a contributor to the first edition, has updated and revised her chapter on factor analysis, which now includes a description of confirmatory factor analysis. Dr. Ellis B. Page, Professor at Duke University and second author of the text, has revised his chapter on path analysis. Additionally, sections on nonparametric techniques and multivariate analysis of variance (MANOVA) have been added, as well as a new chapter on logistic regression.

We would like to thank the users and reviewers of the first edition who made helpful suggestions for this second edition. In particular we would like to thank Dr. Mary E. Duffy, Director of the Center for Nursing Research at Boston College, for her input.

Contents

SECTION 2   SPECIFIC STATISTICAL TECHNIQUES

BIBLIOGRAPHY   321

APPENDICES

INDEX   393

I | UNDERSTANDING THE DATA

1

Organizing and Displaying Data

Barbara S. Jacobsen

OBJECTIVES FOR CHAPTER 1

After reading this chapter you should be able to do the following:

1. **Discuss levels of measurement and their relationship to statistical analysis.**

2. **Interpret a frequency distribution created by a computer program.**

3. **Organize data into a table.**

4. **Interpret data presented in a graph.**

MEASUREMENT SCALES

The raw materials of research are data. To obtain data, researchers must measure characteristics of people or objects. Measurement, in the broadest sense, is the assignment of numerals to objects or events according to a set of rules (Stevens, 1946). For example the width of a piece of paper can be measured by following a set of rules for placing a graduated straightedge and then reading the numeral that corresponds to the concept of *width*. This definition can be broadened to include the assignment of numerals to abstract, intangible concepts such as empathy. After a method of measurement for a concept is decided on, the concept is then called a variable, that is, a measured characteristic that takes on different values.

Stevens (1946) noted four types of measurement scales for variables: nominal, ordinal, interval, and ratio. When analyzing data the first task is to be aware of the type of measurement scale for each of the variables, because this knowledge helps in deciding how to organize and display data.

Barbara Hazard Munro and Ellis Batten Page: STATISTICAL METHODS FOR HEALTH CARE RESEARCH, SECOND EDITION. © 1993, 1986 by J. B. Lippincott Company.

Nominal Scales

The best a researcher can do to measure this type of scale is to classify characteristics of people or objects into categories. Sometimes nominal variables are referred to as categorical or qualitative. Numeric values may be assigned to the categories as labels for computer storage, but the choice of numerals for those labels is absolutely arbitrary. Some examples follow:

Variable	Values
Group membership	1 = Experimental
	2 = Placebo
	3 = Routine
Sex	1 = Male
	2 = Female
Compliance	1 = Kept appointment
	2 = Did not keep appointment

Ordinal Scales

In this case the characteristics can not only be put into categories, but the categories also can be ordered; that is, the assignment of numerals is not arbitrary. The distance between the categories, however, is unknown. For example, in a horse race the results are reported in terms of which horse was first, which was second, and which was third. For the record books and for the bettor, it is irrelevant whether the winning horse won by a nose or by several lengths. Some other examples follow:

Variables	Values
Rank in army	1 = Private
	2 = Corporal
	3 = Sergeant
	4 = Lieutenant
Socioeconomic status	1 = Low
	2 = Middle
	3 = High
Attitude scale	1 = Strongly agree
	2 = Agree
	3 = Neutral
	4 = Disagree
	5 = Strongly disagree

Interval Scales

For this type of scale the distances between the values are equal because there is some accepted physical unit of measurement. In a Fahrenheit thermometer, mercury rises in equal intervals called degrees. However, the zero point is arbitrary, chosen simply because Daniel Gabriel Fahrenheit, the inventor, decided that the zero point on his scale would be 32° below the freezing point of water. Because the units are in equal intervals, it is possible to add and subtract across an interval scale. You can say that 100°F is 50° warmer than 50°F, but you cannot say that 100°F is twice as hot as 50°F.

Interval variables may be continuous (i.e., in theory there are no gaps between the values), or they may be discrete (i.e., there are gaps in the values). The Fahrenheit scale is considered to be continuous because only our eyesight or the quality of the measuring instrument prevents us from reading the scale in more finely graduated divisions. In contrast, parity of a woman is a discrete interval variable, because the number of children borne is obtained by counting indivisible units (children).

Ratio Scales

The zero point for these variables is not arbitrary but determined by nature. On the Kelvin temperature scale, zero represents the absence of molecular motion. Weight and blood pressure are other examples of ratio variables. Because the zero point is not arbitrary, it is possible to multiply and divide across a ratio scale. Thus, it is possible to say that 100°K is twice as hot as 50°K. The distinction between interval and ratio variables is interesting, but for the purposes of this text, these two types of variables are handled the same way in analyzing data.

Issues Concerning Measurement Scales

What type of measurement scale are variables resulting from psychological inventories and tests of knowledge? Certainly they have arbitrary zero points as determined by the inventor of each scale, and they have no accepted unit of measurement comparable to the degree on a temperature scale. Technically, these variables are ordinal, yet in practice researchers often think of them as interval. This has been a controversial issue in the research literature for years. Gardner (1975) reviewed the early literature on this conflict, and Knapp (1990) has commented on more recent literature. In his original article on measurement (1946) and in a later article (1968), Stevens noted that treating ordinal scales as interval or ratio scales may violate a technical canon, but in many instances the outcome had demonstrable use. More recently, Knapp (1990) pointed out that such considerations as measurement perspective, the number of categories that comprise an ordinal scale, and the concept of *meaningfulness* may all be important in deciding whether to treat a variable as ordinal or interval. We recommend the articles by Stevens (1946), Gardner (1975), and Knapp (1990) for further reading on this topic.

Interval or ratio variables can be converted to ordinal or nominal variables. For example diastolic blood pressure, as measured by a sphygmomanometer, is a ratio variable. However, if, for research purposes, blood pressure is recorded as either controlled or uncontrolled, then it is a nominal variable. In this case there is a physiological basis for such a dichotomous division, but when no such reason exists, converting interval or ratio variables to nominal or ordinal variables can be unwise because it results in a loss of information. Cohen (1983) detailed the amount of degradation of measurement as a consequence of dichotomization and urged researchers to fully exploit all of the original measurement information.

UNIVARIATE ANALYSIS

As the first step in organizing data, researchers should examine each variable separately, whether these variables are demographic, prognostic, group membership, or outcomes. Univariate analyses are helpful in cleaning and checking the quality of data, examining the variability of data, describing the sample, and checking statistical assumptions prior to more complex analyses. In some cases data analysis may end here; perhaps your research questions can be answered solely by univariate analyses.

TABLE 1-1
Example of Frequency Distribution Produced by SPSS*:
Stage of Breast Cancer in a Sample of 189 Patients

Program
FREQUENCIES VARIABLES = STAGE.

Output
STAGE   Stage of disease

Value Label	Value	Frequency	Percent	Valid Percent	Cum Percent
Zero	1	8	4.2	4.2	4.1
Stage 1	2	94	49.7	49.7	53.9
Stage 2A	3	50	26.5	26.5	80.4
Stage 2B	4	15	7.9	7.9	88.3
Stage 3A	5	7	3.7	3.7	92.0
Stage 3B	6	9	4.8	4.8	96.8
Stage 4	7.	6	3.2	3.2	100.0
	Total	189	100.0	100.0	

Valid cases, 189; Missing cases, 0

(Lowery, B. J., Jacobsen, B. S., & Ducette, J. [1992]. Causal attributions, control and adjustment to breast cancer. Psychosocial Oncology, 10,4.)
* Statistical Package for the Social Sciences

Tables

When data are organized into values or categories and then described with titles and captions, the result is called a statistical table. A researcher begins to construct a table by tabulating data into a frequency distribution, that is, by counting how frequently each value or category occurs.

For nominal and ordinal variables, the categories should be listed (in some natural order if possible) and then the frequencies indicated for each category. Table 1-1 is an example of such a table, as produced by a computer, for the ordinal variable of stage of breast cancer at diagnosis. It is helpful to have the percentage falling into each category. The reader can then quickly perceive that the majority of subjects in this sample were either stage 1 or stage 2A.

For interval or ratio variables, an ordered array of values (Table 1-2) is usually the first step in constructing a table. This frequency distribution table might be termed a *working table*. If the difference between the maximum and the minimum value is greater than 15, you may want to group the data into classes or categories before

TABLE 1-2
Example of Frequency Distribution (Condensed) Produced by SPSS: Age of 113 Hysterectomy Patients

Program
FREQUENCIES VARIABLES = AGE.

Output
AGE

Value Labels	Frequency	Value Labels	Frequency	Value Labels	Frequency
29	1	44	6	59	1
30	2	45	6	60	3
32	1	46	5	61	1
33	1	47	8	62	1
34	2	48	7	63	1
35	1	49	4	66	1
36	2	50	3	69	1
37	2	51	1	70	1
38	2	52	1	71	2
39	5	53	3	73	1
40	4	54	2	75	1
41	2	56	3	77	1
42	12	57	2	78	1
43	7	58	1		

(Data collected in program grant funded by the National Center for Nursing Research, PO1-NR1859. P.I., D. Brooten, Early Hospital Discharge and Nurse Specialist Followup.)

forming the final table (this also may be true for some ordinal variables). In Table 1-2 the range in age is from 29 to 78 years; therefore, grouping the values will make the data more comprehensible.

As the next step the computer printout for Table 1-3 shows a frequency distribution for the same data, with the values grouped into 11 classes, each having an interval (or width) of 5 years. Note that the top class began with 25, and the bottom class ended with 79, although no one in the sample was that young or that old. This was done to keep the lower limit for each interval divisible by 5 and to keep the classes of equal width. Again, it is most helpful to know the percentage falling into each class.

It is clear from Table 1-3 that the majority of people in this sample were 40 to 49 years of age. In this computer printout, the column labeled "valid percent" gives the

TABLE 1-3
Example of Frequency Distribution Produced by SPSS: Age of 113 Hysterectomy Patients

Program
RECODE AGE (LO THRU 29 = 1) (30 THRU 34 = 2) (35 THRU 39 = 3) (40 THRU 44 = 4) (45 THRU 49 = 5) (50 THRU 54 = 6) (55 THRU 59 = 7) (60 THRU 64 = 8) (65 THRU 69 = 9) (70 THRU 74 = 10) (75 THRU HI = 11).
VALUE LABELS AGE 1 '25–29' 2 '30–34' 3 '35–39' 4 '40–44' 5 '45–49' 6 '50–54' 7 '55–59' 8 '60–64' 9 '65–69' 10 '70–74' 11 '75–79'.
FREQUENCIES VARIABLES = AGE.

Output
AGE

Value Label	Value	Frequency	Percent	Valid Percent	Cum Percent
25–29	1	1	.9	.9	.9
30–34	2	6	5.3	5.4	6.3
35–39	3	12	10.6	10.7	17.0
40–44	4	31	27.4	27.7	44.6
45–49	5	30	26.5	26.8	71.4
50–54	6	10	8.8	8.9	80.4
55–59	7	7	6.2	6.3	86.6
60–64	8	6	5.3	5.4	92.0
65–69	9	2	1.8	1.8	93.8
70–74	10	4	3.5	3.6	97.3
75–79	11	3	2.7	2.7	100.0
		1	.9	MISSING	
	Total	113	100.0	100.0	

Valid cases, 112; Missing cases, 1

(Data collected in program grant funded by the National Center for Nursing Research, PO1-NR1859. P.I., D. Brooten, Early Hospital Discharge and Nurse Specialist Followup.)

percentages for each category with missing data excluded. The column labeled "cum percent" refers to cumulative percentages, again with missing values excluded; this enables the reader to see quickly that approximately 80% of this sample were 54 years of age or younger.

Computer programs can group values for you; however, some programs have defaults for the interval width and the number of classes that can result in an inconveniently constructed table. Most statistical programs allow you to control the choice of interval and the number of classes. Most people find that using a multiple of 5 for the interval width is helpful because it is easier to think about numbers that are divisible by 5. Authorities differ somewhat on their recommendations for the number of classes: Freedman and colleagues (1991) suggest 10 to 15 classes; Freund (1988) suggests six to 15 classes; and Ott and Mendenhall (1990) suggest five to 20 classes. Too few or too many classes will obscure important features of a frequency distribution. Of course some detail is lost by grouping the values, but information is gained about clustering and the shape of the distribution.

The final presentation of the data from Table 1-3 depends on the format requirements of each journal or of the dissertation. Table 1-4 illustrates one possible way of presenting the frequency distribution for the ages of a sample in a research report. Once you have decided that you need a table to present your data, that table should be mentioned in the text of the research report. The discussion of a table should reinforce the major points for which the table was developed (Burns & Grove, 1987). Researchers

TABLE 1-4
Frequency Distribution for Age in a Sample of Hysterectomy Patients From an Urban Medical Center (N = 113)

Age	Frequency	Percent
25–29	1	.9
30–34	6	5.3
35–39	12	10.6
40–45	31	27.4
45–49	30	26.5
50–54	10	8.8
55–59	7	6.2
60–64	6	5.3
65–69	6	5.3
70–74	4	3.5
75–79	3	2.7
	112	100.0

Note. Age was not recorded in the medical chart for one patient.

(Data collected in program grant funded by the National Center for Nursing Research, PO1–NR1859. P.I., D. Brooten, Early Hospital Discharge and Nurse Specialist Followup.)

should comment on the important patterns in the table, as well as the major exceptions (Chatfield, 1988) but should not rehash every fact in the table.

Suggestions for the Construction of Tables for Research Reports

1. Use tables only to highlight major facts. Most of the tables examined by researchers while analyzing their data do not need to be published in a journal. If a finding can be described well in words, then a table is unnecessary. Too many tables can overwhelm the rest of a research report (Burns & Grove, 1987).
2. Make the table as self-explanatory as possible. The patterns and exceptions in a table should be obvious at a glance once the reader has been told what they are (Ehrenberg, 1977). With this goal in mind, the title should state the variable; when and where the data were collected, if pertinent; and the size of the sample. Headings within the table should be brief but clear.
3. Find out the required format for tables in your research report. If you are aiming for a particular journal, examine tables in past issues. Follow the advice about table format for publication in a manual of style, such as the *Publication Manual of the American Psychological Association* (1983).

Graphs

Wainer and Thissen (1981) aptly quote two 19th century scientists as saying, "Getting information from a table is like extracting sunlight from a cucumber." Graphs, on the other hand, can quickly reveal facts about data that might only be gleaned from a table after careful study. They are often the most effective way to describe, explore, and summarize a set of numbers (Tufte, 1983). Graphs are the visual representations of frequency distributions. They give us a global, bird's-eye view of the data and thus help us to gain insight.

There were 75 graphs of data published in *Nursing Research*, *Research in Nursing and Health*, and *Western Journal of Nursing Research* in 1990 and 1991 (excluding charts and diagrams). These 75 graphs were contained in 38 articles, representing 15% of all the research articles published in these journals during that time. Although tables are published much more frequently than graphs, researchers examine many "working" graphs of their data without necessarily attempting to publish them. Some of the most commonly used types of graph for univariate analysis are discussed in this section. More complex graphs are discussed in subsequent sections.

Bar Graph

Bar graphs are the proper type of graph for nominal or ordinal data. When constructing such graphs, the category labels usually are listed horizontally in some systematic order, and then vertical bars are drawn to represent the frequency or percent in each category. A space separates each of the bars to emphasize the nominal or ordinal nature of the variable. The choice of spacing and width of the bars is at the discretion of the researcher, but once chosen, all the spacing and the widths of the bars should be equal.

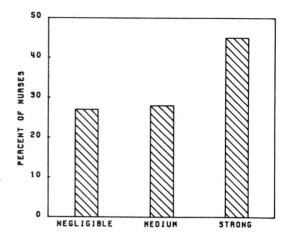

FIGURE 1-1
Degree of emphasis on the nurse as a sex object in motion pictures, 1930–1980 (N = 211). (From Kalisch, B. J., Kalisch, P. A., & McHugh, M. L. [1982]. *Research in Nursing and Health, 5,* 150.)

Figure 1-1 is an example of a bar graph for ordinal data. If the category labels are lengthy, it can be more convenient to list the categories vertically and draw the bars horizontally, as in Figure 1-2. Bar graphs also facilitate comparisons between univariate distributions. Two or more univariate distributions can be compared using a cluster bar graph. Figure 1-3 is an example of such a graph. The current generation of computer graphics, statistics, and spreadsheet programs offer many tempting patterns for filling in the bars, but the researcher should stay away from shading and cross-hatchings that tire the eye or cause illusion effects (Tufte, 1983). Note that the legend explaining Figure 1-3 is outside the graph to avoid clutter (Cleveland, 1985).

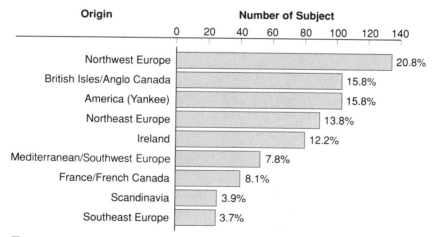

FIGURE 1-2
Claimed region of ethnic origin (N = 645). (From Clinton, J. [1982]. The development of an empirical construct for cross-cultural health research. *Western Journal of Nursing Research, 4,* 281.)

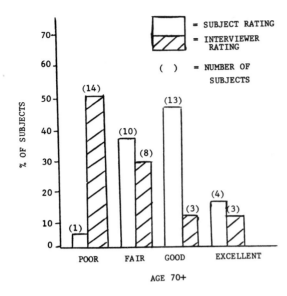

FIGURE 1-3
Subject and interviewer ratings of physical health of the older bereaved. (From Valanis, B. G., & Yeaworth, R. [1982]. Ratings of physical and mental health in the older bereaved. *Research in Nursing and Health, 5*, 142.)

Histogram

Histograms are appropriate for interval and ratio variables and sometimes ordinal variables. These graphs are similar to bar graphs, but the bars are placed side by side. The area of each bar represents frequency or percent; therefore, each histogram has a total area of 100%. The first decision in constructing a histogram is to decide on the number of bars. If there are too few bars, the data will be clumped together; if there are too many bars, the data will be overly detailed. Figure 1-4 shows how the choice for the number of bars affects the appearance of a histogram. The top graph presents a jagged appearance; the bottom graph clumps the data into only five bars and makes the data seem quite skewed. The middle graph, with 10 bars, presents a smoother appearance.

Computer programs are handy for a preliminary graph of a variable, but a researcher should be aware of built-in defaults and should think about the adjustments that are necessary. The advice of the previous section for constructing frequency distributions for interval or ratio variables is helpful here. For example examine the maximum and minimum values, and if the difference is larger than 15, consider grouping the data. Try to choose an interval and a starting point that are divisible by 5. You will find that most histograms have between five and 20 bars.

For discrete interval or ratio variables, the numerals representing the values should be centered below each bar to emphasize the discrete nature of the variable. Figure 1-5 illustrates a histogram for the discrete variable of parity (number of births). For continuous variables the numerals representing the values should be placed at the sides of the bars to emphasize the continuous nature of the distribution.* Figure 1-6 illustrates

---

* *The grouping interval of 25 to 29 has a lower limit of 25 and an upper limit of 29. These are called the written limits. The real or mathematical limits are understood to extend half a unit above and below the written class limits. For convenience, researchers almost always use the written class limits in tables and graphs.*

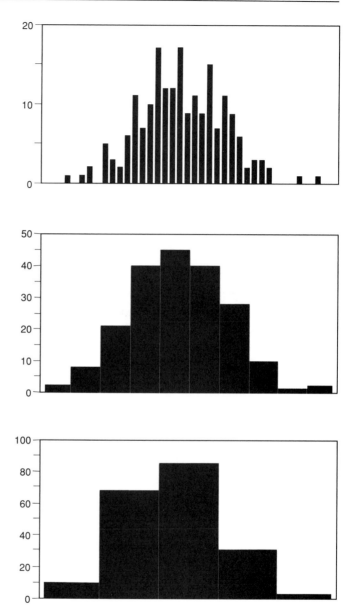

FIGURE 1-4

Illustration of the importance of the number of bars in designing a histogram for a set of data.

a histogram for the continuous variable of age given previously in Table 1-4. Note that tick marks are placed outside the data region to avoid clutter (Cleveland, 1985).

Once the number of bars has been determined, the next decision is the height of the vertical axis. Tufte (1983) recommends, if the graphic is horizontal, a height of approximately half the width. Other authorities, such as Schmid (1983), recommend a height approximately two-thirds to three-fourths the width. The reason for these recommendations is the different effect that can be produced by altering the height of a graph.

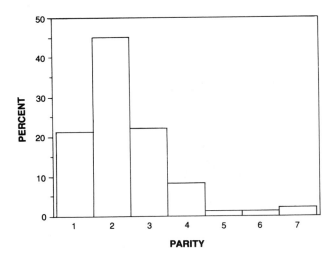

FIGURE 1-5
Number of previous births in a sample of women having cesarean deliveries ($N = 123$). Data collected in program grant funded by National Center for Nursing Research, PO1-NR1859. P.I., D. Brooten: *Early Hospital Discharge and Nurse Specialist Followup*.

Figure 1-7 shows the different impressions that can be created by a tall, narrow graph and a flat, wide graph. The tall, narrow graph seems to emphasize the clustering of the data in the middle, while the flat, wide graph seems to emphasize the scatter of the data to the right. For comparison the graph of the same data in Figure 1-6 is proportioned correctly.

Polygon

A graph for interval or ratio variables, which is equivalent to the histogram but appears smoother, is the polygon. For any set of data the histogram and the polygon will have equivalent total areas of 100%. The polygon is constructed by joining the midpoints of the top of each bar of the histogram and then closing the polygon at both ends by

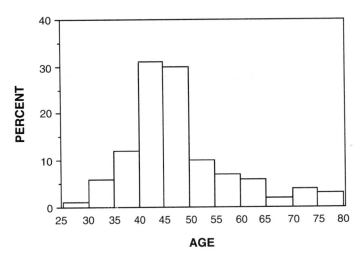

FIGURE 1-6
Histogram of age in a sample of hysterectomy patients from an urban medical center ($N = 112$). Data collected in program grant funded by National Center for Nursing Research, PO1-NR1859. P.I., D. Brooten: *Early Hospital Discharge and Nurse Specialist Followup*.

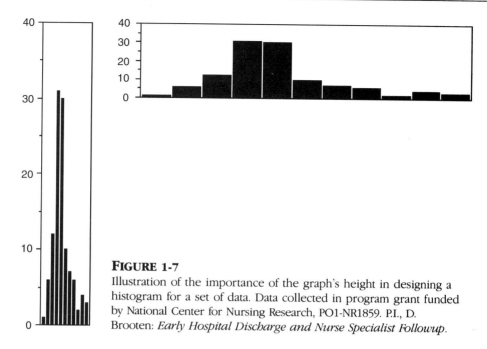

FIGURE 1-7
Illustration of the importance of the graph's height in designing a histogram for a set of data. Data collected in program grant funded by National Center for Nursing Research, PO1-NR1859. P.I., D. Brooten: *Early Hospital Discharge and Nurse Specialist Followup*.

extending lines to imaginary midpoints at the left and right of the histogram. Figure 1-8 illustrates a polygon superimposed on a histogram. In the process of construction, triangles of area were removed from the histogram, but congruent triangles were added to the polygon. Two such congruent triangles are shaded in Figure 1-8 to show why the areas of the two types of graph are equivalent.

Polygons are especially appropriate for comparing two univariate distributions by superimposing them. Figure 1-9 shows such a comparison. Note that percentages were used on the vertical scale because the sizes of the two samples were different.

FIGURE 1-8
Polygon superimposed on histogram shown in Figure 1-6. The two shaded triangles are congruent. Data collected in program grant funded by National Center for Nursing Research, PO1-NR1859. P.I., D. Brooten: *Early Hospital Discharge and Nurse Specialist Followup*.

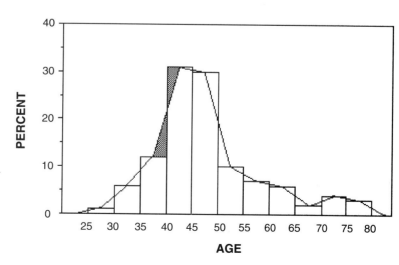

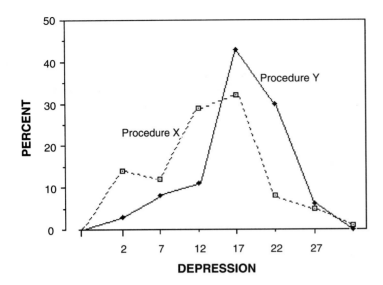

FIGURE 1-9
Comparison of depression scores for patients having surgical procedure X ($N = 104$) and surgical procedure Y ($N = 61$). (Hypothetical data)

What to Look for in a Histogram or Polygon

A graph can help us see quickly the shape of a distribution. Frequency distributions have many possible shapes. Often they have a bell-shaped appearance as in the computer printout in Figure 1-10. In this case heart attack patients were rated for denial on a summated inventory of 24 items, with each item rated for evidence of denial on a seven-point scale. Technically, such a scale is ordinal, because there is no accepted physical unit of "denial," and the zero point is arbitrary. An ordinal scale with such a large range, however, is usually treated as interval in the research literature. In Figure 1-10 the frequency count is given at the left, and the midpoint of each class is listed directly beside each bar. The programmer chose an interval width of 5 with a starting point of 10. Thus, the first class is 10 to 15, and the midpoint of that class is 12.5. In addition, the programmer instructed the computer to plot the bell-shaped (normal) curve atop the histogram with a series of dots. The reader can then visually compare the distribution of denial with the theoretical bell-shaped curve. Distributions also may be skewed, as in Figure 1-11. Occasionally, data may clump at several places, as in Figure 1-12. These graphs also can be helpful in spotting where the data cluster, how the data are scattered around the clustering points, whether there are far-out observations that may be outliers, and if there are gaps in the data. These are the kinds of features that researchers need to know about, and they become immediately evident with simple graphic representation (Cohen, 1990). With the assistance of a computer, a researcher has no excuse for failing to know his or her data (Jacobsen, 1981). As with tables, all graphs included in a research report should be referred to in the accompanying text, and the important features of the distribution should be commented on in the text.

General Suggestions for Constructing Graphs

The purpose of graphing is to promote understanding without distorting the facts; therefore, you should be sure your graph makes the point you want to make *fairly*. Because gross misuses of graphs are not generally found in respected research journals,

Program

FREQUENCIES VARIABLES = DENIAL/HISTOGRAM = NORMAL INCREMENT (5)
MINIMUM (10) MAXIMUM (90).

Output

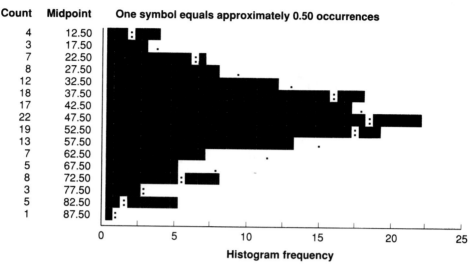

Count	Midpoint	One symbol equals approximately 0.50 occurrences
4	12.50	
3	17.50	
7	22.50	
8	27.50	
12	32.50	
18	37.50	
17	42.50	
22	47.50	
19	52.50	
13	57.50	
7	62.50	
5	67.50	
8	72.50	
3	77.50	
5	82.50	
1	87.50	

Histogram frequency

FIGURE 1-10

Example of histogram produced by SPSS: Denial scores from a sample of 152 heart attack patients. (Jacobsen, B. S., & Lowery, B. J. [1992]. Further analysis of the psychometric properties of the Levine Denial of Illness Scale. *Psychosomatic Medicine, 54*, 372–381.)

some researchers believe that attention to the construction of graphs is not really necessary because editors and reviewers will tell them how to fix them. We urge you to read some of the references on graphing listed at the end of this chapter and follow their advice instead of having your research report rejected. Schmid (1983) listed the following five characteristics of a good graph:

1. *Accuracy*—If you are using computer graphics software, be sure the data have been entered properly. The graph should not be misleading in any way nor be susceptible to misinterpretation. The best advice is to try out the graph on several people, including some who are not involved in your study. Ask them, "What does this graph say to you?"
2. *Simplicity*—The graph should be straightforward, not a puzzle. It should not present a cluttered appearance and should not have any "chartjunk" (Tufte, 1983). Grid lines and tick marks should be kept to a minimum, and elements such as odd lettering or ornate patterns should be avoided.
3. *Clarity*—The graph should be unambiguous and easily understood. The title and axes should be clearly labeled and the scale carefully chosen.
4. *Appearance*—The graph should not be sloppy but should be appealing.
5. *Well-designed structure*—The graph should conform to certain basic principles of perception. The more important elements should be emphasized visually, and the

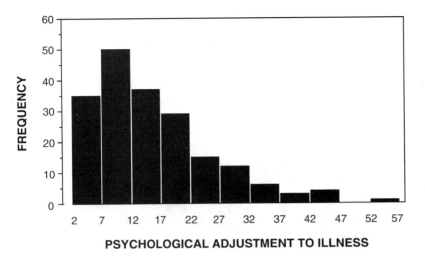

FIGURE 1-11
Histogram for psychological
adjustment to illness by 195
patients with breast cancer
(higher scores indicate poorer
adjustment). (Lowery, B. J.,
Jacobsen, B. S., & Ducette, J.
[1992]. Causal attribution,
control, and adjustment to
breast cancer. *Psychosocial
Oncology*.)

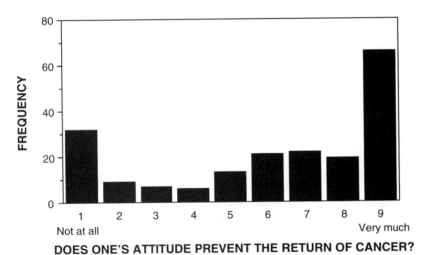

FIGURE 1-12
Responses by 195 breast cancer patients to the question of
whether attitude will help to
prevent a recurrence of
cancer. Data collected in grant
funded by National Center
for Nursing Research, RO1-
NR01897. P.I., B. J. Lowery. *Attributions, control, and adjustment to breast cancer*.

less important should be in the background. For example if you are going to have grid lines, they should be comparatively light. Tufte (1983) suggests that the bars be dark and the grid lines be white (see Fig. 1-10). Tufte (1983) also recommends, if possible, that all lettering be horizontal because it is easier to read.

SUMMARY

Florence Nightingale was able to affect public policy because she appreciated the importance of collecting data and presenting it in an interesting and striking fashion. She even used colored pencils to add emphasis to her graphs. Today, with computer graphics, we have the technology to assist with the organization and presentation of our data.

2

Univariate Descriptive Statistics

Barbara S. Jacobsen

OBJECTIVES FOR CHAPTER 2

After reading this chapter you should be able to do the following:

1. **Define measures of central tendency and dispersion.**
2. **Select the appropriate measures to use for a particular data set.**
3. **Discuss methods to identify and manage outliers.**

INTRODUCTION

Graphs may bring facts to life vividly, but the information they offer for our inspection is often inexact. Frequency distribution tables provide many details, but often a researcher will want to condense a distribution further. After the data have been organized, quantitative measures are frequently calculated to capture the essence of the four basic characteristics of a distribution: central tendency, variability, skewness, and kurtosis. These statistics may be used not only in a descriptive summary, but also in statistical inference. Symbols and formulas for descriptive statistics vary depending on whether one is describing a sample or a population. A *population* includes all members of a defined group; a *sample* is a subset of a population. It is important to distinguish between these. An instructor who is grading an examination given to a class of students ordinarily views that class as a population. A researcher who plans to publish a report on denial in heart attack patients may interview patients from a single urban hospital but may view those patients as a sample of all heart attack patients from that type of hospital or that geographic area.

Characteristics of populations are called *parameters*; characteristics of samples are called *statistics*. To distinguish between them, different sets of symbols are used. Usually, lower case Greek letters are used to denote parameters, and Roman letters are used to denote statistics.

Barbara Hazard Munro and Ellis Batten Page: STATISTICAL METHODS FOR HEALTH CARE RESEARCH, SECOND EDITION. © 1993, 1986 by J. B. Lippincott Company.

MEASURES OF CENTRAL TENDENCY

These statistics, commonly referred to as averages, describe where the values of a distribution cluster. The three measures of central tendency that will be discussed in this text are the mean, the median, and the mode.

Mean

The *mean*, the most widely used average, locates the center of gravity or fulcrum of a distribution. This measure of central tendency does not necessarily imply that 50% of the data are below average, because a center of gravity may not be located in the middle.

The mean of a sample* is represented symbolically by $\overline{X}$, which is read "X bar." Many journals simply use "M" to represent the mean. To compute the mean, add up all the values and divide by the number of values. Expressed as a formula, the sample mean is defined as:

$$\overline{X} = \frac{\Sigma X}{N}$$

The upper case Greek letter sigma (Σ) means "the sum of." If the letter X represents a single quantitative value in a distribution, then ΣX means "sum up all the values."

For example the following list of values for length of stay (in hours) for a sample of cesarean births has 10 entries: 61, 70, 112, 74, 104, 97, 85, 132, 125, and 70. The mean is the sum of the values, or $61 + 70 + 112 + 74 + 104 + 97 + 85 + 132 + 125 + 70 = 930$, divided by the number of values, 10, or $930/10 = 93$. In this example the mean is located near the middle of the 10 values. It is clear from the formula and the example that each value in the distribution contributes to the mean. Because the mean is influenced by all of the data points, it is not appropriate as a descriptive statistic for a variable for which all the data points are not known. For instance not everyone with cancer will have a recurrence of that disease; therefore, some of the values of the variable "time to recurrence" may be absent or "censored."

If there are extreme values in the distribution, these also influence the mean. For example in the previous distribution relating to length of stay in hours for a group of women who underwent cesarean delivery, suppose the value of 132 hours was instead 702 hours. The new mean would be $61 + 70 + 112 + 74 + 104 + 97 + 85 + 702 + 125 + 70 = 1500/10 = 150$ hours. This mean would not be located in the middle of the 10 values. Only one patient would have a length of stay greater than the mean. Thus, the mean works best as an average for symmetrical frequency distributions that have a single peak.

The mean has several other interesting properties. First, for any distribution the sum of the deviations of the values from the mean always equals zero. This helps to explain why the mean is the center of gravity or fulcrum of a distribution. Table 2-1 contains a demonstration of this property. The mean (6) is subtracted from each value to

---

* *The mean of a population is represented by the lower case Greek letter mu (μ). The formula is the same as that for the sample mean.*

TABLE 2-1
Demonstration of Several Important Properties of the Mean

X	$X - \bar{X}$	$(X - \bar{X})^2$
4	$4 - 6 = -2$	$(-2)^2 = 4$
4	$4 - 6 = -2$	$(-2)^2 = 4$
10	$10 - 6 = +4$	$(+4)^2 = 16$
5	$5 - 6 = -1$	$(-1)^2 = 1$
7	$7 - 6 = +1$	$(+1)^2 = 1$
$\Sigma X = 30$	$\Sigma(X - \bar{X}) = 0$	$\Sigma(X - \bar{X})^2 = 26$
$N = 5$		sum of squares
$\bar{X} = 6$		

form *deviations* $(X - \bar{X})$. These deviations from the mean sum to zero. If any value other than the mean is subtracted from each value, the sum of the deviations will not be zero. The reader is invited to try subtracting other values, such as the median or the mode, and summing these deviations.

A second property of the mean relates to the sum of the squared deviations, that is, $\Sigma(X - \bar{X})^2$. In Table 2-1 each of the deviations from the mean has been squared, $(X - \bar{X})^2$, and the sum of these squared deviations equals 26. This sum, referred to in statistics as the *sum of squares*, is at a minimum; that is, it is smaller than the sum of squares around any other value. If any value other than the mean (6) is subtracted from each value and squared, the total will be greater than 26. Again, the reader is invited to try subtracting other values, such as the median or the mode. This characteristic of the mean underlies the idea of *least squares*, which is important in later chapters.

Third, because the mean has a formula, it is algebraic and can be manipulated in equations. For example if two or more means are available from samples of different sizes, a mean of the total group can be calculated. By transposing terms in the formula for the mean, the following shows that the sum of the values is equal to the mean multiplied by the size of the sample.

$$\bar{X}N = \Sigma X$$

Therefore, a formula for a combined mean for two samples (which can be easily extended to include more than two samples) weighted according to sample size, logically follows:

$$\bar{X}_{total} = \frac{\bar{X}_1 N_1 + \bar{X}_2 N_2}{N_1 + N_2}$$

Finally, when repeatedly drawing random samples from the same population, means will vary less among themselves and less from the true population mean than other measures of central tendency. Thus, the mean is the most reliable average when making inferences from a sample to a population.

The mean is intended for interval or ratio variables where values can be added, but many times it is also sensible for ordinal variables. Computers, of course, do not know whether variables are interval or ratio or ordinal and will compute means for nominal data, reporting such uninterpretable facts for a sample as "the mean religion = 2.34."

Median

The median is the middle value of a set of ordered numbers. It is the point or value below which 50% of the distribution falls. Thus, 50% of the sample will be below the median, regardless of the shape of the distribution. The median is sometimes referred to as the 50th percentile and symbolized as P_{50}. It may also be thought of as the bisector of the total area of the histogram or polygon. There is no formula for the median, just a procedure:

1. Arrange the values in order.
2. If the total number of values is odd, count up (or down) to the middle value. If there are several identical values clustered at the middle, the median is that value.
3. If the total number of values is even, compute the mean of the middle values.

In the previous example relating to length of stay in cesarean delivery mothers, the 10 values, arranged in order, were 61, 70, 70, 74, 85, 97, 104, 112, 125, 132. Counting to the center of these 10 entries, the two middle values are 85 and 97. Thus, the median is (85 + 97)/2 = 91. Note that the mean for these data was 93, similar to the median.

From the procedure it is clear that every value does not enter into the computation of the median; only the number of values and the values near the midpoint of the distribution enter into the computation. If the value of 132 is changed to 702 in the previous example, the new distribution is 61, 70, 70, 74, 85, 97, 104, 112, 125, 702. The median of this distribution is still located midway between 85 and 97 and is still 91 hours. Thus, the median is not sensitive to extreme scores. It may be used with symmetrical or asymmetrical distributions, but it is especially useful when the data are skewed. This property of not reflecting all of the values in a distribution also can be a disadvantage in that the median is nonalgebraic. Hence, there is no formula for a weighted median. The median is appropriate for interval or ratio data and for ordinal data but not for nominal data. It can be used for open-end or censored data, such as "time to recurrence," if more than half of the sample have contributed a value to the distribution.

Mode

The mode is the most frequent value or category. It may be interpreted as the fashionable score, as in "a la mode." In the previous example of length of stay in hours, the 10 entries were 61, 70, 70, 74, 85, 97, 104, 112, 125, 132. The mode for this distribution is 70 because that is the score that occurs most frequently. The mode is not calculated but simply spotted by inspection, which is easy with a graph or table of ordered values. If all of the scores are different, the mode does not exist. If several values occur with equal frequency, then there are several modes. If the values of a distribution cluster in several places but with unequal frequency, then there are primary and secondary modes. For example when discussing the graph in Figure 1-12, it would be helpful to note that the primary mode was 9 ("very much") with a secondary mode of 1 ("not at all"). The mode can be used with interval, ratio, or ordinal variables as a rough estimate of central tendency. If it is used as an average for nominal data, it is reported as the modal category. For instance in Figure 1-2 the modal category for ethnic origin is "Northwest Europe."

Comparison of Measures of Central Tendency

The mean is the most common measure of central tendency. It has a formula and is the most trustworthy estimate of a population average. Generally, researchers prefer to use it, unless there is a good reason for not doing so. The most compelling reason for not using the mean is a distribution that is badly skewed. The effect of extreme values on the mean lessens as the size of the sample increases; therefore, another good reason for not using the mean is a small sample with a few extreme values. The mean serves best when used with distributions that are reasonably symmetrical and have one mode.

The median is easy to understand as the 50th percentile of a distribution or the bisector of the area of a histogram. It has no formula but is calculated by a counting procedure. The median may be used with distributions of any shape but is especially useful with very skewed distributions.

The main usefulness of the mode is for calling attention to a distribution in which the values cluster at several places. It can also be used for making rough estimates. In addition the mode is the only average available for nominal data.

Figure 2-1 illustrates the relative positions of these three averages for a polygon that is very skewed. The mode is the value under the high point of the polygon, the mean is pulled to the right by the extreme values in the tail of the distribution, and the median usually falls in between.

Weisberg (1992) points out that it is not always necessary to select only a single

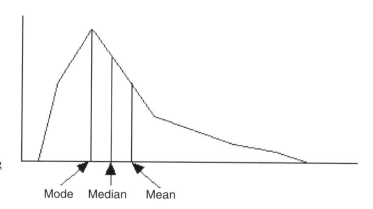

FIGURE 2-1
Sketch of frequency polygon for a distribution skewed to the right, indicating the relative positions of mean, median, and mode.

measure of central tendency because these statistics provide different information. Sometimes it is useful to examine multiple aspects of a distribution. An example from a research journal is presented in Figure 2-2. In this case the mode for delay in seeking treatment was 1 hour, the median was 4 hours, and the mean was 10.6 hours. If the objective of reporting an average is to present a fair view of the data, the reader is asked to consider which average (or averages) should be used here.

MEASURES OF VARIABILITY OF SCATTER

Reporting only an average without an accompanying measure of variability is a good way to misrepresent a set of data. A common story in statistics classes is the woman who had her head in an oven and her feet in a bucket of ice water. When asked how she felt, the reply was, "On the average, I feel fine." Researchers tend to focus on measures of central tendency and neglect how the data are scattered, but variability is at least equally important (Tulman and Jacobsen, 1989). Two sets of data can have the same average but very different variabilities (Fig. 2-3). The three measures of variability that are discussed in this text are the standard deviation, interpercentile measures, and the range. Unlike averages, which are points representing a central value, measures of variability should be interpreted as distances on a scale of values.

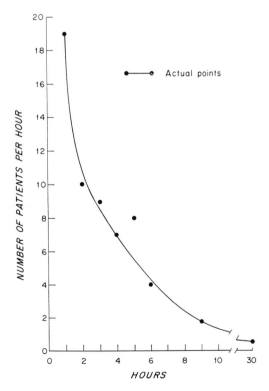

FIGURE 2-2
Graph illustrating a distribution (rate at which patients seek medical care for coronary symptoms as a function of time from onset of symptoms) in which mean, median, and mode are quite different. (From Hackett, T. P., & Cassem, N. H. [1969]. Factors contributing to delay in responding to the signs and symptoms of acute myocardial infarction. *American Journal of Cardiology, 24,* p. 653.) Mean, 10.6 hours; Median, 4 hours; Mode, 1 hour.

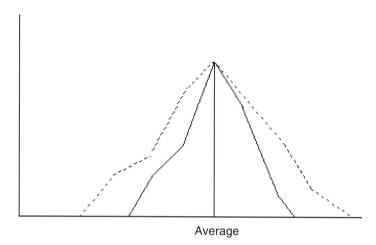

FIGURE 2-3
Two frequency distributions with equal averages but different variabilities.

Average

Standard Deviation

This is the most widely used measure of variability. The sample* standard deviation is defined as:

$$\text{standard deviation} = \sqrt{\sum \frac{(X - \bar{X})^2}{N - 1}}$$

The reason for dividing by the quantity $(N - 1)$ involves a theoretical consideration referred to as *degrees of freedom*. This concept is discussed later in this text. Briefly, it can be shown that using $(N - 1)$ produces, for a random sample, an unbiased estimate of a population variance. This consideration is more important, of course, for small samples.

Table 2-2 illustrates the calculation of the standard deviation for the list of 10 values for length of stay in a sample of cesarean delivery mothers. The first step is to calculate the mean, and then subtract it from each value, making sure that the sum of the deviations is zero. Next, each deviation is squared. The sum of the squared deviations (or "sum of squares") is then divided by $(N - 1)$. The resulting quantity is called the *variance*. Although it is a measure of variability, the variance is not used as a descriptive measure because it is not in the same units as the data. For example the variance of the data in Table 2-2 is 616.67 square hours. Most people would have difficulty interpreting a square hour. Therefore, the square root is taken to return the statistic to its original scale of measurement. The resulting statistic of 24.8 hours is the standard deviation. Again, as with the mean, it is clear that every value in the distribution enters into the calculation of the standard deviation. It is also clear from the formula that the standard deviation is a measure of variability around the mean. The formula in Table 2-2 provides the basic understanding of the sum of squared deviations.

---

* *The standard deviation of a population is represented symbolically by the lower case Greek letter sigma (σ). The formula differs from the sample standard deviation in that the denominator is simply N, not N − 1.*

TABLE 2-2
Demonstration of the Calculation of the Sample
Standard Deviation for Length of Stay (in Hours)
of Cesarean Birth Mothers

X	$X - \bar{X}$	$(X - \bar{X})^2$
61	$61 - 93 = -32$	$(-32)^2 = 1024$
70	$70 - 93 = -23$	$(-23)^2 = 529$
112	$112 - 93 = +19$	$(+19)^2 = 361$
74	$74 - 93 = -19$	$(-19)^2 = 361$
104	$104 - 93 = +11$	$(+11)^2 = 121$
97	$97 - 93 = +4$	$(+4)^2 = 16$
85	$85 - 93 = -8$	$(-8)^2 = 64$
132	$132 - 93 = +39$	$(+39)^2 = 1521$
125	$125 - 93 = +32$	$(+32)^2 = 1024$
70	$70 - 93 = -23$	$(-23)_ = 529$

$\Sigma X = 930$ $\Sigma(X - \bar{X}) = 0$ $\Sigma(X - \bar{X})^2 = 5550 =$
$\bar{X} = 93$ sum of squares

$$\text{variance} = \frac{5550}{9} = 616.67 \text{ square hours}$$

$$\text{standard deviation} = \sqrt{\frac{5550}{9}} = 24.8 \text{ hours}$$

The standard deviation, like the mean, is sensitive to extreme values. For example, in Table 2-2 if the value of 132 is changed to 702, the new standard deviation is 195.1, a large inflation from the original standard deviation of 24.8. Therefore, the standard deviation serves best for distributions that are symmetrical and have a single peak. In general, if it is appropriate to calculate a mean, then ordinarily it is also appropriate to calculate the standard deviation.

The standard deviation has a straightforward interpretation if the distribution is bell-shaped or normal (the normal curve is discussed in detail in the next chapter). For now, if the distribution is perfectly bell-shaped, 68% of the values are within 1 standard deviation of the mean; 95% of the values are within 2 standard deviations of the mean; and more than 99% of the data will be within 3 standard deviations of the mean. For instance Table 2-3 is a computer printout of basic statistics for the approximately bell-shaped distribution of denial scores given in Figure 1-10 in the previous chapter. The mean for denial is 46.5, and the standard deviation is 16.4. By actual count 70% of the denial values fall within the interval of mean ± 1 standard deviation, and 94% of the values are within the interval of mean ± 2 standard deviations.

Even if the distribution is not bell-shaped, however, these percentages hold fairly well. In fact Chebyshev's theorem states that even in oddly shaped distributions at least 75% of the data will fall within 2 standard deviations of the mean (Freund, 1988). Table

TABLE 2-3
Descriptive Statistics Produced by SPSS for the Data in Figure 1-10: Denial Scores From a Sample of 152 Heart Attack Patients

Program
FREQUENCIES VARIABLES = DENIAL/FORMAT = NOTABLE/
STATISTICS = ALL.

Output

Mean	46.533	Std err	1.328	Median	45.500
Mode	45.000	Std dev	16.374	Variance	286.092
Kurtosis	−.249	S E Kurt	.391	Skewness	.195
S E Skew	.197	Range	76.000	Minimum	11.000
Maximum	87.000	Sum	7073.000		

Valid cases	152	Missing cases	0		

Jacobsen, B. S, & Lowery, B. J. (1992). Further analysis of the psychometric properties of the Levine Denial of Illness Scale. Psychosomatic Medicine, 54, 372–381.

2-4 is a computer printout of basic statistics for the very skewed distribution of psychological adjustment scores given in Figure 1-11. The mean for this set of data is 13.8, and the standard deviation is 11.4. By actual count, 82% of the values lie within the interval (mean ± 1 standard deviation). Because this distribution is decidedly not bell-shaped, the percentage in this interval is somewhat different from the expected 68%. Note that trying to subtract 2 standard deviations from the mean of 13.8 leads to the absurd conclusion that some patients had negative denial scores! Based on the rationale of 95% expected to be within 2 standard deviations of the mean for a bell-shaped distribution, Freedman and colleagues (1991) suggest a "quick and dirty" method of

TABLE 2-4
Descriptive Statistics Produced by SPSS for the Data in Figure 1-11: Psychological Adjustment to Illness (PAIS) for a Sample of 195 Patients With Breast Cancer

Program
FREQUENCIES VARIABLES = PAIS/FORMAT = NOTABLE/STATISTICS = ALL.

Output

Mean	13.831	Std err	.814	Median	11.000
Mode	4.000	Std dev	11.366	Variance	129.183
Kurtosis	7.414	S E Kurt	.346	Skewness	2.089
S E Skew	.174	Range	83.000	Minimum	.000
Maximum	83.000	Sum	2697.000		

Lowery, B. J., and Jacobsen, B. S., & Ducette, J. (1992). Causal attribution, control and adjustment to breast cancer. Psychosocial Oncology.

roughly estimating the standard deviation: Compute the difference between the maximum and minimum values, and divide by 4. For the denial distribution this produces an estimated standard deviation of 19, a bit larger than the actual standard deviation of 16.4 but within reason for a rough estimate.

The standard deviation, like the mean, is algebraic. There is, for example, a formula for combining standard deviations from several distributions with different sample sizes (Glass and Stanley, 1970).

If you wish to compare standard deviations between several investigators who have examined the same variable, the coefficient of variation (CV) is useful (Daniel, 1987). This statistic is defined as:

$$CV = \frac{\text{standard deviation}}{\overline{X}} (100)$$

For example Spielberger (1983) reported the following statistics on the State-Trait Anxiety Inventory for a sample of depressed patients: mean = 54.43 and standard deviation = 13.02. For general medical or surgical patients without depression, the statistics were mean = 42.68 and standard deviation = 13.76. The CV for the depressed group was 24%, and the same coefficient for the nondepressed group was 32%. Thus, the nondepressed group was more variable relative to their mean than the depressed group.

Interpercentile Measures

There are several interpercentile measures of variability. Perhaps the most common is the interquartile range (IQR). The first quartile is the 25th percentile, and the third quartile is the 75th percentile. The IQR is defined as the range of values extending from the 25th percentile to the 75th percentile. To locate the first quartile, first locate the median of the distribution. The first quartile is the middle value of all the data points below the median, and the third quartile is the middle value of all the data points above the median. In the example considered previously, the set of 10 ordered values were 61, 70, 70, 74, 85, 97, 104, 112, 125, and 132. The 50th percentile was noted to be 91; there are five values below 91. The median of these five values is 70, and the median of the five values above the 50th percentile is 112. Thus, the IQR is 112 − 70.

This statistic tells how the middle 50% of the distribution is scattered. Other frequently used interpercentile ranges are (P_{10} to P_{90}) and (P_3 to P_{97}). Note that the latter interpercentile range identifies the middle 94% of a distribution, a percentage very similar to that identified in a bell-shaped distribution by the mean ± 2 standard deviations. Table 2-5 contains a printout of selected computer percentiles for the variable of psychological adjustment to illness in a sample of breast cancer patients.

These interpercentile ranges, like the median, are not sensitive to very extreme values. If a distribution is badly skewed and your judgment is that the median (P_{50}) is the appropriate average, then the IQR (or other interpercentile measure) is also appropriate. One of the most common uses of interpercentile measures is for growth charts.

TABLE 2-5
Selected Percentiles Produced by SPSS for the Data in Figure 1-11: Psychological Adjustment to Illness (PAIS) for a Sample of 195 Patients With Breast Cancer

Program
FREQUENCIES VARIABLES = PAIS/FORMAT = NOTABLE/PERCENTILES = 3, 10, 25, 50, 75, 90, 97.

Output

Percentile	Value	Percentile	Value	Percentile	Value
3.00	1.000	10.00	3.000	25.00	6.000
50.00	11.000	75.00	17.000	90.00	27.400
97.00	42.240				
Valid cases	195	Missing cases	0		

Lowery, B. J., Jacobsen, B. S., & Ducette, J. (1992). Causal attribution, control and adjustment to breast cancer. Psychosocial Oncology.

Range

The range is the simplest measure of variability. It is the difference between the maximum value of the distribution and the minimum value. In the example of the 10 values (see Table 2-2) the range is (132 − 61) = 71. If the range is reported in a research journal, it would ordinarily be given as a maximum and a minimum, without the subtracted value.

The range can be unstable because it is based on only two values in the distribution and because it tends to increase with sample size. It is sensitive to very extreme values. For example, in Table 2-2 if the single value of 132 is changed to 702, the range would then be 702 − 61 = 641, a tremendous increase.

The main use of the range is for making a quick estimate of variability; however, the range can be informative in certain situations. For example an engineer planning a dam may want to know what the *worst* flood that ever occurred in the area was. Also, an investigator who is considering a case study may be interested in knowing the most extreme values. A researcher who intends to report a standard deviation or an IQR also may choose to report the range for the additional information it provides about the two endpoints of a distribution.

Comparison of Measures of Variability

The standard deviation is the most widely reported measure of variability. It has a formula and is the most reliable estimate of population variability. Generally, researchers prefer to use the standard deviation, unless there is a good reason for not doing so. Like the mean, the most compelling reason for not using the standard deviation is a distribution that has extreme values. The standard deviation serves best with distributions that are reasonably symmetric and have one mode.

Interpercentile measures are easy to understand. In a histogram they mark off a certain percentage of area around the median. For instance the IQR, extending from P_{25} to P_{75}, delineates the middle 50% of a distribution. These measures have no formulas but are calculated by a counting procedure. They can be used with distributions of any shape but are especially useful with very skewed distributions.

The main uses of the range are to call attention to the two extreme values of a distribution and for quick, rough estimates of variability. To choose the appropriate measures, you must know the distribution. All of the previous measures of variability are intended for use with interval or ratio variables, and often they are sensible for ordinal values. There are no measures of variability for nominal data in common use (Weisberg, 1992).

MEASURES OF SKEWNESS OR SYMMETRY

In addition to central tendency and variability, symmetry also is an important characteristic of a distribution. Sets of data can have the same mean and standard deviation but different skewness (Fig. 2-4). Two measures of symmetry are considered here: Pearson's measure and Fisher's measure.

Pearson's Skewness Coefficient

This measure of skewness is nonalgebraic but is easily calculated and is useful for quick estimates of symmetry. It is defined as:

$$\text{Skewness} = \frac{(\text{mean} - \text{median})}{\text{standard deviation}}$$

For a perfectly symmetrical distribution, the mean will equal the median, and the skewness coefficient will be zero. If the distribution is skewed to the right, the mean will be greater than the median, and the coefficient will be positive (Fig. 2-5). If the

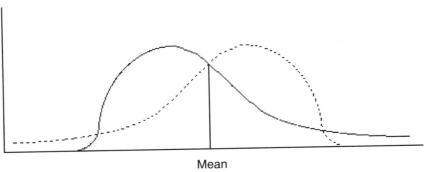

Mean

FIGURE 2-4
Two frequency distributions with the same mean and standard deviation but different symmetry.

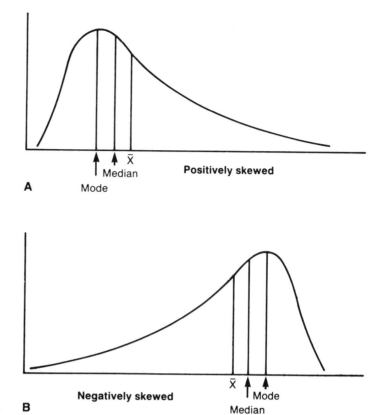

FIGURE 2-5
(*A* and *B*) Skewed distributions.

coefficient is negative, then the distribution is skewed to the left. In general the values will fall between −1 and +1. It would be an odd distribution if the mean differed from the median by more than 1 standard deviation.

For the denial data of Table 2-3 the coefficient is (46.5 − 45.5)/16.4. The resulting value of 0.06 is close to zero. Hildebrand (1986) states that skewness values above 0.2 or below −0.2 indicate rather severe skewness. Therefore, the value of 0.06 indicates little skewness. For the psychological adjustment data of Table 2-4, the story is different. The coefficient is (13.8 − 11.0)/11.4, which results in a value of 0.24, indicating severe skewness.

Fisher's Measure of Skewness

This statistic is based on deviations from the mean to the third power. The formula can be found in Hildebrand (1986). The calculation is tedious and is ordinarily done by a computer program. A symmetrical curve will result in a value of 0. If the skewness value is positive, then the curve is skewed to the right, and vice versa for that skewed to the left. For the denial data in Table 2-3, Fisher's skewness measure is 0.195, a value close to zero. Dividing the measure of skewness by the standard error for skewness (0.195/0.197

= 0.99) results in a number that is interpreted in terms of the normal curve. (This concept is explained further in the next chapter.) Values above $+1.96$ or below -1.96 are significant at the 0.05 level because 95% of the scores in a normal distribution fall between $+1.96$ and -1.96 standard deviations from the mean. Our value of 0.99 indicates that this distribution is not significantly skewed. Because this statistic is based on deviations to the third power, it is very sensitive to extreme values.

MEASURES OF KURTOSIS OR PEAKEDNESS

Fisher's Measure of Kurtosis

This statistic indicates whether a distribution has the right bell-shape for a normal curve. It measures whether the bell-shape is too flat or too peaked. Fisher's measure is based on deviations from the mean to the fourth power. The formula can be found in Hildebrand (1986). Again, the calculation is tedious and is ordinarily done by a computer program. A curve with the right bell-shape will result in a value of zero. If the kurtosis value is positive, the distribution is too peaked to be normal; if the kurtosis value is negative, the curve is too flat to be normal. For the denial data in Table 2-3, the kurtosis statistic is given as -0.249, a value close to zero, indicating that the shape of the bell for this distribution can be called "normal." Dividing this value by the standard error for kurtosis ($-0.249/0.391 = -0.64$), we see that our distribution is not significantly kurtosed; that is, the value is not beyond ± 1.96. Because this statistic is based on deviations to the fourth power, it is very sensitive to extreme values. If a distribution is asymmetric, there is no particular need to examine kurtosis, the distribution is not normal.

ROUNDING STATISTICS FOR TABLES

When reporting descriptive statistics in a table, too many digits are confusing. Because a computer program has provided the statistic to the fourth decimal place, this does not mean that you have to report all those digits. If diastolic blood pressure is measured to the nearest whole number, why report descriptive statistics for blood pressure to the nearest 10,000th?

Chatfield (1988) suggests the two effective digits rule for rounding summary statistics. An effective digit varies over the full range from 0 to 9. For example a set of diastolic blood pressures is recorded as 70, 74, 85, 96, 100, 102, and 108. The digit in the hundreds place is either 0 or 1, and the digit in the 10s place is either 0, 7, 8, or 9. Neither of these digits is an effective digit. The remaining digit in the ones place is an effective digit. Therefore, a descriptive statistic for blood pressure should be rounded to one decimal place. For example the mean for the example should be reported as 90.7, and the standard deviation as 14.6.

In rounding to the nearest 10th (or 100th), if the last digit to be dropped is less than 5, round to the lower number; if it is higher than 5, round to the higher number. If the last digit to be dropped is exactly 5, no change is made in the preceding digit if it is even, but if it is odd, it is increased by 1. Thus, 4.25 to the nearest 10th is 4.2, but 4.35 becomes 4.4.

GRAPHS USING DESCRIPTIVE STATISTICS

Line Graphs

A frequently used type of graph in health-care research is the line graph, which is often used to display longitudinal trends. Time points are placed on the horizontal axis, and the scale for the statistic is on the vertical axis. Dots representing the statistic (e.g., means, medians, or percentages) at each time point are then connected. This type of graph presents a smoother appearance than drawing bars over each time point. Frequently, vertical error bars are added to each time point to indicate the accuracy of the statistic as an estimate of a population parameter. These error bars represent standard errors, which are discussed in detail later in this text. Examples of line graphs from research journals showing change with time are given in Figures 2-6 and 2-7. When several groups are being compared in the same line graph, Tufte (1983) recommends that labels be integrated into the graph rather than having a separate legend, so the eye is not required to go back and forth.

We are frequently told that graphs should include zero on the vertical axis, but sometimes this wastes a lot of space (Cleveland, 1985). For example the graph in Figure 2-7 has been redrawn in Figure 2-8 so that zero is included on the vertical axis. Editors of research journals do not appreciate graphs such as Figure 2-8, which has a lot of blank space. Choose the scale for the vertical axis so that the data "fill up" the graph. You may assume that the reader of a scientific journal will look at tick mark labels and breaks in the axes or line plot and understand them (Cleveland, 1985).

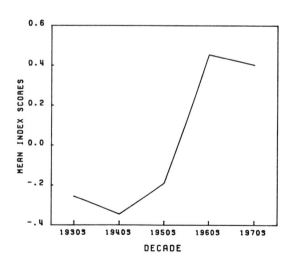

FIGURE 2-6

Mean sex object index scores by decade ($N = 211$). (From Kalisch, B. J., Kalisch, P. A., & McHugh, M. L. (1982). The nurse as a sex object in motion pictures, 1930–1980. *Research in Nursing and Health, 5*, 151.)

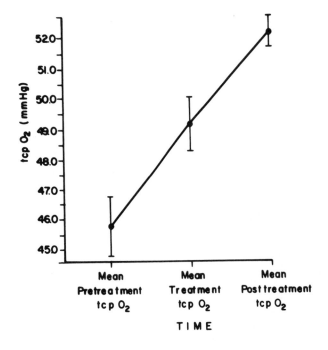

FIGURE 2-7

Effect of non-nutritive sucking on tcp O_2 level as demonstrated by 26 sets of measurements on preterm neonates. Values (means ± standard errors) are the averaged readings for each 8-minute observation period. (From Burroughs, A. K., Asonye, U. O., Anderson-Shanklin, G. C., & Vidyasagar, D. [1978]. The effect of non-nutritive sucking on transcutaneous oxygen tension in noncrying, preterm neonates. *Research in Nursing and Health, 1,* 69–75.)

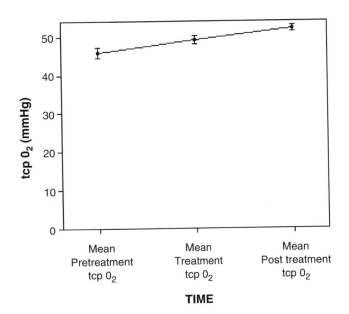

FIGURE 2-8

Data from Figure 2-6 with vertical scale redrawn to include zero.

Box Plots

A box plot is a graphical display that uses descriptive statistics based on percentiles (Tukey, 1977). The first step in constructing this plot is to draw the box. Its length corresponds to the IQR; that is, the box begins with the 25th percentile and ends with the 75th percentile (Fig. 2-9). A line (or other symbol) within the box indicates the location of the median or 50th percentile. Thus, the box provides information about central tendency and the variability of the middle 50% of the distribution.

The next step is to locate the wild values of the distribution, if any. Calculate the IQR ($P_{75} - P_{25}$), and then multiply this value by 3. Individual scores that are more than 3 times the IQR from the upper and lower edges of the box are extreme outlying values and are denoted on the plot by a symbol such as E. Next, multiply the IQR by 1.5. Individual scores that are between 1.5 and 3 times the IQR away from the edges of the box are minor outlying values. Denote them on the boxplot with a different symbol,

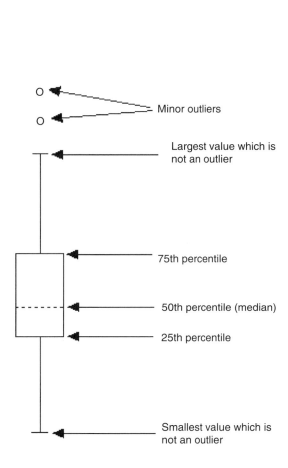

FIGURE 2-9
Schematic diagram of the construction of a boxplot.

such as O. Finally, draw the whiskers of the box. These lines should extend to the smallest and largest values that are not minor or extreme outlying values. Thus, the whiskers and designation of the outlying values provide more detail about how the lower 25% and upper 25% of the distribution are scattered. The boxplot is particularly well suited for comparisons among several groups. Examples of boxplots are given in Figure 2-10, which compares psychological adjustment to illness in a sample of breast cancer patients according to stage of cancer. From this figure you can readily see that as the stage of cancer became higher, adjustment worsened (i.e., the average score increased). Also, it is clear that the variability of the adjustment scores was greater as the stage became higher. Note that the subject identification numbers can be placed on the plot for convenient reference.

OUTLIERS

Outliers are values that are extreme relative to the bulk of the distribution. They appear to be inconsistent with the rest of the data. The source of an outlier may be any of the following:

1. An error in the recording of the data
2. A failure of data collection, such as not following sample criteria (e.g., inadvertently

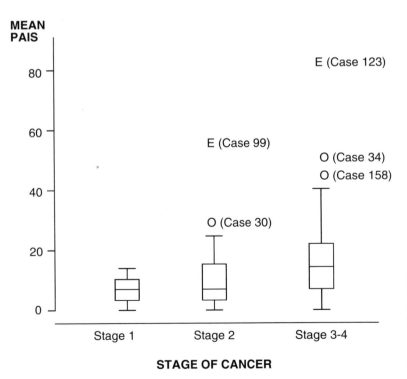

FIGURE 2-10
Boxplots of psychological adjustment to illness (PAIS) in a sample of breast cancer patients by stage of cancer (hypothetical data): Higher scores indicate poorer adjustment.

admitting a disoriented patient into a study), a subject not following instructions on a questionnaire, or equipment failure
3. An actual extreme value from an unusual subject

The first step is to identify outliers by an objective method. A traditional way of labeling outliers has been to locate any values that are more than 3 standard deviations from the mean. The problem with this method is that outliers inflate the standard deviation, making it less likely that a value will be 3 standard deviations away from the mean. A more recent recommendation by Tukey (1977) was described in connection with the boxplot. Values that are more than 3 IQRs from the upper or lower edges of the box are extreme outliers. Values that are between 1.5 and 3 IQRs from the upper and lower edges of the box are minor outliers. The reason for having an objective method rather than judgment only is to prevent undue (perhaps unethical) data manipulation, such as pruning very high or very low values that are not really outliers.

Once outliers have been identified, the next step is to try to explain them. If they represent errors in coding or a failure in data collection, then usually these observations are discarded or occasionally corrected. If the outliers represent actual values or the explanation is unknown, a researcher must decide how to handle them. One frequent suggestion is to analyze the data two ways: with the outliers in the distribution and with the outliers removed. If the results are similar, as they are apt to be if the sample size is large, then the outliers possibly may be ignored.

If the results are not similar, then a statistical analysis that is resistant to outliers can be used (e.g., median and IQR). If a researcher wishes to use a mean with outliers, then the *trimmed mean* is an option. This statistic is calculated with a certain percentage of the extreme values removed from both ends of the distribution. For example if the sample size is 100, then the 5% trimmed mean is the mean of the middle 90% of the observations. Special formulas for using the trimmed mean in statistical inference are given in Koopmans (1987).

Another alternative is a *winsorized mean*. In the simplest case the highest and lowest extremes are replaced, respectively, by the next-to-highest value and the next-to-lowest value. If the sample size is 100, the resulting 100 data points are then processed as if they were the original data. Winer (1971) outlines the special techniques for handling statistics computed from winsorized samples. Further details on the treatment of outliers can be found in Barnett and Lewis (1985). A researcher also can view these actual outliers as case material and adopt the advice of Skinner (1972): "When you run onto something interesting, drop everything else and study it."

SUMMARY

Measures of central tendency and variability are necessary for describing and understanding our variables. Examination of these measures must precede use of variables in statistical analyses.

3

Introduction to Inferential Statistics and Hypothesis Testing

Barbara Hazard Munro

Barbara S. Jacobsen

Leonard E. Braitman

OBJECTIVES FOR CHAPTER 3

After reading this chapter you should be able to do the following:

1. **Describe the characteristics of the normal curve.**

2. **Explain statistical probability.**

3. **Differentiate between a Type I and a Type II error.**

4. **Explain the relationship between one- and two-tailed tests and the power of a test.**

5. **Interpret a confidence interval.**

NORMAL CURVE

The *normal curve* is a theoretically perfect frequency polygon in which the mean, median, and mode all coincide in the center and which takes the form of a symmetrical bell-shaped curve (Fig. 3-1). De Moivre, a French mathematician, developed the notion of the normal curve based on his observations of games of chance. It has been found that many human traits, such as intelligence, attitudes, and personality, are distributed among the population in a fairly "normal" way. That is, if you measure

Barbara Hazard Munro and Ellis Batten Page: STATISTICAL METHODS FOR HEALTH CARE RESEARCH, SECOND EDITION. © 1993, 1986 by J. B. Lippincott Company.

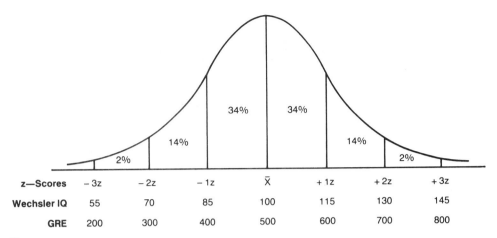

FIGURE 3-1
The normal curve.

something, such as an IQ test, in a representative sample of sufficient size, the resulting scores will assume a distribution that is similar to the normal curve. Most of the scores will fall around the mean (an IQ of 100), and there will be relatively few extreme scores, such as an IQ below 55 or one above 145.

The concept of the normal curve is very useful. For example, when we discuss hypothesis testing, we will talk about the probability (or the likelihood) that a given difference or relationship could have occurred by chance alone. Understanding the normal curve prepares you for understanding the concepts underlying hypothesis testing.

The baseline of the normal curve is measured off in standard deviation units. These are indicated by the lower case letter z in Figure 3-1. A score that is 1 standard deviation above the mean is symbolized by $+1z$, and $-1z$ indicates a score that is 1 standard deviation below the mean. For example, the Wechsler IQ test has a mean of 100 and a standard deviation of 15. Thus, 1 standard deviation above the mean ($+1z$) is 115, and one standard deviation below the mean ($-1z$) is 85.

In a normal distribution, approximately 34% of the scores fall between the mean and 1 standard deviation above the mean. Because the curve is symmetrical, 34% also fall between the mean and 1 standard deviation below the mean. Therefore, 68% of the scores fall between $-1z$ and $+1z$. With the Wechsler IQ test, this means that 68%, or approximately two thirds of the scores, will fall between 85 and 115. Of the one third of the scores remaining, one sixth will fall below 85, and one sixth will be above 115.

Of the total distribution, 28% fall between 1 and 2 standard deviations from the mean. Fourteen percent fall between 1 and 2 standard deviations above the mean, and 14% fall between 1 and 2 standard deviations below the mean. Thus, 96% of the scores (14 + 34 + 34 + 14) fall between ±2 standard deviations from the mean. For the Wechsler IQ test this means that 96% of the population receive scores between 70 and 130.

Most of the last 4% fall between 2 and 3 standard deviations from the mean, 2% on each side. Thus, 99.7% of those taking the Wechsler IQ test score between 55 and 145.

There are two other z-scores that are important because we will use them when constructing confidence intervals (CIs). They are $z = \pm 1.96$ and $z = \pm 2.58$. Of the scores in a distribution, 95% fall between $\pm 1.96z$, and 99% fall between n $\pm 2.58z$. For additional practice with the normal curve, look at the graduation requirement examination (GRE) scores in Figure 3-1. Each section of the GREs was scaled to have a mean of 500 and a standard deviation of 100. Someone who scored 600 on this test would be 1 standard deviation above the mean, or at the 84th percentile. (The 50th percentile is the mean, and 34% above the mean equals the 84th percentile.)

PERCENTILES

In the discussion of the interquartile range, we pointed out that percentiles allow us to describe a given score in relation to other scores in a distribution. A percentile tells us the relative position of a given score. It allows us to compare scores on tests that have different means and standard deviations. A percentile is calculated as:

$$\frac{\text{number of scores less than a given score}}{\text{total number of scores}} \times 100$$

Suppose that you received a score of 90 on a test given to a class of 50 people. Of your classmates, 40 had scores lower than 90. Your percentile rank would be:

$$\frac{40}{50} \times 100 = 80$$

You achieved a higher score than 80% of the people who took the test, which also means that almost 20% of those who took the test did better than you.

The 25th percentile is referred to as the *first quartile*; the 50th percentile, the *second quartile*, or more commonly, the *median*; and the 75th percentile, the *third quartile*. The quartiles are points, not ranges like the interquartile range. Therefore, the third quartile is not from 50 to 75, it is just the 75th percentile. One does not usually say that a score fell within a quartile, because the quartile is only one point.

As demonstrated with the GRE score of 600, we also can determine percentile rank by using the normal curve. For another example, note Figure 3-1. The IQ score of 85 exceeds the IQ score of 16% of the population, so a score of 85 is equal to a percentile rank of 16. To test your understanding, determine the percentile rank of a GRE score of 700.

Tables have been established that make it possible to determine the proportion of the normal curve found between various points along the baseline. They are set up as in Appendix A. To understand how to read the table, go down the first column until you come to 1.0. Note that the percent of area under the normal curve between the mean and a standard score (z-score) of 1.00 is 34.13. This is where the 34% came from in Figure 3-1. Moving down the row to the right, note that the area under the curve between the mean and 1.01 is 34.38, between the mean and 1.02 is 34.61, and so forth.

Suppose you have a standard score of +1.86 (we demonstrate how to calculate the z-scores in the next section). Finding this score in the table, we see that the percent of the curve between the mean and 1.86 is 46.86. A plus z-score is above the mean, so 50% of the curve is on the minus z side, and another 46.86% is between the mean and +1.86; the percentile rank is 96.86 (50 + 46.86). If the z-score were −1.86, the score falls below the mean, and the percentile rank would be 3.14 (50 − 46.86).

In summary to calculate a percentile when you have the standard score, you first look up the score in the table to determine the percent of the normal curve that falls between the mean and the given score. Then, if the sign is positive, you add the percentage to 50. If the sign is negative, you subtract the percentage from 50.

When using percentiles to determine relative position, it is important to remember the following factors:

1. Because so many scores are located near the mean and so few at the ends, the distance along the baseline in terms of percentiles varies a great deal.
2. The distance between the 50th and 55th percentile is much smaller than the distance between the 90th and the 95th.

What this means in practical terms is that if you raise your score on a test, there will be more impact on your percentile rank if you are near the mean than if you are near the ends of the distribution.

As an example suppose three people retook the GRE quantitative examination in hopes of raising their score and thus their percentile rank (Table 3-1). All three subjects raised their score by 10 points. For subject one, who was right at the mean, that meant an increase of 4 points in percentile rank, whereas for subject three, who was 2 standard deviations above the mean to start with, the percentile rank only went up 0.5 of a point.

STANDARD SCORES

Standard scores are a way of expressing a score in terms of its relative distance from the mean. A z-score is one such standard score. As has been pointed out, the meaning of an ordinary score varies, depending on the mean and the standard deviation of the

TABLE 3-1
Relationship of Scores to Percentiles at Varying Distances from the Mean

Subject	Scores	GRE-Q	Percentile
1	1st score	500	50
	2nd score	510	54
2	1st score	600	84
	2nd score	610	86
3	1st score	700	97.7
	2nd score	710	98.2

distribution from which it was drawn. In research standard scores are used more often than percentiles. Thus far, we have used examples when the z-score was easy to calculate. The GRE score of 600 is 1 standard deviation above the mean, so the z-score is $+1$. The formula used to calculate z-scores follows:

$$z = \frac{X - \bar{X}}{\text{standard deviation}}$$

As you can see, the numerator is a measure of the deviation of the score from the mean of the distribution. The following is for the GRE example:

$$z = \frac{600 - 500}{100} = \frac{100}{100} = 1$$

Now let us try another example. Suppose an individual obtained a score of 48 on a test in which the mean was 35 and the standard deviation was 5:

$$z = \frac{48 - 35}{5} = \frac{13}{5} = 2.6$$

Using the table in Appendix A, we find that 49.53% of the curve is contained between the mean and 2.6 standard deviations above the mean, so the percentile rank for this score would be 99.53 (50 + 49.53).

Suppose the national mean weight for a particular group is 120 pounds, and the standard deviation is 6 pounds. An individual from the group, Mary, weighs 112 pounds. What is Mary's z-score and percentile rank?

$$z = \frac{112 - 120}{6} = \frac{-8}{6} = -1.33$$

Mary's percentile rank is 50 − 40.82, or 9.18.

If all the raw scores in a distribution are converted to z-scores, the resulting distribution will have a mean of zero and a standard deviation of 1. If several distributions are converted to z-scores, the z-scores for the various measures can be compared directly. Although the new distributions have a new standard deviation and mean (1 and 0), the shape of the distribution is not altered.

Transformed Standard Scores

Because calculating z-scores results in decimals and negative numbers, some people prefer to transform them into other distributions. One distribution that has been widely used is one with a mean of 50 and a standard deviation of 10. Such *transformed standard scores* are generally referred to as *T-scores*, although some authors call them *Z*-scores. Some standardized test results are given in *T*-scores. To convert a z-score to a *T*-score, use the following formula:

$$T = 10z + 50$$

For example, with a z-score of 2.5, the T-score would be:

$$T = (10)(2.5) + 50$$
$$T = 25 + 50$$
$$T = 75$$

In the new distribution the mean is 50 and the standard deviation is 10, so a score of 75 is still 2.5 standard deviations above the mean.

In the same way other distributions can be established. This is the technique used to transform z-scores into GRE scores with a mean of 500 and a standard deviation of 100. The basic formula for transforming z-scores is to multiply the z-scores by the desired standard deviation and add the desired mean.

transformed z-scores = (new standard deviation)(z-score) + (new mean)

Suppose you wanted to transform your z-scores into a scale with a mean of 70 and a standard deviation of 5. Then your formula would be $5z + 70$.

Transforming scores in this way does not change the original distribution of the scores. In some circumstances, however, a researcher may wish to change the distribution of a set of data. This might occur when you have a set of data that is not normally distributed. There are several ways to accomplish this, but it is not within the scope of this book to detail such transformations. One simple method, however, is to square all the numbers in the distribution. Logarithmic transformations also are used.

CENTRAL LIMIT THEOREM

If you draw a sample from a population and calculate its mean, how close have you come to knowing the mean of the population? Statisticians have provided us with formulas that allow us to determine just how close the mean of our sample is to the mean of the population.

It has been shown that when many samples are drawn from a population, the *means* of these samples tend to be normally distributed; that is, when they are graphed along a baseline, they tend to form the normal curve. The larger the number of samples, the more the distribution approaches the normal curve. Also, if the average of the means of the samples is calculated (the mean of the means), this average (or mean) is very close to the actual mean of the population. Again, the larger the number of the samples, the closer this overall mean is to the population mean.

If the means form a normal distribution, we can then use the percentages under the normal curve to determine the probability statements about individual means. We would know, for example, that the probability of a given mean falling between $+1$ and -1 standard deviation from the mean of the population is 68%.

To calculate the standard scores necessary to determine position under the normal curve, we need to know the standard deviation of the distribution. You could calculate the standard deviation of the distribution of means by treating each mean as a raw score and applying the regular formula. This new standard deviation of the means is called the *standard error of the mean*. The term *error* is used to indicate the fact that due to sampling error, each sample mean is likely to deviate somewhat from the true population mean.

Fortunately, statisticians have used these techniques on samples drawn from known populations and have demonstrated relationships that allow us to estimate the mean and standard deviation of a population given only the data from *one sample*. They have demonstrated that there is a constant relationship between the standard deviation of a distribution of sample means (the standard error of the mean), the standard deviation of the population from which the samples were drawn, and the size of the samples. We do not usually know the standard deviation of the population. If we had measured the entire population, we would have no need to infer its parameters from measures taken from samples. The formula for the standard error of the mean can be written as:

$$\frac{\text{standard deviation}}{\sqrt{n}}$$

The formula indicates that we are estimating the standard error given the standard deviation of a sample of n size. It has been shown that a sample of 30 is enough to estimate the population mean with reasonable accuracy.

Given the standard deviation of a sample and the size of the sample, we can estimate the standard error of the mean. For example given a sample of 100 and a standard deviation of 20, we would estimate the standard error of the mean to be:

$$\frac{20}{\sqrt{100}} = \frac{20}{10} = 2$$

Two factors influence the standard error of the mean: the standard deviation of the sample and the sample size. Note that the sample size has a large impact on the size of the error, because the square root of n is used in the denominator. As the size of n increases, the size of the error decreases. Suppose we had the same standard deviation as just demonstrated, but a sample size of 1000 instead of 100. Now we have

$$\frac{20}{\sqrt{1000}} = \frac{20}{31.62} = 0.63,$$

a much smaller standard error. From this, we see that the larger our sample, the less error there is. If there is less error, we can estimate more precisely the parameters of the population.

If there is more variability in the sample, the standard error increases. If there is much variability, it is harder to draw a sample that is representative of the population. Given wide variability, we need larger samples. Note the effect of variability (standard deviation) on the standard error of the mean.

$$\frac{20}{\sqrt{100}} = \frac{20}{10} = 2$$

$$\frac{40}{\sqrt{100}} = \frac{40}{10} = 4$$

As is shown in a later section in this chapter, the standard error of the mean underlies the calculation of confidence intervals. First, though, let us take a look at the overall notion of probability.

PROBABILITY

Ideas about probability are of fundamental importance for health-care researchers. The use of data in making decisions is a hallmark of our information world, and probability provides a means for translating observed data into decisions about the nature of our world (Kotz & Stroup, 1983). For example, probability helps us to evaluate the accuracy of a statistic and to test a hypothesis. Thus, research findings in journals often are stated in probabilistic terms, and often communicated to patients using probabilistic language. The approach to probability in this chapter is practical, with special attention given to concepts that are important later in this text.

In the everyday life of a health-care professional, questions about probability frequently occur in connection with a patient's future. For example suppose patient X's mammogram revealed a cluster of five calcifications with no other signs of breast abnormality. The patient is told she should have a breast biopsy based solely on these x-ray findings. If the patient enquires about the probability that the biopsy will reveal a malignancy, health-care professionals refer to the literature. Powell, McSweeney, and Wilson (1983) studied 251 consecutive patients who received a breast biopsy with mammographic calcifications as the only reason for the biopsy. Everyone in the sample had at least five microcalcifications in a well-defined cluster; cancer was found in 45 of these patients (17.9%). Consequently, the health-care professional might tell patient X that the probability of cancer was 17.9%.

What has really been stated? The health-care practitioner has presumably imagined that the names of the 251 patients in the study were placed in a hat, and one name was drawn by lot. The chances of drawing the name of one of the 45 patients with cancer is

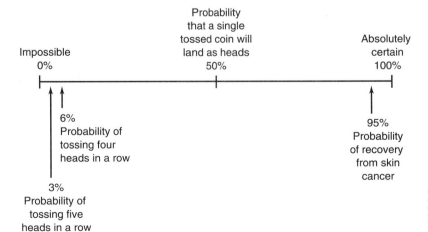

FIGURE 3-2
Diagram of the scale of probabilities.

45/251, or 17.9%. Patient X, of course, is not one of the 251 names in the hat, but the practitioner is thinking along the lines of, "What if she were?" This way of thinking, while hypothetical, is reasonable if patient X can at least be considered to be similar to the group of 251 patients in the study. Powell et al. (1983) described the sample of 251 patients as consecutively chosen over a period of 18 years from the practice of one surgeon at one hospital. While this information implies a fairly broad sample, it does not provide any breakdown by prognostic variables.

Yet an outcome may vary according to membership in a certain subset of a total group. For example, in 1982 a male patient was diagnosed with a rare form of abdominal cancer (Gould, 1985). A trip to the library by the patient revealed that the median mortality was 8 months after diagnosis; therefore, he reasoned that his chances of living longer than 8 months were 50%. On reading further, he decided that his chances of being in that 50% who lived longer were good: he was young, the disease was discovered early, and he was receiving the best treatment.

Self-Evident Truths (Axioms) About Probabilities

All probabilities are between 0% and 100%, as illustrated in Figure 3-2. There are no negative probabilities. If the probability of something happening is 0%, then it is impossible. One has to be careful about assigning probabilities of 0% to an event; after all, the Titanic was advertised as an unsinkable ship! At the moment, however, it does appear that the probability is 0% for a 90 year old to run a 4-minute mile. If the probability of an event is 100%, then we are absolutely certain that it will occur. The eventual death of a person currently has a probability of 100%.

The probability of an event is 100% minus the probability of the opposite event. Perhaps a different health-care worker would have preferred to report the probability for the biopsy of patient X as an 82.1% chance that the calcifications would *not* be malignant. This would be accurate, too, because 100% − 17.9% = 82.1%.

Table 3-2 lists the four possibilities for the sample of 45 women who were diagnosed with cancer after a biopsy based on a suspicious mammogram, as given by Powell

TABLE 3-2
Malignant Pathology of X-Ray Calcifications

Pathology	N
Duct cancer, in situ	25
Lobular cancer, in situ	9
Duct, invasive	9
Lobular, invasive	2
	45
	(100%)

(Data from Powell, R. W., McSweeney, M. B., & Wilson, C. E. (1983). X-ray calcifications as the only basis for breast biopsy. Annals of Surgery, 197, 555–559. Modified slightly to represent individual patients rather than 47 breasts from 45 patients.)

et al. (1983). The sum of all the possibilities for an event is 100%. Note that the sum of the four outcomes in Table 3-1 is 100%, indicating that it is certain that one of these possibilities will occur.

Definitions of Probability

Frequency Probability

If scientists were asked about the meaning of probability, they would give many different answers (Carnap, 1953). Most health-care professionals, however, think of probability in the sense of a frequency or statistical probability. That is, they think of probability as a percentage based on empirical observation, which allows them to make an intelligent guess about the future. Their definition for such a probability, based on observations from a sample, is given below:

$$\text{sample probability} = \frac{\text{number of times the event occurred}}{\text{total number of people in the sample}} \times 100$$

In the previously noted case of patient X with the suspicious mammogram, the health-care worker would substitute as follows:

$$\text{probability of cancer} = \frac{45}{251} \times 100 = 17.9\%$$

Patient X was not a member of the group of 251 patients, but the hypothetical type of thinking "What if patient X were from that group?" is at least reasonable as a practical type of probability. Of course it helps to be able to argue logically that patient X might have been a member of the total group of 251 patients.

In mathematical theory, however, probabilities are only meaningful in the context of chance. In the previous example we also have to imagine that patient X was chosen "by lot" from the total sample, which implies a random choice. There are two criteria for a random process. First, every item must have an equal chance of being chosen. In the case of drawing from a hat, this means that attention must be given to details such as whether each name was written on the same size slip of paper, whether the slips were well stirred, whether the person who drew from the hat was blindfolded, and so forth.* Second, each choice must be independent of every other choice. This means that we must not be able predict whose name will be drawn after patient X.

These criteria for a random process also are important when we consider the larger question of whether the 17.9% probability of cancer would still be the same if more patients were followed. The mathematical definition for a frequency probability invokes the law of averages. That is, we must think of drawing more and more patients at random. As the sample becomes larger and larger, the percentage will converge to the true or population value.

---

* Health-care researchers who wish to draw a random sample avoid having to deal with such details by using a random number table.

$$\text{population probability} = \frac{\text{total number of times the event occurred}}{\text{total number of people in the population}} \times 100$$

Thus, the sample probability is an estimate of the population probability. A random sample provides, in theory, a better estimate of the population probability.

In a brief discussion section following the article by Powell et al. (1983), A. H. Letton reported on a second sample of 269 patients, collected for 10 years. A mammogram indicated calcium deposits, and subsequent biopsies revealed that 46 patients (17.1%) had cancer. Thus, a second study, again with a nonrandom sample, produced remarkably similar results to those of Powell et al.

The reader might protest, "But this has no connection to mathematical theory because there was no random process here." The 251 women in the first sample were not chosen at random, nor were the 269 women in the second sample, nor was patient X. Random sampling or random assignment to groups is infrequently used in health-care research (Brown, Tanner, & Padrick, 1984; Fletcher & Fletcher, 1979; Jacobsen & Meininger, 1985). Patients who arrive for care become the sample, and health-care researchers take all they can get rather than drawing random samples. These sample probabilities, though not based on a chance process, remain as our only estimates of the true or population probabilities.

Frequency probabilities are based on empirical observations and can thus be termed objective. However, not all probabilities that can be considered objective are determined empirically. For example when tossing a fair coin, the probabilities of heads or tails can be deduced logically without ever actually tossing the coin. These are called a priori (before the fact) probabilities. Derdiarian and Lewis (1986) provided an illustration of how a priori probabilities could be used in health-care research. Each of three raters was asked to code an item from an interview transcript as belonging to category 1 or category 2. There are eight possible outcomes as listed in Table 3-3. All three raters could agree that the item belonged in category 1 (1-1-1), or they could disagree, for example, with the first rater coding the item as category 1 and the other two coding the item as category 2 (1-2-2). If all of these outcomes are equally likely by chance, then each will have a probability of $\frac{1}{8}$ (see Table 3-3). Derdiarian and Lewis (1986) show how comparing actual results to the tabled probabilities can provide a measure of inter-rater agreement.

Subjective Probability

Another definition for probability is a percentage that expresses our personal, subjective belief that an event will occur. Kotz and Stroup (1983) stress that these judgments are rational assessments, not arbitrary beliefs. In the example of patient X with the suspicious mammogram, what about the health-care professional's opinion of the probability of 17.9% that the calcifications are cancer? If the patient were told that the probability was close to zero that the biopsy was malignant, then we would be surprised if it turned out to be cancer. On the other hand, a probability of 17.9% would not be viewed as "close to zero" by most health-care professionals. A practitioner would not to be very surprised if the calcifications turned out to be cancer, and that is why patient X

TABLE 3-3
*Probability of Eight Possible Outcomes for Three Raters
Coding an Item Into Dichotomous Categories (1 or 2)
by Chance*

	Outcome		
Rater #1	*Rater #2*	*Rater #3*	**Probability**
1	1	1	$1/8$
1	1	2	$1/8$
1	2	1	$1/8$
2	1	1	$1/8$
1	2	2	$1/8$
2	1	2	$1/8$
2	2	1	$1/8$
2	2	2	$1/8$

(Derdiarian, A. K., & Lewis, S. [1986]. The D-L test of agreement: A stronger measure of interrater reliability. Nursing Research, 35, 375–378)

with five or more calcifications in a cluster was recommended for biopsy instead of ignoring the x-ray.

With regard to the topic of testing hypotheses, which is discussed later in this text, researchers focus on probabilities (often referred to as *p* values) that fall at the lower end of the continuum in Figure 3-2. Generally, probabilities that are 5% or less are considered unusual in research. The reasons for this are partly intuitive and partly historical. As part of my statistics classes for many years, I would toss a coin and "arrange" for it to turn up heads all the time. Intuitively, students begin to laugh and be skeptical after seeing four or five heads in a row. The probability of four heads in a row by chance is approximately 6%, and the probability of five heads in a row is approximately 3%. Note that 5% falls between the two.

The historical reasons for the 5% cutoff are partly based on the preference of Sir Ronald Fisher. Moore (1991) quotes Fisher as writing in 1926 that he preferred the 5% point for marking off the probable from the improbable. Because Fisher was an enormously influential statistician, others adopted this rule too. Also, the past inconveniences of calculating have influenced the choice of the 5% mark. Before the computer age, the tables for probabilities for various distributions in textbooks were constructed with handy columns such as 20%, 10%, 5%, and 1%—presumably because we have five fingers, and our number system is based on 10. Today these tables and the use of the 5% level are "almost obsolete" (Freedman, Pisani, Purves, & Adhikari, 1991, p. 494) because the computer can produce an exact probability based on a mathematical equation. Many researchers and editors of journals, however, persist in using the 5% mark as a cutoff for "unusual" simply because it is convenient to have some general standard that is easy to grasp.

Instead of using the 5% criterion, however, researchers often adopt probability cutoffs that are more generous (e.g., 10%) or more strict (e.g., 1%) based on their own intuition or the purposes and design of their research. With regard to intuition, the Nobel physicist, Enrico Fermi, reportedly believed that the 10% level was the cutoff for separating a miracle from a commonplace event. Meininger (1985) used a cutoff of 20% because the purpose of her research was exploratory—testing potential items for a behavior scale; Jacobsen and Lowery (1992) used a cutoff of 1% for statistical reasons—several hypotheses were tested using one dataset.

At the higher end of the probability continuum, probabilities of 95% or more are commonly considered by researchers as evidence for reporting potential events that they are quite confident will occur. The oft-quoted probability of 95% for recovery from skin cancer is empirically derived, and most health-care workers would be surprised if recovery did not occur. Additionally, probabilities near the upper end of the probability scale frequently are used to express confidence in a statistic. For example a poll reported that 38% of a pre-election random sample favored candidate A. The margin of error was given as 3%, with 95% confidence.

Probability Rules

Conditional Probability

The site of malignant breast calcifications can be ductal or lobular. Does the probability of invasive breast cancer vary according to site? The answer to this question can be found in Table 3-4, a crosstabulation of site and invasiveness based on the data in Table 3-2. Given that the site is lobular, what is the probability of invasive cancer? Table 3-4 shows that a total of 11 patients had lobular calcifications, and two of these were invasive. Therefore, the probability of invasive breast cancer, *on the condition* that the site is lobular, is 2/11 or 18.2%. What is the probability of invasive cancer, given that the site was ductal? Table 3-4 shows that a total of 34 patients had duct calcifications, and nine of these were invasive. Therefore, the probability of invasive breast cancer, *on the condition* that the site was ductal, is 9/34 or 26.5%. Notice that the two probabilities are

TABLE 3-4
Crosstabulation of Malignant Pathology of X-Ray
Calcifications by Site and by Whether the Cancer Was Invasive

Site	Invasive		Totals
	Yes	No	
Duct	9	25	34
Lobular	2	9	11

(Based on Table 3-2.)

different, indicating that invasiveness depends, to some extent, on site. A formula for conditional probability is given below:

$$\text{probability of event B, given event A} = \frac{100(\text{total number with event A and event B})}{\text{total number with event A}}$$

In the previous example, relative to the lobular site, the formula would be:

$$\text{probability of invasive, given lobular} = \frac{100(\text{total number with lobular invasive})}{\text{total number with lobular cancer}}$$

The substitutions would be as follows:

$$\text{probability of invasive, given lobular} = \frac{100(2)}{2 + 9} = \frac{2}{11} = 18.2\%$$

Multiplication Rule

Earlier in this chapter the idea of independence in choosing a random sample was defined as lack of ability to predict what person will be chosen next. More formally, independence means that given knowledge of event A, the probability of event B does not change. In coin tossing the a priori probability of a head on a single toss of a fair coin is $1/2$ (event A). If you are told that a person has obtained a head on the first toss of a coin, what is the probability of a head on the second toss (event B)? Because a fair coin has no memory, the probability of a head on the second toss is still $1/2$. That is, the probability of a head on the second toss remains the same, in spite of the fact that you have been given information about the first toss. Therefore, successive tosses of a fair coin are independent. In the previous example regarding breast biopsies for calcifications, the probabilities for invasive breast cancer changed according to site; therefore, the variables of site and invasiveness were not independent.

When two events are independent, the probability that both events will occur is equal to the product of their probabilities. What is the probability of tossing two heads in a row? Because each coin toss is independent, the answer may be obtained simply by multiplying together the probabilities for two separate coin tosses: $1/2 \times 1/2 = 1/4$ or 25%. Thus, when events are independent, one does not have to think about conditional probabilities. The formula for the probability of two events both occurring, *if the two events are independent*, follows:

probability of event A *and* event B = the probability of A times the probability of B

This formula, of course, can easily be extended to include more than two events. For the probability of tossing four heads in a row, the substitutions would be:

$$\text{probability of four heads in a row} = 100\left(\frac{1}{2} \times \frac{1}{2} \times \frac{1}{2} \times \frac{1}{2}\right) = \frac{100(1)}{16} = 6\%$$

The ideas of independence and dependence are very important in statistics. If the events are dependent, then the formula for conditional probability is used. If they are independent, then the probabilities may simply be multiplied. It is sometimes difficult to tell in health-care situations whether events are independent or not. Indeed, the fundamental aim of many research projects is to learn whether two variables are independent. Also, many statistical procedures require the assumption of independence of events. If a sample is chosen at random or assigned to groups at random, then this assumption of independence is much easier to defend.

Addition Rule

Two events are said to be mutually exclusive when they cannot occur simultaneously; that is, the occurrence of one prevents the other. For instance in the example of breast biopsies for women with a cluster of five or more calcifications, the site of the clustered calcifications is either ductal or lobular—it cannot be both. *If two events are mutually exclusive*, the probability that either one event or the other will occur is the sum of their probabilities, as given in the following formula:

probability of event A *or* event B = probability of A + probability of B

In Table 3-2 if we wish to compute the probability that a cluster of cancerous calcifications is invasive, the substitutions follow:

probability of ductal invasive or lobular invasive =
100(9/45 + 2/45) = 11/45 = 24%

As another example in Table 3-3, the raters can agree perfectly in two ways. All three can assign the interview item to category 1, or all three can assign it to category 2. Thus, the outcomes of 1-1-1 and 2-2-2 are mutually exclusive because the three raters cannot do both simultaneously. Therefore, the probability of perfect agreement by chance is:

probability of 1-1-1 or 2-2-2 = 100(1/8 + 1/8) = 100(2/8) = 25%

In statistics the probability of two such mutually exclusive events, both located at the extremes of a distribution, is called a "two-tailed probability." If our interest is in only one extreme of a distribution, such as all three raters assigning the interview item to category 1, then the substitutions are:

probability of 1-1-1 = 100(1/8) = 12.5%

This probability is referred to as "one-tailed" and is exactly half of the two-tailed probability.

For events that are not mutually exclusive, the addition rule is somewhat more complicated. This more complex rule is omitted because it is not used in later sections of this text. The interested reader can find the addition rule for nonmutually exclusive events in Freund (1988).

HYPOTHESIS TESTING

Given an underlying theoretical structure, a representative sample, and an appropriate research design, the researcher is able to test hypotheses. We test to see whether or not the data support our hypothesis. We do not claim to "prove" that our hypothesis is true, because one study can never prove anything. It is always possible that some error has distorted the findings.

Null Hypothesis

The *null hypothesis* is often written H_o. It proposes that there is no difference. The null hypothesis is the basis of the statistical test. If a "significant" difference is found, the null hypothesis is *rejected*, but if no difference is found, the null hypothesis is *accepted*. In older studies hypotheses were usually stated in null form; however, this is not done as often today. When you hypothesize, you are stating that you believe there is a difference or a relationship. It is clearer if you state what differences or relationships you expect, rather than write a string of null hypotheses. It is important to understand the null hypothesis, however, because without it, there is no significance test. Suppose you stated that there is "no significant difference" between breast- and bottle-fed babies in terms of weight gain. If you really had no idea about this issue, you would not be stating a hypothesis but would simply ask the question: Is there a difference in weight gain between breast- and bottle-fed babies? If you had rationale for a hypothesis, you might state a research hypothesis (H_1), such as breast-fed babies gain more weight in the first week of life than bottle-fed babies.

Types of Error

Types of "error" are defined in terms of the null hypothesis. After analyzing the data, the researcher *accepts* the null hypothesis if there are no significant results or *rejects* the null hypothesis if there are indeed significant results. Rejecting a null hypothesis means that significant differences *have* been found. Because no study is perfect, there is always a chance for error; perhaps this is one of the five chances in 100 ($p < 0.05$) that such an extreme result has happened by chance.

Two potential errors could be made. They are called *Type I* and *Type II*. Before describing these errors, the possibilities related to decisions about the null hypothesis are presented through use of the following diagram:

	Null hypothesis	
Decision	**True**	**False**
Accept H_o	ok	Type II
Reject H_o	Type I	ok

If we have a null hypothesis that is true and we accept that hypothesis, we have responded correctly. The incorrect response would be to reject a true null hypothesis (Type I error). If the null hypothesis is false and we reject it, we have responded correctly. The wrong response would be to accept a false null hypothesis (Type II error).

Suppose you compared two groups taught by different methods (A and B) on their knowledge of statistics, and the data indicated that group A scored significantly higher than group B. You would then reject the null hypothesis. Suppose, however, that group A had people with higher math ability in it and that actually the method did not matter at all. Rejecting the null hypothesis is a Type I error.

The probability of making a Type I error is called alpha (α) and can be *decreased* by altering the level of significance. That is, you could set the p at 0.01, instead of 0.05. Then there is only 1 chance in 100 that the result termed "significant" could occur by chance alone. If you do that, however, you will make it more difficult to find a significant result; that is, you will decrease the *power* of the test and increase the risk of a *Type II error*.

A Type II error is accepting a *false* null hypothesis. If the data showed no significant results, the researcher would accept the null hypothesis. If there were significant differences, a Type II error would have been made. To avoid a Type II error, you could make the level of significance less extreme. There is a greater chance of finding significant results if you are willing to risk 10 chances in 100 that you are wrong ($p = 0.10$) than there is if you are willing to risk only 5 chances in 100 ($p = 0.05$). Other ways to decrease the likelihood of a Type II error are to increase the sample size, decrease sources of extraneous variation, and increase what is known as the *effect* size. The effect size is the impact made by the independent variable. For example if group A scored 10 points higher on the statistics final than group B, the effect size would be 10 divided by the standard deviation of the measure (Cohen, 1987). Of course there is a trade-off: Decreasing the likelihood of a Type II error increases the chance of a Type I error. If decreasing the probability of one type of error increases the probability of the other type, the question arises as to which type of error you are willing to risk. As might be expected that depends on the study. Suppose you had a test for a particular genetic defect, and if the defect really exists and is diagnosed early, it can be successfully treated; however, if it is not diagnosed and treated, the child will become severely retarded. On the other hand if a child is erroneously diagnosed as having the defect and treated, no physical damage is done.

In terms of the types of errors, a Type I error would be diagnosing the defect when it does not exist. In that case the child would be treated but not harmed by the treatment. A Type II error would be declaring the child to be normal, when he or she is not. In that case irreparable damage would be done. In such a situation it is obvious that you would make every attempt to avoid the Type II error.

On the other hand suppose a federal study was conducted to determine whether a particular approach to preschool preparation of underprivileged children leads to increased success in school. This approach would cost a great deal of money to implement nationwide. Those responsible for deciding whether or not to implement this approach would certainly want to be sure that a Type I error had not been made. They would not want to institute a costly new program if it did not really have any effect on success in school.

We have found that the notion of Type I and II errors is hard for some people to grasp, so we will give a few examples to allow you to determine whether or not you have grasped the concept.

It is hypothesized that two groups are equal in their knowledge of statistics. Has an error been made, and if so, what type of error, if the researcher does the following?

1. Accepts the hypothesis when the groups are really equal in statistics knowledge
2. Rejects the hypothesis when the groups are really equal in statistics knowledge
3. Rejects the hypothesis when the groups are really different in terms of their knowledge of statistics
4. Accepts the hypothesis when one group has much more knowledge of statistics than the other

These four examples summarize the possibilities surrounding these errors. First, if we are given a situation in which the null hypothesis is true, that is, there is no difference, we can either accept it and make the correct decision (#1), or reject it and make an incorrect decision, or a Type I error (#2). Second, if the null hypothesis is false, we can reject it, making a correct decision (#3), or accept it and make an incorrect decision, or a Type II error (#4).

Power of a Test

As previously mentioned, a more *powerful* test is one that is more likely to reject a null hypothesis; that is, it is more likely to indicate a statistically significant result when such a difference exists in the population. The level of significance (probability level) and the power of the test are important factors to consider.

One- and Two-Tailed Tests

The "tails" refer to the ends of the probability curve. When we test for statistical significance, we are asking if the difference or relationship is so extreme, so far out in the tail of the distribution, that it is unlikely to have occurred by chance alone. When we hypothesize the direction of the difference, we are indicating in which tail of the distribution we expect to find the difference.

Although there is some controversy about this, the practice among many researchers is to use a *one-tailed* test of significance when a directional hypothesis is stated and a *two-tailed* test in all other situations. The advantage of using the one-tailed test is that it is more powerful, because the value yielded by the statistical test does not have to be so large to be significant at a given level. To gain this advantage, however, you must have a sound theoretical basis for the directional hypothesis. You cannot base it on a hunch.

Let's look at some examples to see why this is so. Because you are familiar with the normal curve, we will use that to demonstrate the difference between one- and two-tailed tests (Fig. 3-3). Recall from our discussion of CIs that 95% of the distribution fall

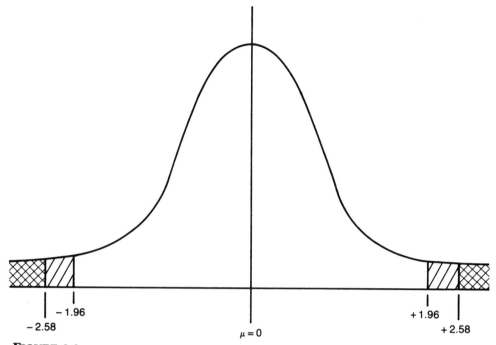

FIGURE 3-3
Two-tailed test of significance using the normal curve.

between ±1.96 standard deviations from the mean. Thus, only 5% fall beyond these two points. Two and one-half percent of the distribution fall below a z-score of -1.96, and 2.5% fall above $+1.96z$. To be so "rare" as to occur only 5% of the time, a z-score would have to be $-1.96z$ or less or $+1.96z$ or greater. Note that we are using both tails of the distribution. Because 99% of the distribution fall between ±2.58 standard deviations from the mean of the normal curve, a score would have to be -2.58 or less or $+2.58$ or more to be declared significant at the 0.01 level.

Figure 3-4 shows what occurs when a directional hypothesis is stated. We look at only one tail of the distribution. In this example we will look at the positive side of the distribution. Fifty percent of the distribution fall below the mean, and 45% fall between the mean and a z-score of $+1.65$ (see Appendix A). Thus, 95% (50 + 45) of the distribution fall below $+1.65z$. To score in the upper 5% would require a score of $+1.65$ or greater. Given a one-tailed test of significance, you would need a score of $+1.65z$ to be significant at the 0.05 level, whereas with a two-tailed test, you needed a score of $+1.96z$. This is an example of the concept of power. With an a priori hypothesis, a lower z-score would be considered significant.

For the 0.01 level of significance and a one-tailed test, a z-score of $+2.33$ or greater is needed for significance. This is because 49% of the distribution fall between the mean and $+2.33$, and another 50% fall below the mean.

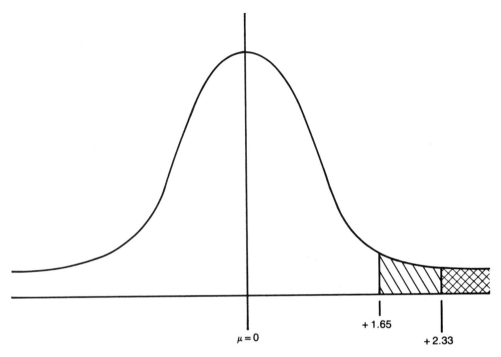

FIGURE 3-4
One-tailed test of significance using the normal curve.

Degrees of Freedom

We have already shown the effects of degrees of freedom (*df*) when we discussed the denominator in the computation of the standard deviation. We pointed out that in the sample formula, the denominator is $n - 1$, thus correcting for the possible underestimation of the population parameter. In describing the calculation of various statistics, we will discuss dividing by the degrees of freedom and looking up levels of significance in tables using *df*s. Because this is sometimes a confusing concept, a simple example of degrees of freedom follows.

Degrees of freedom are related to the number of scores, items, or other units in a data set and to the idea of freedom to vary. Given three scores (1, 5, 6), we have three degrees of freedom, one for each independent item. Each score is "free to vary"; that is, before collecting the data we do not know what any of these scores will be. Once we calculate the mean, however, we lose one *df*. The mean of these three scores is four. Once you know the mean and two of the three scores, you can figure out what the third score is. It is no longer free to vary. In calculating the variance or standard deviation, you are calculating how much the scores vary around the sample mean. Because the sample mean is known, one *df* is lost, and the *df*s become $n - 1$, the number of items in the set less one.

STATISTICAL INFERENCE

In statistics a sample (part) is used to obtain results that are representative of a target population (whole) to which one wants to generalize. For example the average birth weight of newborns in a hospital in 1991 (population) can be estimated using observations from a sample of those newborns. Suppose there were 810 infants born in the hospital in 1991, and the birth weights of the first 81 newborns (starting January 1) were recorded and averaged. Would the average (mean) birthweight in that sample of 81 be a good estimate of the mean birth weight in the 810 (the population of interest)? It would not be if birth weight depends on time of year or if an effective prenatal nutrition program to improve birth weight had begun in the surrounding community near that time. How can a sample that *is* representative of that population of 810 be selected? One way is by random selection.

A *random sample* is drawn from the population of interest so that every member of the population has the same probability (chance) of being selected in the sample. To make this possible, one must have a list of everyone in the population. A table of random numbers can then be used to select a random sample of any size (Remington & Schork, 1970). Note that samples of convenience or samples drawn in a haphazard manner are *not* random samples. Suppose a 10% random sample was selected from the population of 810. It is extremely unlikely that the resulting random sample would be the first 81 infants born in 1991. Because the process of random sampling does not play favorites, random samples are likely to be representative of the target population. On the other hand it is impossible to know that "judgment samples" (such as the first 81 newborns of 1991) are representative of the population of interest. Random samples are unbiased in that, on average, the process of random sampling produces samples that are representative of the population. Most important, the statistical theory on which this book is based assumes random sampling (or random assignment, discussed later).

STATISTICAL ESTIMATES

When an estimate of the population parameter is given as a single number, it is called a *point estimate*. The sample mean is a point estimate. A *confidence interval* (CI) or *interval estimate* is a range or interval of values. Point estimates and CI estimates are types of statistical estimates that allow us to *infer* the true value of an unknown population parameter using information from a *random* sample of that population.

Confidence Intervals

When the means (point estimates) are normally distributed, we can use the standard error of the mean to calculate interval estimates. Typically, the 95% and 99% intervals are used. Recall from our discussion of the normal curve earlier in this chapter that 95% of the curve is contained between ± 1.96 standard deviations from the mean, and that 99% of the curve is contained between ± 2.58 standard deviations from the mean.

The following formulas are used to calculate the CIs for the population means when the sample size is adequate (generally greater than 30). (For small samples the *t* distribution may be used to calculate CIs.)

$$95\% = \bar{X} \pm 1.96 \text{ (standard error)}$$
$$99\% = \bar{X} \pm 2.58 \text{ (standard error)}$$

The following hypothetical examples are designed to illustrate point estimates and CI estimates derived from a random sample. Suppose that a random sample of 81 newborn infants from a hospital in a poor neighborhood during the last year had a mean birth weight of 100 oz with a standard deviation of 27 oz.

1. What is the point estimate for the unknown true value of the average (mean) birth weight of all infants born in that hospital in the last year (called the population parameter)?

    Answer: The mean value of 100 oz (computed from the 81 observations) is the best single number estimate (the point estimate) of the unknown value (parameter) for the population of interest. Remember that another random sample of 81 would have given a sample mean different from 100 oz, so the mean value depends on the particular sample that was taken. The difference between the sample mean of 100 oz and the unknown population mean (which it estimates) is called sampling error. "It is not an error in the sense of a blunder or mistake, but a calculated error we make because we do not collect data on the entire population" (Remington & Schork, 1970).

    Because the point estimate, 100 oz, is a single number, it gives no indication of its sampling error. CIs computed from random samples enable us to measure sampling error in numerical terms.

2. What is the value of the 95% CI estimate for mean birth weight?

    Answer: First, we must calculate the standard error. Remember that the formula is the standard deviation divided by the square root of the sample size:

$$\frac{\text{standard deviation}}{\sqrt{n}}$$

For our example this is:

$$= \frac{27}{\sqrt{81}} = \frac{27}{9} = 3$$

Next, we calculate the 95% CI:

$$\bar{X} \pm 1.96 \text{ (standard error)}$$
$$100 \pm (1.96)(3)$$
$$100 \pm 5.88$$
$$94.12 \text{ and } 105.88$$

The 95% CI ranges from 94.12 to 105.88. It is a range or interval of estimates for the unknown true value. Thus, a CI consists of an entire interval of estimates for the population parameter.

3. How do we interpret the 95% CI?

> *Answer*: First, another sample of 81 would almost surely yield a different point estimate. The width of the 95% CI reflects the sampling error resulting from using an estimate based on a random sample of 81 rather than the entire population. In other words the width of the 95% CI indicates the range of variation for point estimates that may be expected by chance differences from one random sample of the hospital population to another. It is a 95% CI because about 95% of such CIs (obtained from different random samples of that size) will include the true mean value of hospital birth weights. Because that parameter value is usually unknown, we use statistical estimates, the point estimate and the CI estimate, to approximate it. However, if the parameter value (the true mean birth weight for *all* newborn infants born in that hospital during the last year) were known, approximately 95% of the 95% CIs computed from different random samples of 81 would include that true value.
>
> It is important to understand that the value of the point estimate and the CI estimate depend on the birth weights in the particular sample that was taken, and those estimates will vary from sample to sample. Therefore, we may *not* conclude that the probability is 95% that the mean hospital birth weight is between 94 and 106 oz.
>
> Either the parameter (the mean of all birth weights in the hospital during 1991) is between 94 and 106 oz or it is not; we do not know which. "Thus, the 95% refers to the average accuracy of the procedure for constructing the varying confidence intervals, and not to the one interval that is itself presented" (Hahn & Meeker, 1991). However, the width of the CI provides useful information about the sampling error or uncertainty of the point estimate unavailable from the point estimate itself. To interpret the specific CI we computed from our sample (here, 95% CI, 94.12 to 105.88), it is necessary to understand the relationship between CIs and significance tests.

The Relationship Between Confidence Intervals and Significance Tests

To help explain the relationship between CIs and the levels of significance (p values) derived from statistical tests, we will use the following four questions that might be asked in relation to our sample mean:

1. Is the mean birth weight in this hospital sample (100 oz) statistically significantly different from 88 oz (5.5 lb, the definition of low birth weight)?
2. Is the mean birth weight in this sample statistically significantly different from 106 oz (6.6 lb, the mean birth weight in that city)?
3. Is the mean birth weight in this sample statistically significantly different from a birth weight of 103 oz?
4. Is the mean birth weight in this sample statistically significantly different from 100 oz, the sample estimate itself?

To test the null hypothesis that there is no statistically significant difference between the mean of 100 oz and each of the other values, we apply the *t* test. The results are:

Question	Null Hypothesis	Difference Between Values	*p* Value
1.	88	12 oz	0.0006
2.	106	6 oz	0.0456
3.	103	3 oz	0.3174
4.	100	0 oz	1.0000

For the first question the null hypothesis is rejected. The observed mean of 100 oz is statistically significantly higher than the hypothesized value of 88 oz; that is, the 12-point difference is a significant difference. The *p* value indicates that a difference that large would occur by chance alone only 6 times in 10,000! The null hypothesis is also rejected for question 2, that is the hospital mean of 100 oz is statistically significantly lower than the city mean of 106 oz. A difference that large would occur by chance alone only $4\frac{1}{2}$ times in 100 random samples of equal size. For questions 3 and 4 the null hypothesis is not rejected; that is, the observed mean of 100 oz is not statistically significantly different from the values of 103 or 100 oz. In the case of the 3-oz difference (question 3), if there really was no difference between the population means, a difference at least that large could be expected to occur by chance in 32% of the random samples. In question 4 the point estimate and the null hypothesis are numerically indistinguishable (both 100 oz), and also statistically indistinguishable ($p = 1$), because the difference between the two values being compared is zero.

From the chart of the *p* values, it can be seen that the further a particular null hypothesis is from the point estimate (100 oz), the lower the *p* value. In other words hypotheses become less compatible with the mean of the observed values (here 100 oz) the larger the difference between the point estimate and the hypothesized or comparison score.

Figure 3-5 summarizes our results. The null hypotheses are numbered and indicated by H_o. For example our first null hypothesis compared our mean of 100 with a value of 88. The CI of 94.12 to 105.88 is included in the figure. What can be said about the *p* values for null hypotheses that fall outside the 95% CI? The two that fall outside of the CI are 88 and 106 from questions 1 and 2, and in both cases the *p* was <.05. Notice that $H_o: 106$ is just outside the 95% CI, and its *p* value is barely below 0.05. If a null hypothesis falls at either end of a 95% CI, $p = 0.05$.

Because all numbers outside of the CI have *p* values less than 0.05, we would expect that all numbers within the CI would have *p* values greater than 0.05. This leads to a characterization of a 95% CI in terms of *p* values. A 95% CI contains all the (null hypothesis) values for which $p \geq .05$. In other words a 95% CI contains values (hypotheses) that are statistically compatible (will not be rejected at the 0.05 level) with the point estimate (observed value).

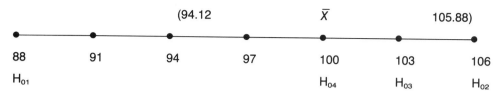

FIGURE 3-5
Relationship of confidence intervals to hypothesis testing.

Consistency Checks for Evaluating Research Reports

The relationships between point estimates, CI estimates, and significance tests make it possible to uncover inconsistencies in manuscripts. The point estimate cannot be outside of the CI. A value for a null hypothesis within the 95% CI should have a p value greater than 0.05, and one outside of the 95% CI should have a p value less than 0.05.

Value of Confidence Intervals

Levels of significance (p values) ascertain whether a particular hypothesis is statistically compatible with the observed sample value, while 95% CIs specify all the population values that are statistically indistinguishable from the observed sample value. "The confidence interval contains more information (than the p value) because it is equivalent to performing a significance test for all values of the parameter, not just a single value" (Berry, 1986).

A Word of Caution

Statistical tests and statistical estimates assume random sampling. When using either significance tests or CIs, clear-cut conclusions regarding the entire population apply only when the study sample is a random sample of that population. Because study patients are rarely random samples from a population, we should be wary about statistical inferences and ask "From what population might this group constitute a random sample?"(Remington & Schork, 1970, p. 93). If the sample appears to be representative of some population (but not a random sample), the width of the CI is often conceived of as a lower bound (minimum) for the uncertainty in the point estimate. However, clinical judgment must supplement statistical analysis whenever nonrandom samples are used to generalize to individuals not studied (Riegelman, 1981, p. 205).

When reading a research report, it is essential to determine if there is an explicitly defined population of interest and to ascertain if and how the study sample was selected. Although a representative (nonrandom) sample from an explicitly defined population falls short of a random sample, it is superior to a nonrepresentative sample or to a situation in which the population or the study sample is not clearly defined. When inferences about the population are drawn using statistical tests or CIs in such situations, let the reader beware! Descriptions of the study sample (e.g., using point estimates) provide useful information in all situations. When the population is ill defined, the study sample unrepresentative, or the relation of the study sample to the population unclear, point estimates and other statistics describing the sample may provide the only reliable information.

SAMPLE SIZE

In planning research the question always arises as to how large a sample is needed. Determination of sample size involves ethical and statistical consideration. If the sample size is too small to detect significant differences or relationships or includes far more subjects than necessary, the cost to subjects and researchers cannot be justified. Sample size is addressed as it relates to the specific statistics covered in this book. Here, we cover only the main determinants of sample size. A major contribution to sample size determination was made by Jacob Cohen (1987). His book provides tables that help us determine the appropriate sample size for a particular statistical test.

Sample size is related to power, effect size, and significance level. Power is the likelihood of rejecting the null hypothesis (i.e, avoiding a Type II error). An 80% level is generally viewed as an adequate level. As noted, effect size is the difference between the groups or the strength of the relationship. For example, for the t test, which compares the means of two groups, Cohen (1987) defines a small effect as 0.2 of a standard deviation, a moderate effect as 0.5 of a standard deviation, and a large effect as 0.8. In relation to GRE scores with a standard deviation of 100, a small effect would be 20 points (100 × 0.2); a moderate effect, 50 points; and a large effect, 80 points.

The significance level is the probability of rejecting a true null hypothesis (making a Type I error); it is called alpha and is often set at 0.05. Given three of these parameters, the fourth can be determined. Cohen's book has both power and sample size tables. If we know the sample size, effect size, and significance level, we can determine the power of the analysis. This can be particularly helpful when critiquing research, as nonsignificant results may be related to an inadequate sample size, and significant results may be related to a very large sample, rather than to a meaningful result. When planning a study one determines the desired power, acceptable significance level, and expected effect size and uses these three parameters to determine the necessary sample size. In addition to Cohen's book, software programs have been developed to assist with the determination of sample size.

SUMMARY

Topics covered in this chapter are basic to understanding the use of the specific statistical techniques contained in the second section of this book. Please take time to be sure that you understand these topics before proceeding.

4

Confidence Interval Estimates and Significance Tests for Percentages:
Examples to Aid Understanding of Statistical Inference

Leonard E. Braitman

OBJECTIVES FOR CHAPTER 4

After reading this chapter you should be able to do the following:

1. Explain the relationships between point estimates, confidence intervals, and probability values.

2. Distinguish between a random sample and randomization.

3. Differentiate between statistical significance and clinical significance.

Barbara Hazard Munro and Ellis Batten Page: STATISTICAL METHODS FOR HEALTH CARE RESEARCH, SECOND EDITION. © 1993, 1986 by J. B. Lippincott Company.

Data are usually collected on a sample of people selected from a larger group (population) to which the researchers want to generalize their findings. The two major approaches to statistical inference from sample to population are significance tests and statistical estimates (point estimates and confidence intervals). Point estimates and confidence intervals can address the general question: How large is the difference between groups? This subsumes the question addressed by significance tests, whether there is a nonzero (statistically significant) difference. In this section statistical estimates, including point estimates and confidence interval estimates of percentages, are discussed through the use of examples.

CONFIDENCE INTERVALS FOR PERCENTAGES

Example 1

None of 20 healthy study subjects younger than 65 years fell during the last year. The point estimate is the percentage, $0/20 = 0\%$, of subjects in the study sample who actually fell. If the study sample is representative of the population of interest, the point estimate, 0%, is the best single number that approximates the unknown true percentage of people who fell during the last year in the population of interest (healthy people younger than 65 years). However, "if nothing goes wrong [in the sample], is everything all right [in the population of interest]?" (Hanley & Lippman-Hand, 1983, p. 1743). Obviously, we cannot conclude that no one in the population of interest fell just because no one fell in the sample of 20. We need to know the margin of error of the point estimate (0%) in estimating the unknown true percentage.

A rough idea of the uncertainty in a point estimate will be provided using a confidence interval. The 95% confidence interval (CI) of the percentage $0/20 = 0\%$ ranges from 0% to 17%. The values, 0% to 17% in the 95% CI, provide a range of values that is reasonably compatible with the observed result: 0 out of 20 fell in the study group (sample). The point estimate of 0% and values nearby are most compatible with the observed data. However, we cannot be certain that the true percentage of interest is 0% or even near it. The CI provides a range of plausible estimates. Because repeated samples from the same population usually give different results, the point estimate from that sample (0%) is unlikely to be exactly equal to the unknown population value (parameter). Thus, a range of estimated values is needed.

How is a confidence interval for a single percentage determined? It can be found using a computer program, Confidence Interval Analysis (CIA) (available from *Annals of Internal Medicine*, 6th and Race streets, Philadelphia, PA 19106-1657) or read from tables for groups up to size $N = 100$ (Lentner, 1982). However, when the point estimate is 0 (0%), a simple approximate method called the rule of three applies. The rule of three gives an approximate 95% CI from 0 to $3/N$ when the point estimate is $0/N$ (Hanley & Lippman-Hand, 1983). For this sample of $N = 20$, the 95% CI ranges from 0 to $3/20$ (from 0% to 15%), close to the correct answer 95% CI of 0% to 17%. The numbers in this 95% CI are the values from the population that are reasonably compatible with the observed sample percentage (0%). Candidates for the unknown population value (parameter) become less compatible with the sample value (0%), the further they are from 0%; those outside the 95% CI are unlikely candidates but still possible.

Example 2

Suppose none of 100 normal subjects younger than 65 years fell during the last year. Find the point estimate and 95% CI for the percentage that fell.

Answer: The point estimate is 0% ($^0/_{100}$ = 0%). The rule of three shortcut results in a 95% confidence interval of 0 to 3% ($^3/_N$ = $^3/_{100}$ = 3%). (Using the table or the computer program yields 0% to 3.6%.) This 4-percentage-point interval is much smaller than the 0% to 17% in example 1. Although no one fell in either group, the larger sample of 100 in example 2 has a narrower 95% CI and is a more reliable statistical estimate of the unknown percentage of subjects who fell.

Why? The width of the 95% CI reflects the sampling error resulting from using an estimate based on a random sample rather than using the entire population. In two random samples with the same point estimate (in this case, 0%), the larger sample yields a more reliable estimate (a narrower 95% CI, indicating less sampling error) than the smaller sample. In other words if other things are equal, a statistical estimate derived from a larger random sample has a smaller margin of error.

Example 3

Of 100 people at least 65 years old, 34 fell in the last year. Find the point estimate and 95% CI for the percent that fell.

Answer: The point estimate is $^{34}/_{100}$ = 34%. The table and computer program both give 95% CI of 25% to 48%. (The rule of three does not apply here because p is not 0%.)

Now compare the uncertainty in statistical estimates based on two groups (samples) of the same size that are representative of the population of interest. In examples 2 and 3, groups of 100 people were followed. Despite the same size sample, the 95% CI is much wider in example 3 (48% to 25% = 23 percentage points) than in example 2 (3.6 percentage points). This is because in example 2, 0 of 100 fell, so there is no variability in the response (falling or not falling). This extreme uniformity of response facilitates a precise generalization to the population of interest. However, in example 3 there was substantial variability; approximately $^1/_3$ (34%) fell and $^2/_3$ did not. This greater variability results in a more uncertain estimate (of the true but unknown percentage) indicated by the wider 95% CI in example 3. "This difference exemplifies a property of confidence interval for percentages (proportions): For a given sample size, percentages near 50% have wider confidence intervals (more uncertainty) than percentages near either 0% or 100%" (Braitman, 1988). Greater variability of response leads to greater random sampling errors in predictions from sample data to the population of interest.

Example 4

Suppose that in a group of people at least 65 years old and taking benzodiazepines daily, 60% fell during the last year. Find the point estimate and confidence interval estimate for the percent that fell. The point estimate is 60%. However, the confidence interval estimate cannot be determined without knowledge of the size of the group.

ASSUMPTIONS UNDERLYING CONFIDENCE INTERVALS OF SINGLE PERCENTAGES

Confidence intervals for percentages depend on underlying assumptions about the process of sampling:

1. Within-sample independence: Observations within the sample must be independent of one another for a confidence interval to be valid.
2. The sample is a random sample of the population of interest

Example 5

Suppose there were 35 falls in the last year in 50 patients at least 65 years old taking benzodiazepines daily. Find the point estimate and 95% CI for the percentage that fell.

Answer: Note that 35 falls in 50 patients does not mean that 35 of 50 patients fell. We need to know how many times each patient fell because multiple falls by the same person are not independent observations. By using the number of patients who fell (rather than the 35 falls), we would eliminate the multiple falls, which are the nonindependent observations.

Example 6

Suppose there were 35 falls in 50 patients at least 65 years old and taking benzodiazepines daily. One person fell six times, and everyone else fell once during the last year. Find the point estimate and 95% CI.

Answer: The patient, not the fall, is the phenomenon of clinical interest. In addition, patients who fall once are more likely on average to fall again, so falls are not independent observations. Because the patient, not the fall, represents an independent observation, the patient (not the fall) is a proper unit of statistical analysis. One patient fell six times, and each of the remaining 29 falls occurred to a different patient. Thus, $1 + 29 = 30$ patients out of 50 fell at least once during the last year for a point estimate of $30/50 = 60\%$ (not $35/50 = 70\%$). The percentage of patients who fell *one or more times* is 60% (95% CI is 45% to 74%). Because 29 patients fell once and one patient fell 6 times, the percentage of patients who fell *more than once* is $1/50 = 2\%$ (95% CI of 0.5% to 14%). Which estimate is appropriate depends on the substantive question being addressed.

Notice that 95% CI of 0.5% to 14% is much narrower (13.5 percentage points wide) than 95% CI of 45% to 74% (approximately 29 percentage points wide) because $1/50$ has less variability of response (one fell, 49 did not) than $30/50$ (30 fell, 20 did not), despite both percentages being based on groups of 50.

STATISTICAL MISTAKES VS. STATISTICAL ERRORS

Example 6 illustrated that unless the assumption of within-sample independence of observations is satisfied, the computed point estimate and associated confidence interval will not be correct. A similar mistake involves using the percentage of serum samples (with nonindependent multiple serum samples for some patients) with a particular characteristic to draw conclusions about the percentage of patients with that characteristic. Another example of a statistical *mistake* is using statistical formulas when the sample size is too small. Such mistakes are avoidable and are completely different from sampling errors and type I and type II errors (see Chapter 3), all of which can be minimized but cannot be entirely avoided. If a result is obviously wrong, for example a probability greater than 1 or a percentage less than 0, we would check our calculations and our assumptions to determine where the error lies. An inconsistency gives us valuable information that leads us to correct our mistakes. However, unrecognized statistical mistakes (e.g., when the answer is incorrect but not inconsistent or otherwise obviously wrong) are common and more dangerous. Many statistical mistakes result from assuming that answers generated by computers are necessarily correct. Most computer programs do not check any assumptions before providing results, and no computer program checks all assumptions. Thus, it is essential to verify all calculations and assumptions underlying statistical tests.

ASSUMPTIONS OF RANDOM SAMPLING AND RANDOMIZATION UNDERLYING CONFIDENCE INTERVALS AND SIGNIFICANCE TESTS

Significance tests and confidence intervals assume random sampling (or random assignment, which is discussed later). The random sampling assumption is an integral part of the interpretation of confidence intervals. The term *random sample* often is used incorrectly to denote a convenience sample of whatever patients are available. In random sampling a relevant population (from which the sample will be selected) must be carefully listed. Suppose that a sample of 100 was randomly selected from the population of patients receiving a new treatment. That means every sample of 100 has the same chance of being selected from a listing of the population (Wonnacott & Wonnacott, 1985).

The uncertainty that results from making an estimate using a part (sample) rather than the entire population of interest is called sampling error. Such uncertainty in the point estimate depends on the amount of sampling variability (chance variation from sample to sample) expected in random samples of that size. Because we expect more sampling variability in small samples than large samples, we were not surprised that $0/20$ has a 95% CI of 0% to 17%, approximately five times as wide as the 95% CI of 0% to 3.6% for $0/100$ in example 2. The margin of error expressed by the width of a confidence interval includes random or chance error (sampling error) that accompanies choosing a random sample rather than the entire population but does not include observer errors of measurement or classification or any other systematic errors. Such systematic errors often are larger than random (sampling) errors and are difficult to detect. Thus, appropriate measurement and careful study design and study execution remain crucial to control systematic (nonrandom) errors in clinical studies (Rothman, 1986).

RANDOMIZATION AS AN ALTERNATIVE ASSUMPTION TO RANDOM SAMPLING

Randomization is the "allocation of individuals to groups, e.g., to experimental and control regimens, by chance. Within the limits of chance variation, randomization should make the control and experimental groups similar at the start of an investigation and ensure that personal judgement and prejudices of the investigator do not influence allocation. Randomization or random assignment should not be confused with haphazard assignment. The pattern of assignment may appear to be haphazard, but this arises from the haphazard nature with which digits occur in a table of random numbers, and not from the haphazard whim of the investigator in allocating patients" (Last, 1983). Using randomization, chance differences between treatment groups can be measured using probabilities, and nonchance differences are minimized.

Random assignment facilitates fair comparisons. By randomly assigning patients to treatment so that each patient is equally likely to receive either treatment (randomization), treatment groups are formed that differ (before treatment) only by chance, not by human choice. Methods such as keeping subjects and observers unaware of treatment assignments (blinding) and giving placebos to controls are intended to keep other things (besides treatment) equal in the groups during the execution of the study. When carefully performed, such maneuvers make it likely that any observed group differences in response to treatment are due to actual differences between treatments (if sample size is sufficiently large) and not to other differences between the groups.

Randomization (random assignment) also justifies the use of hypothesis tests and confidence intervals. If patients are randomized (randomly assigned) to treatment and control groups, but the entire study group is not a random sample of the population of interest, statistical inferences apply to differences in treatment effects between the study samples but *not* necessarily to the population. This is because such random assignment is equivalent to selecting two random samples from the total study sample (not from the population).

TAILORING THE STATISTICAL ANALYSIS TO THE SUBSTANTIVE PROBLEM

Example

Suppose 15 of 25 patients (60%) responded to a new treatment compared to 7 of 25 (28%) on a standard treatment. Before beginning a study to collect such data, the investigators should decide what specific substantive or clinical question(s) is to be addressed? At least four separate substantive questions can be addressed using these data:

1. What percent of patients responded to the new treatment?
2. What percent of patients responded to the standard treatment?
3. Is there a statistically significant difference between the percentages that responded to the two treatments?
4. What is the size of the difference between the percentages of patients that responded to the new and the standard treatment?

Possible Approaches to the Four Questions

To address question 1 and question 2, estimate separate percentages responding to the new and the standard treatments without comparing them. The percentage that responded to the new treatment was $^{15}/_{25} = 60\%$ (95% CI of 39% to 79%). The percentage that responded to the standard treatment was $^7/_{25} = 28\%$ (95% CI of 12% to 49%).

To address question 3, compare the percentages responding to the new and standard treatments using a statistical test and report the p value. Because the expected cell sizes in the 2 × 2 table are all above five, the chi-squared test is used to compare the percentages (Norusis, 1990c). The chi-squared test (discussed in the next chapter) yields $p = 0.046$. Thus, we say that there is a statistically significant (detectable) difference between the percentages.

To address question 4, estimate the difference between those two percentages by determining the point and confidence interval estimates of the difference. The point estimate of the difference is $60\% - 28\% = 32\%$ or 32 percentage points. Because the difference between two percentages is itself not a percentage but is instead measured in percentage points, we should *not* use the method for the confidence interval of a percentage that was used in the previous examples.

The *confidence interval for the difference between two percentages* is used to find the appropriate 95% CI. The computer program, CIA, gives the 95% CI of 6% to 58% (differences between 6 and 58 percentage points). In sum 32% (percentage points) is the best single number estimate of the magnitude of the difference in the population of interest, and 95% CI of 6% to 58% provides a range of estimates (interval estimate) that is statistically compatible with the observed difference of 32%.

A common misconception holds that statistical significance can be determined by observing whether the individual 95% CIs for the two groups overlap. However, we saw that the two percentages, 60% and 28%, are statistically significantly different despite the overlap in their individual confidence intervals (from 39% to 49%). The statistical significance of the difference can be correctly determined from the confidence interval of the difference, 95% CI of 6% to 58%, but not from the two separate confidence intervals found in addressing questions 1 and 2 above. However, the 95% CI of the difference provides much information in addition to statistical significance. The 95% CI of 6% to 58% provides a set of estimates (indeed, an entire interval) that is statistically compatible with the observed 32-percentage-point difference. Thus, it addresses the size of the difference, not just whether there is a statistically significant difference. The four examples in the next section show the advantages of the confidence interval of the difference when the substantive question of interest is the size of the difference between responses to two treatments.

CONFIDENCE INTERVALS OF DIFFERENCES BETWEEN PERCENTAGES

Authors of papers reporting tests of new treatments often address only statistical significance (or p values) and not the question of a real clinical advantage. In this section we distinguish clinical (practical) significance from statistical significance and show how confidence intervals of differences can assess them both (Braitman, 1991). Hypothetical examples comparing the percentages of arthritis patients responding to two treatments provide interpretations of p values, point estimates, and confidence intervals.

Example 1

Suppose in a multicenter clinical trial, 156 of 400 patients (39%) responded to a new treatment for arthritis, and 128 of 400 different patients (32%) responded to the standard treatment. Significance tests and statistical estimates address distinct but related questions using these data. A significance test addresses the question, "*How likely* was the difference to occur by chance?" Statistical estimates of differences (point estimates and confidence intervals) address, "*How large* is the difference in the population of interest?" (Wonnacott & Wonnacott, 1985).

Whether a difference in the percentages responding to the two treatments exists in the *population* of arthritis patients is ascertained using a significance level or p value. The null hypothesis, H_0, states that there is really no difference between the percentages responding in the population of interest. The alternative hypothesis is that such a difference (in either direction) exists. The significance test uses the p value to weigh the evidence that there is a real difference (the alternative hypothesis) against the null hypothesis that the observed difference is due to chance variation. The p value, $p = 0.046$, comes from a chi-squared test comparing $156/400$ (39%) with $128/400$ (32%). $p = 0.046$ is the probability of obtaining the observed difference (7% = 39% − 32%) or one larger in the study sample *assuming* H_0: no difference in the percentages responding in the population of interest. A low p value suggests incompatibility between the observed data and H_0. Because $p = 0.046 < 0.05$ (0.05 is the conventional cutoff point), the observed difference is called statistically significant at the $\alpha = 0.05$ level. While this p value indicates a statistically detectable difference between the populations of interest, it provides no information on the size of that difference.

Two statistical measures estimating the size of the unknown population difference are the point estimate and the confidence interval. The point estimate of the difference in this example is the difference between the observed percentages responding in the two groups (samples), 39% − 32% = 7%. Because the observed difference, 7% (7 percentage points), is unlikely to be exactly equal to the unknown true difference between the percentages of all arthritis patients responding to these two treatments (called the parameter), a range or confidence interval estimate is needed. The method for the 95% CI of the difference between percentages (proportions) yields a 95% CI ranging from 0.4% to 14% (see example 1 in Fig. 4-1). A 95% CI means that approximately 95% of such intervals constructed from repeated (random) samples of that size will include the parameter (the unknown true population difference). This definition focuses on the average accuracy (95%) of the CI estimation process but does not help us interpret the single 95% CI of 0.4% to 14% that was computed. Each value in the 95% CI is not statistically significantly different from the observed difference (in this case, 7%).

"Experienced clinicians weigh the side effects, long-term complications and other costs against the benefits of the two treatments to judge the size of the smallest clinically important difference" (Braitman, 1991, p. 515). Assume that the *smallest* clinically important difference is 20% (20 percentage points) in all the examples. Because *every* value in the 95% CI of 0.4% to 14% is below 20% (example 1 in Fig. 4-1), the difference is considered "not clinically significant." Thus, this statistically significant difference is not clinically significant.

Example 2

In a smaller study in which 15 of 25 patients (60%) responded to a new treatment compared with 7 of 25 (28%) on a standard treatment, the p value = 0.046. The point estimate of the difference is 60% − 28% = 32% (32 percentage points). Because the same p value (0.046) corresponds to highly disparate differences of 32% in example 2 and 7% in example 1 (see Fig. 4-1), the p value gives no information on the size of the

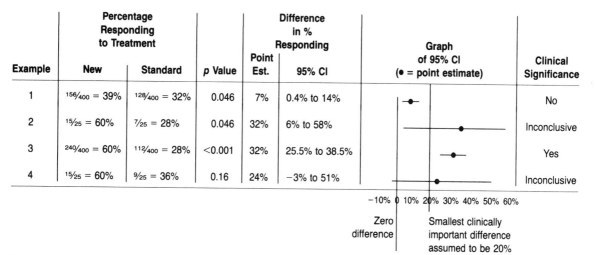

Example	Percentage Responding to Treatment		p Value	Difference in % Responding		Graph of 95% CI (• = point estimate)	Clinical Significance
	New	Standard		Point Est.	95% CI		
1	$^{156}/_{400}$ = 39%	$^{128}/_{400}$ = 32%	0.046	7%	0.4% to 14%		No
2	$^{15}/_{25}$ = 60%	$^{7}/_{25}$ = 28%	0.046	32%	6% to 58%		Inconclusive
3	$^{240}/_{400}$ = 60%	$^{112}/_{400}$ = 28%	<0.001	32%	25.5% to 38.5%		Yes
4	$^{15}/_{25}$ = 60%	$^{9}/_{25}$ = 36%	0.16	24%	−3% to 51%		Inconclusive

−10% 0 10% 20% 30% 40% 50% 60%

Zero difference

Smallest clinically important difference assumed to be 20%

FIGURE 4-1
Confidence intervals of differences.

difference. This point estimate and the 95% CI (6% − 58%) estimate the size of the unknown "true" difference.

How are hypothesis tests and confidence intervals related to one another? When comparing two groups, the usual null hypothesis (H_o) is zero (no) difference between the two groups. If zero is outside the 95% CI of a difference, the observed difference is statistically significantly different from zero ($p < 0.05$). In Figure 4-1 the 95% CIs do not include zero in examples 1 through 3, and the associated p values are less than 0.05. In example 4, zero is included in the 95% CI (−3% to 51%) and $p = 0.16$. Thus, a 95% CI can be viewed as the set of values hypothesized for the parameter that cannot be rejected at the $\alpha = 0.05$ level (Braitman, 1991). In other words a 95% CI contains values that are not statistically significantly different ($p \geq 0.05$) from the observed value.

Example 3

Suppose that 240 of 400 patients (60%) responded to a new treatment compared with 112 of 400 (28%) on the standard. In this larger study the same percentages as in example 2 respond to the new (60%) and standard (28%) treatments, respectively. Using a chi-squared test, $p < 0.001$. Because $p < 0.05$, the difference is statistically significant; however, is it clinically significant? Remember that a p value does not address the size or importance of the difference.

The statistical estimates of the difference, the point estimate and confidence interval estimate, address these issues. Define a difference as clinically significant when the entire 95% CI is above the predetermined smallest clinically important difference (Braitman, 1991). Because all of the 95% CI of 25.5% to 38.5% is above 20%, the difference is clinically significant. Confidence intervals permit readers to assess clinical significance using their own value for the smallest clinically important difference rather than having to depend on the author's interpretation (Berry, 1986).

In example 1 the difference is not clinically significant because the whole 95% CI is below the smallest clinically important difference of 20%. When the smallest clinically important difference is included within the 95% CI, as in example 2, no definitive conclusion about clinical significance is possible. Nevertheless, the point estimate and confidence interval suggest trends in the data. Because in example 2, the point estimate (32%) and more than 2/3 of the 95% CI exceeds 20%, these data do tend toward clinical significance.

When two groups receive different treatments, a commonly used (but less informative) alternative statistical analysis presents two separate 95% CIs, one for the percentage responding to each treatment. If the relevant question is the percentage that respond to each treatment separately without providing a treatment comparison, these two confidence intervals suffice. However, if they overlap, they do not enable us to conclude whether the difference is statistically significant. The 95% CI of the difference enables us to assess statistical significance and clinical significance. In example 2 the difference of 32 percentage points (95% CI of 6% to 58%) is statistically significant and tends toward clinical significance. Thus, only the 95% CI of the difference, not the two single sample 95% CIs, makes the assessment of statistical and clinical significance possible.

INTERPRETATION OF CONFIDENCE INTERVALS

The 95% CI means that approximately 95% of such varying random confidence intervals (one for each random sample), if constructed, would include the population parameter, and 5% would not. The words "95% confidence" refer to the 95% average accuracy of the estimation process and *not* to a probability of 95% for a single computed confidence interval (Wonnacott & Wonnacott, 1985). Either the 95% CI includes the parameter (the unknown true value) or it does not; we cannot tell which. The single 95% CI may be interpreted as the set of hypotheses for parameter values that cannot be rejected at $p \geq 0.05$.

Although 32% is the point estimate for the unknown parameter in examples 2 and 3, its value is more uncertain in the smaller sample. The narrower 95% CI of 25.5% to 38.5% (13 percentage points wide) from the larger sample is more precise than 95% CI of 6% to 58% (52 percentage points wide). The width of a 95% CI indicates the amount of uncertainty (called sampling variability or sampling error) about the population parameter inherent in examining only a random sample rather than the population. The 95% CI's combined information on the size of the "true" difference and how precisely that size is known (Rothman, 1986) helped us assess clinical and statistical significance.

Although confidence intervals and significance tests can help us assess the impact of sampling or random error, other methods involving the design and analysis of research studies are needed to deal with nonrandom systematic errors. Neither the p value nor the statistical estimates enable us to decide what caused the observed difference in response. A careful analysis of the experimental design and execution of the study is necessary before alternative explanations for the results can be discarded. Confidence intervals communicate only the effects of sampling error on the precision of point estimates; they cannot control for systematic (nonsampling) errors, such as unmeasured confounders or measurement error. To limit the effects of systematic errors and biases, careful attention must be given to study design (e.g., randomization) and epidemiologic methods (Rothman, 1986; Wonnacott & Wonnacott, 1985). In the analysis phase multivariable regression models can address the net effect of treatment on study outcome by controlling statistically for confounding variables (see Chapter 12, Regression).

Although inferences about the population of interest actually presume random (or probability) sampling, point and confidence interval estimates and p values generally are considered to be useful approximations to the extent that the study sample is representative of the population.

INFORMATION CONTENT OF COMMON FORMS OF STATISTICAL PRESENTATIONS

The next example illustrates the relevance of statistical estimates of the difference between treatment response rates even when the difference is not statistically significant. In addition, it demonstrates the different types of information provided by p values, point estimates, and confidence intervals.

Example 4

Suppose a study produced results similar to those in example 2, with 15 of 25 responding to the new treatment but 9 of 25 responding to the standard treatment. In other words the same number responded to the new treatment, but two additional patients responded to the standard treatment.

Intuitively, we would expect the statistical presentation to lead to an interpretation similar to the one in example 2. However, traditional presentations too often state only that the difference was "significant ($p < 0.05$)" in example 2 and "not significant ($p > 0.05$)" in example 4. Such presentations incorrectly suggest very different conclusions in examples 2 and 4. Although all of examples 1 through 3 contain statistically significant results, the $p < 0.001$ in example 3 provides a much greater weight of evidence against H_o (the hypothesis of zero difference) than $p = 0.046$. Thus, more specific information is provided by an exact p value than by a statement of statistical significance or by $p < 0.05$. However, by themselves, p values yield *no* information on the size of the difference. Indeed, among these examples, the highest p value (0.16) does not correspond to the smallest difference (7%). That shows how a large difference between two small samples can yield a large (nonsignificant) p value.

p values cannot be used to gauge the size of differences because they also depend on sample size. p values address the existence of a real nonzero difference between treatments but not the size of that treatment difference. Thus, they cannot be used to assess clinical (practical) significance. The point estimate of the difference measures the magnitude of differences in the observed samples.

The point estimates in examples 2 through 4 are all large differences (of at least 24 percentage points) contrasted with a small difference of 7 percentage points in example 1. The point estimate *describes* the observed data (the size of the difference between *samples*) and estimates the unknown difference parameter. Point estimates and confidence intervals of differences estimate the size of the treatment effect. However, being a single number, a point estimate cannot indicate its own sampling error as a confidence interval does. The 95% CI provides two related types of information: the uncertainty in their respective point estimates and the clinical significance of the differences.

The larger group sizes of 400 in examples 1 and 3 yield more precise confidence interval estimates (width approximately 14 percentage points) than the smaller groups of 25 in examples 2 and 4, in which 95% CIs are more than 50 percentage points wide. Assuming that the smallest clinically important difference is 20 percentage points, the observed difference is clinically significant in example 3 and not clinically significant in example 1. In examples 2 and 4 the clinical significance of the differences is inconclusive. However, in example 2 the point estimate, 32%, and almost 3/4 of the 95% CI of 6% to 58% are above the smallest clinically important difference (20%), so the difference tends toward clinical significance. Although the difference in example 4 is not statistically significant, it may be real and even clinically important because the point estimate (24%) and more than 1/2 of the 95% CI correspond to clinically important differences. Thus, using confidence intervals to evaluate practical significance avoids the common fallacy of "equating non-significance with no (difference)" (Berry, 1986). It is important to include a 95% CI of any substantial difference even if that difference is not statistically significant.

SUMMARY OF ROLES OF POINT ESTIMATES, CONFIDENCE INTERVALS, AND P VALUES

p values, point estimates, and confidence intervals are used to make statistical inferences about a population parameter. Both p values and confidence intervals are defined in terms of the compatibility of hypothesis with the sample difference, while the point estimate is that sample difference. Only the point estimate describes what is actually observed in the sample. Thus, it is a descriptive and an inferential statistic. When there is no random assignment and the sample is neither random nor representative, statistical inference using either the p value or confidence interval is problematic; the point estimate still accurately describes the sample difference. Thus, the point estimate of a difference should be reported because it extracts the most fundamental and consistently meaningful information from a statistical comparison. Point estimates, confidence intervals, and p values extract complementary information from study data and should be reported for major results.

II | SPECIFIC STATISTICAL TECHNIQUES

5 Selected Nonparametric Techniques

Barbara Hazard Munro

OBJECTIVES FOR CHAPTER 5

After reading this chapter you should be able to do the following:

1. **Identify situations in which the use of nonparametric techniques is appropriate.**

2. **Interpret a computer printout containing a chi-square analysis.**

3. **Relate the results of the analysis to the research question posed.**

The nonparametric techniques to be covered in this chapter are contained in Table 5-1, which was adapted from Hinkle, Wiersma, & Jurs (1988, p. 550). This is not intended to be comprehensive, but rather a discussion of the commonly used nonparametrics. The parametric analogs that are covered in later chapters also are included.

PARAMETRIC VS. NONPARAMETRIC TESTS

When we use *parametric* tests of significance, we are estimating at least one population parameter from our sample statistics. To be able to make such an estimation, we must make certain assumptions; the most important one is that the variable we have measured in the sample is normally distributed in the population to which we plan to generalize our findings. With *nonparametric* tests, there is no assumption about the distribution of

Barbara Hazard Munro and Ellis Batten Page: STATISTICAL METHODS FOR HEALTH CARE RESEARCH, SECOND EDITION. © 1993, 1986 by J. B. Lippincott Company.

TABLE 5-1
Nonparametric Tests and Corresponding Parametric Analogs

| | Nonparametric Tests | | |
	Nominal Data	Ordinal Data	Parametric Analog
One-Group Case	Chi-square goodness of fit	—	—
Two-Group Case	Chi-square	Mann-Whitney U	t test
k-Group Case	Chi-square	Kruskal-Wallis H	One-way ANOVA
Dependent Groups (Repeated Measures)	McNemar test for significance of change	Wilcoxon matched-pairs signed rank test Friedman Matched samples	Paired t tests Repeated measures ANOVA

the variable in the population. For that reason nonparametric tests often are called *distribution free.*

At one time, level of measurement was considered an important element in deciding whether to use parametric or nonparametric tests. It was believed that parametric tests should be reserved for use with interval- and ratio-level data. Now, however, it has been shown that the use of parametric techniques with ordinal data rarely distorts the results.

Parametric techniques have several advantages. They are more *powerful* and more *flexible* than nonparametric techniques. They not only allow the researcher to study the effect of many independent variables on the dependent variable, but also make possible the study of their interaction. Nonparametric techniques are much easier to calculate by hand than parametric techniques, but that advantage has been eliminated by the use of computers. Small samples and serious distortions of the data should lead one to explore nonparametric techniques.

CHI-SQUARE

Chi-square is the most commonly reported nonparametric statistic. It is used when the data are nominal (categorical). In later chapters we discuss how the chi-square is used to test the fit of models in techniques such as logistic regression and path analysis.

Chi-square can be used with one or more groups. It compares the actual number (or frequency) in each group with the "expected" number. The "expected" number can be based on theory, previous experience, or comparison groups.

CARDIAC CATH		SEX		Row totals
		MALE	FEMALE	
	NO	15	16	31
	YES	45	24	69
	Column totals	60	40	100

FIGURE 5-1
Data for chi-square analysis.

For example suppose we were interested in the question of whether men are treated more aggressively for cardiovascular problems than women. We select people for our sample who have similar results on initial testing. We then record the sex of the patient and whether or not a cardiac catheterization was recommended. Figure 5-1 contains the fictitious results. We see that 69 people were referred for cardiac catheterization, 45 men and 24 women.

The null hypothesis is that recommendation for cardiac catheterization is not related to the sex of the patient. If the data support the null hypothesis, there will be no difference in the rates between men and women. Because the numbers of men and women in our sample are different, it is not easy to tell whether there were differences by sex. To clarify matters we could calculate percentages (Fig. 5-2). Seventy-five percent of the men and 60% of the women were referred. Thus, it does appear that men are more likely to be referred than women. The statistical question is whether or not this difference is significant, that is, if it is unlikely to occur by chance alone. In most studies people judge significance at the 0.05 level, which means if there are less than 5 chances in 100 that a difference this large would have occurred by chance alone, the difference is significant. Sixty-nine of the 100 subjects or 69% were referred. If the rates of referral are the same for men and women, then 69% of the 60 men ($60 \times 0.69 = 41.4$) and 69% of the women (27.6) should have been referred. The numbers 41.4 for men and 27.6 for women are the *expected frequencies*, that is, the numbers we would expect if the rates were the same. Because it is much more likely these days that data will be analyzed by the computer rather than by hand, we will present the computer output first, followed later by the hand calculations. See Figure 5-3 for the output.

CARDIAC CATH		SEX		Row totals
		MALE	FEMALE	
	NO	15 (25%)	16 (40%)	31
	YES	45 (75%)	24 (60%)	69
	Column totals	60	40	100

FIGURE 5-2
Percentage of males and females referred for cardiac catheterization.

(1) CROSSTABS /TABLES= CATH BY SEX /CELLS= COUNT COLUMN /STATISTICS= CHISQ PHI CC
LAMBDA UC.

(2) CATH   cardiac cath   by   SEX

```
                            SEX
            Count
            Col Pct    MALE     FEMALE
                                          Row
                         1        2       Total
      CATH
            NO    0      15       16        31
                       25.0     40.0      31.0

            YES   1      45       24        69
                       75.0     60.0      69.0

            Column       60       40       100
            Total      60.0     40.0     100.0
```

(3)
Chi-Square	Value	DF	Significance
Pearson	2.52454	1	.11209
Continuity Correction	1.87198	1	.17125
Likelihood Ratio	2.49898	1	.11392
Mantel-Haenszel test for linear association	2.49930	1	.11390

Minimum Expected Frequency -   12.400

(4)
Statistic	Value	ASE1	T-value	Approximate Significance
Phi	.15889			.11209 *1
Cramer's V	.15889			.11209 *1
Contingency Coefficient	.15692			.11209 *1
Lambda :				
symmetric	.01408	.07784	.17963	
with CATH dependent	.00000	.00000		
with SEX dependent	.02500	.13744	.17963	
Goodman & Kruskal Tau :				
with CATH dependent	.02525	.03197		.11390 *2
with SEX dependent	.02525	.03192		.11390 *2
Uncertainty Coefficient :				
symmetric	.01934	.02444	.79030	.11392 *3
with CATH dependent	.02018	.02549	.79030	.11392 *3
with SEX dependent	.01857	.02348	.79030	.11392 *3

*1 Pearson chi-square probability
*2 Based on chi-square approximation
*3 Likelihood ratio chi-square probability

FIGURE 5-3
Computer output of chi-square analysis.

Computer Output for Chi-Square Analysis

The output was produced by SPSS-PC. It was edited slightly to remove page numbers, dates, and so forth, and the numbers in circles have been added to help us describe the content.

① These are the commands that produced the output. The procedure used was CROSSTABS, and the table requested will have CATH (cardiac catheterization) as the row variable and SEX as the column variable. Within each cell, the COUNT (number of subjects) and the COLUMN (column percents) are requested. All the statistics that are appropriate for nominal level variables were selected. These include CHISQ (chi-square), PHI, CC (contingency coefficient), LAMBDA, and UC (uncertainty coefficient).

② The contingency table looks very much like Figure 5-2. Within each cell, the percent is given below the number of subjects.

③ These are the chi-square values, degrees of freedom (*df*), and significance (probability levels). But which one do you use? All you wanted was a chi-square, and what you see are four different chi-square values, each with its own level of significance. Maybe life was simpler when we did this by hand! A good place to decipher your printout is the manual that comes with the software. Let's look at these in the order in which they appear. The *Pearson value* is what you would get if you did this by hand using the usual formula. It is based on the differences between the observed and expected frequencies. For example the actual (or observed) number of men referred is 45, but the expected number (based on an overall referral rate of 69%) is 41.4. The difference between these two values is 3.6. The chi-square value based on the differences between observed and expected frequencies in each of the four cells in our design is 2.52454. There is one degree of freedom, and the significance level is 0.11209. Therefore, we would say that the null hypothesis of no difference between men and women in the rates of referral has been supported. Degrees of freedom in chi-square analyses are explained in a subsequent section.

The *continuity correction* is often referred to as the Yates' correction. Although nominal data are used to calculate a chi-square, chi-square values have a distribution (see Appendix B). The distribution is continuous, but when the expected frequency in any of the cells in a 2 × 2 table is less than 5, the sampling distribution of chi-square for that analysis may depart substantially from normal (Hinkle, Wiersma, & Jurs, 1988). In those cases the continuity correction is recommended. The correction consists of subtracting 0.5 from the difference between each pair of observed and expected frequencies. In our example the difference of 3.6 would be reduced to 3.1 by subtracting 0.5. This results in an overall lower chi-square value. On the output we see that the Pearson value is 2.52454, but with the continuity correction, this drops to 1.87198. Thus, applying the correction reduces the power of the analysis. In our example the *minimum expected frequency* is 12.4; therefore, we would report the Pearson result. If this value had been less than 5, the continuity correction value should have been reported.

The *likelihood ratio* chi-square is based on maximum likelihood theory (Norusis, 1990c) and is of more interest when we discuss the fitting of models, such as with structural equation models. When the sample is large the likelihood ratio is very similar to the Pearson, which is evident in our example.

Although the *Mantel-Haenszel test for linear association* is given automatically when chi-square is requested, it is not appropriate for nominal data because it is based on the relationship between the two variables as measured by the Pearson correlation coefficient.

④ These are the other statistics that are appropriate with nominal data.

Phi is a shortcut method of calculating a correlation coefficient that can be used when both variables are dichotomous (have only two levels). It is used as a measure of the association between the two variables. It is only appropriate when the chi-square value is significant. In our example, because there is no significant relationship between sex and referral for catheterization as measured by chi-square, phi would not be reported. When it is appropriate to use, it is interpreted as a measure of association; that is, the correlation between these two variables is 0.15889. It allows us to interpret the strength of the relationship. It is most useful with 2 × 2 tables in which the values of phi range from 0 to 1. With tables with more cells, the value can be greater than 1, decreasing its usefulness. It is complementary to chi-square because it is less sensitive to sample size. It could be used to compare the strength of the relationship across studies.

Cramer's V is a slightly modified version of phi that can be used with larger tables. Phi is adjusted for the number of rows and columns. Thus, given a significant chi-square, report phi for 2 × 2 tables and Cramer's V for larger tables.

Contingency coefficient also is used to measure the relationship between two nominal level variables. It is a nonparametric technique, not a shortcut version of the parametric correlation coefficient. It can be used with a table of any size, but its value is affected by the number of cells. With a 2 × 2 table, the maximum value is 0.707; with a 4 × 4, it is 0.87. Thus, if it is used to compare across studies, it should only be used when the tables have the same number of rows and columns.

Lambda measures how much the error rate decreases when additional information is added. In our example if you did not know the sex of the individual, and you wanted to predict whether or not someone would be referred, you would choose the most frequently occurring event. Because 69 of the 100 people were referred, your "best guess" would be that a given individual would be referred. You would be wrong 31 times.

Does knowing the sex of the individual improve your "guess"? For men and women you would predict referral. For men you would be wrong 15 times, and for women 16 times. Lambda is the percentage by which the error rate is reduced with knowledge of the second variable. The calculation is the simplest way to explain this. Lambda is calculated as the number misclassified when you do not have information about one variable (one) minus the number misclassified when you have information on the second variable (two) divided by the number misclassified in one.

$$\frac{\text{misclassified in one} - \text{misclassified in two}}{\text{misclassified in one}}$$

In our example that would be:

$$\frac{31 - (15 + 16)}{31} \text{ or } \frac{31 - 31}{31}$$

There is obviously no improvement, because we would have been wrong 31 times whether or not we knew the sex of the individual. We could look at this the other way around. Suppose we tried to predict the sex of the individual. Then we would guess male and be wrong 40 times. If we added knowledge of whether or not the person was referred, we would guess female for no and be wrong 15 times, and we would guess male for yes and be wrong 24 times. Lambda would then equal:

$$\frac{40 - (15 + 24)}{40} \text{ or } \frac{40 - 39}{40} = 0.0250$$

In that case we have decreased our error by 2.5%.

The values are not the same; that is, they vary by which variable is considered dependent. They are not symmetric. If you have no reason to consider one variable dependent and the other independent, you can calculate a symmetric lambda. You predict the first from the second and then the second from the first, as we have done, and enter both into the formula as:

$$\frac{(31 - 31) + (40 - 39)}{31 + 40} = \frac{0 + 1}{71} = 0.0141$$

As you can see on the printout, we are given symmetric lambda when neither variable is considered dependent and then the asymmetric lambdas, first with CATH as the dependent variable and then with SEX. Lambda ranges from 0 to 1; 0 means knowledge of the variable is no help in reducing the error of prediction, and one means it is perfect in enabling correct prediction. ASE1 is the asymptotic standard error and can be used to construct confidence intervals.

Goodman & Kruskal Tau. With lambda, the same prediction is made for all cases in a row or column. In our example our best guess is referral for cardiac catheterization, and our error is 31. Instead, using Goodman and Kruskal Tau, the prediction can be randomly made in the same proportion as the marginal totals. We could randomly select 31% as no and 69% as yes for referral. We would then expect to correctly predict 31% of the 31 noes (9.61) and 69% of the 69 yesses (47.61) for a total of 57.22 correct choices (42.78 incorrect).

Adding in our knowledge of sex, we could then predict that for men 75% would be referred, and for women 60% would be referred. When these numbers are applied, we have a correct prediction rate of 58.30 (incorrect of 41.70). Subtracting the error rate when both variables are known from the rate when only one variable is known, we have:

$$\frac{0.4278 - 0.4170}{0.4278} = 0.0252$$

This indicates that knowledge of the sex of the patient reduces the error rate by 2.5%. This same type of reasoning can be applied with sex as the dependent variable. As you can see on the printout the error rate remains the same. The *uncertainty coefficient* is a measure of how much the uncertainty in the dependent variable is reduced by knowledge of the independent variable. The calculation of this coefficient is similar to that of lambda, but the uncertainty coefficient is based on the entire distribution, not just the mode (Nie, Hull, Jenkins, Steinbrenner, & Bent, 1975). The coefficient ranges from 0 to 1, with 0 being complete uncertainty and 1 being complete certainty.

Assumptions Underlying Chi-Square

1. Frequency data
2. Adequate sample size
3. Measures independent of each other
4. Theoretical basis for the categorization of the variables

The first assumption is that the data are frequency data, that is, a count of the number of subjects in each condition under analysis. The chi-square cannot be used to analyze the difference between scores or their means. If data are not categorical, they must be categorized before being used. Whether or not to categorize depends on the data and the question to be answered.

If the data are not normally distributed and violate the assumptions underlying the appropriate parametric technique, then categorization might be appropriate. The categories developed must adequately represent the data and be based on sound rationale. If you had the ages of subjects, you could categorize them as 20 to 29, 30 to 39, and 40 to 49. However, you have treated all people within one of your three categories as being equal in age. Does a 29 year old belong in the same group as a 20 year old, or is he or she more like the 30 year old? Specificity and variability are decreased through this categorization, and as a result the analysis will be less powerful.

The question addressed affects the categorization of subjects. Suppose the researcher was interested in whether or not being in school affects some categorical outcome measure. Then grouping the children as preschool and in school would make sense, rather than using their actual ages.

Another example is a study of children's tonsillectomies (Visintainer & Wolfer, 1975; Wolfer & Visintainer, 1975). In that study children who received systematic psychological preparation before surgery were compared to children who received no such preparation on a variety of outcome measures. One measure was temperature, which was recorded for each child 4 hours after he or she returned from the recovery room. The first analysis studied mean temperatures for each group of children. (The technique used was the *t* test, which is described in Chapter 6.) That analysis showed that children who had the preparation showed a significantly lower temperature than those who did not have the preparation.

Consider the group means. The children who received the preparation had a mean temperature of 98.9°F; the children who did not receive the preparation had a mean temperature of 99.5°F. The means differed by just 0.6 degree, large enough, given the sample size, to show statistical significance.

Was such a statistical difference *clinically* relevant as well? In caring for children the importance of a change in tenths of a degree is determined first by the *category of temperature*: The first and most relevant clinical question is, "Does the child have a fever?" If so, tenths of a degree may be relevant in showing that the temperature is rising or falling. However, if the child is in the normal category for temperature, tenths of a degree are not especially relevant.

In that research, therefore, a more clinically useful analysis was the 2 × 2 chi-square classifying children into "preparation" and "no preparation" by "fever" and "no fever" groups. By the chi-square analysis, the presence of fever was not different between the groups; that is, preoperative preparation had no demonstrated effect on fevers, even though the groups differed on mean temperature.

When categories have clinical relevance, statistical analyses that preserve these categories are more likely to give us useful interpretations. They are less likely to give us "differences that do not make a difference."

The second assumption is that the sample size is adequate. As already mentioned, expected frequencies of less than five in 2 × 2 tables present problems. In larger tables a cell with an expected frequency of less than five is less of a problem, but when more than 20% of the cells have less than five, or if one of the cells has no frequencies, the researcher is advised to reduce the number of cells in the analysis by grouping the subjects into a smaller number of categories (Hinkle, Wiersma, & Jurs, 1988).

It is important to consider power when planning sample size. If you have 40 subjects, 10 in each of the four cells in a 2 × 2 design, set your probability level at 0.05, and expect a moderate effect—your power is only 0.47 (Cohen, 1987, p. 235). You have less than a 50% chance of finding a significant relationship between the two variables.

The third assumption is that the measures are independent of each other. This means that the categories created are mutually exclusive; that is, no subject can be in more than one cell in the design, and no subject can be used more than once. It also means that the response of one subject cannot influence the response of another. This seems relatively straightforward, but difficulties arise in clinical research situations when data are collected for a period of time. If you are testing subjects in a hospital, you must be sure that a person who is readmitted does not get enrolled in the study for a second time. You also must be sure that subjects in one condition are not communicating with subjects in their own or different conditions in such a way that responses are "contaminated."

The fourth assumption is that there is some theoretical reason for the categories. This ensures that the analysis will be meaningful and prevents what is known as "fishing expeditions." The latter would occur if the researcher kept recategorizing subjects, hoping to find some relationship between the variables. Research questions and methods for analysis are established prior to data collection. While these may be modified to suit the data actually obtained, the basic theoretical structure remains.

Calculation of Chi-Square

For those who are interested in the actual calculations, we will use the same example.

Expected Frequencies

We have already demonstrated that in our example, because 69% of all the subjects are referred, we would expect 69% of men and 69% of women to be referred if the null hypothesis is supported. For men, for example, 69% of 60 gives an expected frequency of 41.4. The expected number of nonreferrals is 31%, which means that we would expect that 31% of the 60 men (18.6) would not be referred. In Figure 5-4 the expected frequencies are in parentheses.

SEX

CARDIAC CATH		MALE	FEMALE	Row totals
	NO	15 (18.6)	16 (12.4)	31
	YES	45 (41.4)	24 (27.6)	69
Column Totals		60	40	100

FIGURE 5-4

Contingency table with expected frequencies.

The following formula calculates an expected frequency (*fe*) for a given cell:

$$fe = \frac{\text{number of subjects in row} \times \text{number of subjects in column}}{\text{total number of subjects}}$$

For the cell male/no,

$$fe = \frac{31 \times 60}{100} = 18.6$$

Similarly, the expected frequencies for the other cells are:

$$\text{female/no, } fe = \frac{31 \times 40}{100} = 12.4$$

$$\text{male/yes, } fe = \frac{69 \times 60}{100} = 41.4$$

$$\text{female/yes, } fe = \frac{69 \times 40}{100} = 27.6$$

Although we have gone through the calculation of each expected frequency, it is only necessary to calculate one; the others can be derived by subtraction, because the expected frequencies add up to their respective row and column totals. *This will always be the case in calculating a chi-square: The sum of the expected frequencies and the sum of the observed frequencies must be equal.* Once we had the expected frequency of 18.6 for male/no, the rest could be derived by subtraction as follows:

$$\text{female/no} = 31 - 18.6 = 12.4$$
$$\text{male/yes} = 60 - 18.6 = 41.4$$
$$\text{female/yes} = 40 - 12.4 = 27.6 \text{ (or } 69 - 41.4 = 27.6)$$

Chi-Square Formula

Once the expected frequencies for all the cells have been calculated, they are compared to the observed frequencies using the chi-square formula, which follows:

where: Σ = sum of all cells

fo = observed frequency in a given cell

fe = expected frequency in a given cell

In our example, the formula becomes:

$$\Sigma \frac{(15 - 18.6)^2}{18.6} + \frac{(16 - 12.4)^2}{12.4} + \frac{(45 - 41.4)^2}{41.4} + \frac{(24 - 27.6)^2}{27.6}$$

First, we *subtract* each expected frequency from its respective observed frequency to obtain the difference. The result is:

$$\Sigma \frac{(-3.6)^2}{18.6} + \frac{(3.6)^2}{12.4} + \frac{(3.6)^2}{41.4} + \frac{(-3.6)^2}{27.6}$$

Second, we *square* each difference. Note that this eliminates the negatives. The difference between the two values is measured, not the direction of the difference. The result is:

$$\Sigma \frac{12.96}{18.6} + \frac{12.96}{12.4} + \frac{12.96}{41.4} + \frac{12.96}{27.6}$$

Third, we *divide* the result by the appropriate expected frequency. The result is:

$$0.69677 + 1.04516 + 0.31304 + 0.46957$$

Finally, we *sum* the results to obtain the chi-square value.

$$\text{chi-square} = 2.52454$$

If the expected frequency had been less than five in any of the cells, we would have applied the Yates' continuity correction by subtracting 0.5 from the absolute value of each difference. This would result in:

$$\Sigma \frac{(-3.1)^2}{18.6} + \frac{(3.1)^2}{12.4} + \frac{(3.1)^2}{41.4} + \frac{(-3.1)^2}{27.6} = \Sigma \frac{9.61}{18.6} + \frac{9.61}{12.4} + \frac{9.61}{41.4} + \frac{9.61}{27.6}$$

Application of the correction resulted in a decrease in the chi-square value from 2.52454 to 1.87198.

Degrees of Freedom in Chi-Square

In Chapter 3 the concept of degrees of freedom (*df*) is defined as the extent to which values are free to vary given a specific number of subjects and a total score. In chi-square analysis, however, frequencies are used rather than scores. The number of cells that are free to vary depends on the number of cells found in the table. How many cell frequencies would we need to know to derive the others? The answer to that question will be equal to the *df*. We have already demonstrated that given one expected frequency, we can determine the other frequencies by simple subtraction. Similarly, if we are given the row and column totals and know one of the cell frequencies, we could calculate the others. By knowing one cell value in a 2 × 2 table, we know all the other cell values. Therefore, only one cell is free to vary; the others are dependent on that value. The *df* for a 2 × 2 chi-square analysis is always 1, regardless of sample size. The formula for calculating the *df* for any size table in a chi-square analysis follows:

$$df = (r - 1)(c - 1)$$

where r = number of rows

c = number of columns

For our 2 × 2 table this becomes $df = (2 - 1)(2 - 1) = 1$.

Interpreting the Chi-Square

We look up the value of chi-square using the appropriate degrees of freedom in a table of chi-square values. In Appendix B with one degree of freedom, a chi-square value of 3.841 is significant at the 0.05 level; a value of 6.635 is significant at the 0.01 level. The chi-square value of 2.5246 is not significant at the 0.05 level. Thus, the null hypothesis cannot be rejected, and we would say that there is no difference in referral for cardiac catheterization between men and women.

Calculation of Other Statistics Related to Chi-Square

The phi coefficient has been described. Phi (ϕ) is only interpreted when there is a significant chi-square. The formula is:

$$\text{phi} = \sqrt{\frac{\text{chi-square value}}{\text{number in sample}}}$$

First, the chi-square value is *divided* by the number of subjects in the sample. Then the *square root* is taken. For our example, phi is:

$$\sqrt{\frac{2.52454}{100}}$$

$$\phi = 0.15889$$

Cramer's V is a modification of phi based on the number of rows and columns. In a 2 × 2 table, phi and Cramer's V are the same.

$$V = \sqrt{\frac{\text{chi-square value}}{n(k - 1)}}$$

n = number in sample

k = smaller number of rows and columns

$$V = \sqrt{\frac{2.52454}{100(2 - 1)}}$$

$$V = 0.15889$$

The contingency coefficient, which can be used with a table of any size, is calculated as:

$$C = \sqrt{\frac{\text{chi-square value}}{\text{chi-square} + n}}$$

$$C = \sqrt{\frac{2.52454}{2.52454 + 100}}$$

$$C = 0.15692$$

SUMMARY FOR CHI-SQUARE

Chi-square is the appropriate technique when variables are measured at the nominal level. It may be used with one or more groups. In the *one-group* case comparison data may be provided from a theoretical perspective, norms, or past experience. Suppose a hospital had a cesarean section rate of 30%. This percentage could be compared with reported rates (locally, regionally, or nationally) through the use of chi-square.

Although only a 2 × 2 design has been used as an example, this *two-group* case with two levels in each group can be extended to larger designs. It was pointed out that the groups in a chi-square analysis must be mutually exclusive. However, an adaptation of chi-square is the *McNemar* test for use with repeated measures at the nominal level.

NOMINAL-LEVEL DATA, DEPENDENT MEASURES

The *McNemar test* can be used with two-dichotomous measures on the same subjects. It is used to measure change. Figure 5-5 contains an example of a computer printout produced by SPSS/PC.

① The command line requests the nonparametric program, NPAR, and the specific nonparametric procedure, MCNEMAR. The two variables are PRETEST and POSTTEST.

② This contains the output from the program.

The marginal values have been added to the printout for ease of interpretation. Suppose an investigator went to a high school to talk with boys about nursing as a career.

③ PRETEST: Before the talk, the boys were asked whether or not they would consider nursing for a career. One hundred and seventy-five said no, and 25 said yes.

④ POSTTEST: After the talk, 50 boys said yes, and 150 said no. Looking at the cells in the table, we see that 30 boys who originally said no changed to yes, and five boys who

```
            SPSS/PC+ The Statistical Package for IBM PC
```

① NPAR TESTS /MCNEMAR PRETEST WITH POSTTEST.

```
      - - - - - McNemar Test
②        PRETEST
      with POSTTEST
```

			④ POSTTEST					
			YES 1	NO 0		Cases	200	
③ PRETEST	NO	0	30	145	175	Chi-Square	16.4571	
	YES	1	20	5	25	Significance	.0000	
			50	150				

FIGURE 5-5
McNemar test.

originally said yes, changed to no. The other boys did not change their minds. One hundred and forty-five said no on both occasions, and 20 said yes on both occasions.

The McNemar test uses an adaptation of the chi-square formula to test the direction of the change. Only the two cells that include changes from pretest to post-test are included in the analysis; therefore, the degrees of freedom equal one. The chi-square value of 16.4571 has a significance level of less than 0.0001 and indicates that significantly more boys became positive about nursing than negative after listening to the talk.

ORDINAL DATA, INDEPENDENT GROUPS

Two commonly used techniques are the *Mann-Whitney U*, which is used to compare two groups and is thus analogous to the *t* test, and *Kruskal-Wallis H*, which is used to compare two or more groups and is thus analogous to the parametric technique analysis of variance. An example of these techniques comes from analysis of data collected from three groups in a program grant supported by the National Center for Nursing Research (Jacobsen, Munro, & Brooten, 1991). The Multiple Affect Adjective Checklist Revised (MAACL-R) was used to collect data from three groups of subjects: cesarean section mothers, diabetic pregnant women, and hysterectomy patients. In our preliminary check of the data, we found that the measure of anxiety seriously violated the assumptions underlying the use of parametric techniques. We elected, therefore, to compare the three groups through the use of the nonparametric technique, the Kruskal-Wallis one-way analysis of variance (ANOVA). In this technique scores for subjects are converted into ranks, and the analysis compares the mean rank in each group. Figure 5-6 contains the computer printout.

①The command line requests the KRUSKAL-WALLIS procedure. ANXIETY is the dependent variable, and GROUP is the independent variable.

②With 277 subjects, rankings can go from 1 to 277. The actual scores on the anxiety scale ranged from 0 to 10.

③Two chi-square values are given; one is corrected for ties in rankings. Because 56% of our subjects scored 0 or 1 on this measure, the correction for ties is important. With a significance of 0.0026, we know that the three groups differ, but further analysis must be done to determine which pairs of groups differ.

We used the Mann-Whitney U for the post-hoc comparisons. It does not require normally distributed data but is sensitive to the central tendency and the distribution of the scores. To protect against a Type I error, we used a *Bonferroni correction*. We divided our level of significance by the number of comparisons we would make. (0.05/3 = 0.0167) was 0.05/3 or 0.0167. For a comparison to be considered significant, it must have a significance level of 0.0167, not 0.05. Figure 5-7 contains the three analyses.

①MANN-WHITNEY is requested. ANXIETY is the dependent variable, and the GROUPs being compared are 1 and 2.

②As with the Kruskal-Wallis analysis, ranks are assigned and compared.

③U is a measure of how often ranks in one group are lower than ranks in the other group. U is calculated for each group, and the printout contains the smaller of the two U's. W is the sum of the ranks for the group with the smaller number of subjects, here the

SPSS/PC+

① NPAR TESTS /KRUSKAL-WALLIS ANXIETY BY GROUP (1,3).

- - - - - Kruskal-Wallis 1-way ANOVA

     ANXIETY
  by GROUP

②   Mean Rank   Cases

        128.73   121   GROUP = 1   CESAREAN
        135.88   112   GROUP = 2   HYSTERECTOMY
        175.19   44   GROUP = 3   DIABETIC
                ---
                277   Total

③   Corrected for Ties
      CASES   Chi-Square Significance   Chi-Square Significance
       277   11.1416   .0038   11.8730   .0026

FIGURE 5-6
Kruskal-Wallis test. (Data collected in program grant funded by the National Center for Nursing Research, PO1-NR1859. P.I., D. Brooten. *Early Hospital Discharge and Nurse Specialist Followup*.)

hysterectomy group. The significance level is obtained by transforming the score into a standard score, Z (Norusis, 1990d). The cesarean and hysterectomy groups did not differ significantly on their anxiety scores.

④ The second analysis compares groups 1 and 3. The diabetic group scored significantly higher (mean rank = 103.10) than the cesarean group (mean rank = 75.69), $p = 0.0007$.

⑤ In the third analysis groups 2 and 3 are compared, and we see that the diabetic group scored significantly higher than the hysterectomy group.

To summarize, the post-hoc tests demonstrated that the diabetic pregnant women had significantly higher anxiety scores than either the cesarean or hysterectomy women. The latter two groups did not differ significantly from each other.

ORDINAL DATA, DEPENDENT GROUPS

The last two nonparametric techniques to be presented are the *Wilcoxon matched-pairs signed rank test* and the *Friedman matched samples*. The Wilcoxon matched-pairs is analogous to the parametric paired *t* test, and the Friedman matched samples is analogous to a repeated measures analysis of variance. We will start with the Friedman to demonstrate once more how initial analysis and post-hoc tests might be done using nonparametric techniques.

This is a fictitious example of a repeated measures design in which subjects serve as their own controls. Each subject is exposed to each treatment. The order of their

① NPAR TESTS /MANN-WHITNEY ANXIETY BY GROUP (1,2).

- - - - - - Mann-Whitney U - Wilcoxon Rank Sum W Test

```
      ANXIETY
   by GROUP
```

②   Mean Rank   Cases

```
          114.04      121  GROUP = 1   CESAREAN
          120.20      112  GROUP = 2   HYSTERECTOMY
                      ---
                      233  Total
```

③   Corrected for Ties
```
         U              W              Z      2-tailed P
       6417.5        13462.5        -.7258       .4680
```

④ NPAR TESTS /MANN-WHITNEY ANXIETY BY GROUP (1,3).

- - - - - - Mann-Whitney U - Wilcoxon Rank Sum W Test

```
      ANXIETY
   by GROUP
```

```
       Mean Rank    Cases

           75.69      121  GROUP = 1   CESAREAN
          103.10       44  GROUP = 3   DIABETIC
                      ---
                      165  Total
```

```
                                        Corrected for Ties
         U              W              Z      2-tailed P
       1777.5         4536.5        -3.3717      .0007
```

⑤ NPAR TESTS /MANN-WHITNEY ANXIETY BY GROUP (2,3).

- - - - - - Mann-Whitney U - Wilcoxon Rank Sum W Test

```
      ANXIETY
   by GROUP
```

```
       Mean Rank    Cases

           72.18      112  GROUP = 2   HYSTERECTOMY
           94.59       44  GROUP = 3   DIABETIC
                      ---
                      156  Total
```

```
                                        Corrected for Ties
         U              W              Z      2-tailed P
       1756.0         4162.0        -2.8604      .0042
```

FIGURE 5-7

Mann-Whitney.

(Data collected in program grant funded by the National Center for Nursing Research, PO1-NR1859. P.I.D. Brooten. *Early Hospital Discharge and Nurse Specialist Followup.*)

exposure to the three treatments is random, and adequate time is allowed between treatments to prevent carryover effects. The subjects are in a nursing home, and the three treatments are a group that goes outside and walks for 30 minutes each day, a discussion group that meets during the same 30 minutes, and a control group that has no special attention during the 30 minutes. After 1 week of treatment, the subject is rated on his or her orientation on a scale from one (disorientation) to four (completely oriented). Figure 5-8 contains the computer output.

① The command line requests the FRIEDMAN test and specifies three variables: WALKING, GROUPMTG, and CONTROL. Each subject has a score on each of these variables representing his or her level of orientation after completing 1 week of the intervention. The question is whether or not the subjects' levels of orientation differed across the three treatments.

② We see that the chi-square has a significance level of 0.0066. Because the initial analysis is significant, we will conduct comparisons of each pair of ranks. The Wilcoxon matched-pairs is used for the three comparisons, and the Bonferroni correction is $0.05/3$ or 0.0167. Figure 5-9 contains the results.

① The command line requests a WILCOXON and indicates that all possible comparisons should be made among the three variables: WALKING, GROUPMTG, and CONTROL.

② In the first comparison ranks in the walking condition are compared with ranks in the group meeting condition. In 12 cases the subject's level of orientation was less in the group meeting than under the walking condition. Two subjects had higher levels of orientation with walking, and there was one tie; that is, the subject had the same rank under both conditions. The p value of 0.0132 is less than our level of significance of 0.0167, so subjects had significantly higher levels of orientation after 1 week in the walking group than after 1 week of group meetings. Similarly, after walking, they scored significantly higher than after the control condition, but there was no difference between the group meeting and control conditions.

```
                                        SPSS/PC+
① NPAR TESTS /FRIEDMAN WALKING GROUPMTG CONTROL.

    - - - - - Friedman Two-way ANOVA


        Mean Rank    Variable

            2.67     WALKING
            1.70     GROUPMTG
            1.63     CONTROL

②           Cases         Chi-Square        D.F.    Significance
             15            10.0333            2         .0066
```

FIGURE 5-8
Friedman.

(1) NPAR TESTS /WILCOXON WALKING GROUPMTG CONTROL.

SPSS/PC+

- - - - - Wilcoxon Matched-pairs Signed-ranks Test

    WALKING
with GROUPMTG

(2)
    Mean Rank   Cases

       7.67   12 - Ranks (GROUPMTG Lt WALKING)
       6.50   2 + Ranks (GROUPMTG Gt WALKING)
                1   Ties (GROUPMTG Eq WALKING)
              --
              15   Total

      Z =   -2.4797   2-tailed P = .0132

- - - - - Wilcoxon Matched-pairs Signed-ranks Test

    WALKING
with CONTROL

    Mean Rank   Cases

       6.68   11 - Ranks (CONTROL Lt WALKING)
       4.50   1 + Ranks (CONTROL Gt WALKING)
                3   Ties (CONTROL Eq WALKING)
              --
              15   Total

      Z =   -2.7064   2-tailed P = .0068

- - - - - Wilcoxon Matched-pairs Signed-ranks Test

    GROUPMTG
with CONTROL

    Mean Rank   Cases

       4.00   4 - Ranks (CONTROL Lt GROUPMTG)
       4.00   3 + Ranks (CONTROL Gt GROUPMTG)
                8   Ties (CONTROL Eq GROUPMTG)
              --
              15   Total

      Z =   -.3381   2-tailed P = .7353

FIGURE 5-9
Wilcoxon.

SUMMARY

A few of the more commonly reported nonparametric techniques have been presented. It is important that investigators examine their data prior to analysis to determine which techniques are appropriate.

6

t Tests: Measuring the Differences Between Group Means

Barbara Hazard Munro

OBJECTIVES FOR CHAPTER 6

After reading this chapter you should be able to do the following:

1. Determine when the *t* test is the appropriate technique to use.

2. Discuss how mean difference, group variability, and sample size are related to the statistical significance of the *t* statistic.

3. Discuss how the results of the homogeneity of variance test are related to choice of *t* test formula.

4. Select the appropriate *t* test formula (separate, pooled, or correlated) for a given situation.

5. Interpret computer printouts of *t* test analyses.

Many research projects are designed to test the differences between two groups. When the differences involve interval or ratio data, the analysis requires an evaluation of means and distributions of each group.

In this chapter a statistical method for testing the difference between two groups is presented. This method is the *t* test, or Student's *t* test. It is named after its inventor, William Gosset, who published under the

Barbara Hazard Munro and Ellis Batten Page: STATISTICAL METHODS FOR HEALTH CARE RESEARCH, SECOND EDITION. © 1993, 1986 by J. B. Lippincott Company.

pseudonym of Student. Gosset invented the *t* test as a more precise method of comparing groups. He described a set of distributions of *means* of randomly drawn samples from a normally distributed population. These distributions are the *t* distributions.

The shape of the distributions varies depending on the size of the samples drawn from the populations. However, all the *t* distributions have a normal distribution with a mean equal to the mean of the population. Unlike the *z* distributions, which are based on the normal curve and estimate the theoretical population parameters, the *t* distributions are based on the sample size and vary according to the degrees of freedom. The use of the *t* distribution is based on the concepts presented in Chapter 3. Theoretically, when an infinite number of samples of equal size are drawn from a normally distributed population, the mean of the sampling distribution will equal the mean of the population. If the sample sizes were large enough, the shape of the sampling distribution would approximate the normal curve.

THE RESEARCH QUESTION

When we compare two groups on a particular characteristic, we are asking whether the groups are different. The statistical question asks *how different* the groups are; that is, is the difference we find greater than that which could occur by chance alone? The null hypothesis for the *t* test states that any difference that occurs between the means of two groups is a difference in the sampling distribution. The means are different not because the groups are drawn from two different theoretical populations, but because of different random distributions of the samples from such a population. The null hypothesis is represented by the *t* distributions constructed by the random sampling of one population. When we use the *t* test to interpret the significance of the difference between groups, we are asking the statistical question, "What is the probability of getting a difference of this magnitude in groups this size if we were comparing random samples drawn from the same population?" That is, "*What is the probability of getting a difference this large by chance alone?*"

An example of the *t* test used to compare two groups is the study of Youngblut, Loveland-Cherry, and Horan (1991) who investigated "the effects of maternal employment status and the mother's degree of choice and satisfaction regarding her employment status on family functioning and on the preterm infant's development at three months chronologic age" (p. 272). Mothers were classified into two groups. One group consisted of women whose attitude toward employment and employment status were congruent, and the other group included women whose employment status was incongruent with their attitude. These two groups were compared on outcome measures using *t* tests. Mothers in the congruent group scored significantly higher on measures of choice and satisfaction, but there were no differences between the two groups on measures of cohesion, adaptability, relationships, and mental or motor development.

To answer research questions through use of the *t* test, we compare the difference we obtained between our means with the sampling distribution of such differences. In general the larger the *difference* between our two means, the more likely it is that the *t* test will be significant. When we look at the formula for *t*, we see that this difference appears in the numerator. However, two other factors are taken into account: the variability and the sample size. In the *t* formula the denominator is the standard error of the *t* statistic. In Chapter 3 the standard error of the mean is discussed and it is pointed out that the standard deviation (variability) and *n* (sample size) are used in calculating that error term. An increase in variability is shown to lead to an increase in error, and an increase in sample size is shown to lead to a decrease in error. These same principles apply to the *t* test.

Given the same mean difference, groups with less variability will be more likely to be significantly different than groups with wide variability. This is because in groups with more variability, the error term will be larger, reflecting the fact that if the groups have scores that vary widely, there is likely to be considerable overlap between the two groups; thus, it will be difficult to ascertain whether a difference exists. Groups with less variability and a real mean difference will have distributions more clearly distinct from each other; that is, there will be less overlap between their respective distributions. With *more* variability (thus, larger error), we need a *larger difference* to be reasonably "sure" that a real difference exists.

TYPE OF DATA REQUIRED

For the *t* test we need one nominal-level variabie, with two levels as the independent variable. A simpler way to say this is that we must have two groups. The dependent variable should be interval or ratio level, although as previously indicated, ordinal-level data often can be treated as interval-level data and used in *t* test analysis.

The *t* test has been commonly used to compare two groups. The mathematics involved are simpler than those required for analysis of variance, which is discussed in Chapter 7. However, note that when comparing two groups on an interval- or ratio-level variable, it does not matter whether one uses a *t* test or a one-way analysis of variance. The results will be mathematically identical. The *t* statistic (derived from the *t* test formula) is equal to the square root of the *F* statistic (derived from the one-way analysis of variance). Symbolically then, $t = \sqrt{F}$ and $F = t^2$.

With the use of the computer, ease of calculation is not an issue, so some people use analysis of variance to compare two groups. Either way is correct; it is a matter of individual preference. The typical *t* test table has the advantage of clearly presenting the means being compared in the analysis.

ASSUMPTIONS

The four assumptions underlying the *t* test concern the type of data used in the test and the characteristics of the distribution of the variables.

First, the *t* test requires at least *interval-level* data for the dependent measure.

Second, the test assumes that each subject will contribute one score to the distribution of one specific group; that is, each subject can belong to one and only one of the two groups and contributes one and only one score. This is the assumption of independence. When this assumption is violated, as when subjects are measured twice, a correlated or paired *t* test may be appropriate.

A *third* assumption of the *t* test is that the distribution of the dependent measure is normal. If the distribution is seriously skewed, the *t* test may be invalid.

The fourth requirement for a valid *t* test interpretation is that the groups that we are comparing are similar in their *variances*. This is related to the assumption implied by the null hypotheses that the groups are from a single population. This assumption is referred to as the requirement of *homogeneity of variance*.

Meeting this last assumption protects against Type II errors—incorrectly accepting the null hypothesis. When the variances are unequal, that is, when the variation in one sample is significantly greater than the variation in the other, we are less likely to find a significant *t* value. Therefore, we might incorrectly conclude that the groups were drawn from the same population when they were not.

What if the variances are significantly different? Occasionally, groups that we wish to compare do not have equal variances. Fortunately, a statistical method approximates the *t* test and can be interpreted in the same way using a different calculation for the standard error.

Actually, three different formulas based on the *t* distribution can be used to compare two groups.

First, the basic formula, sometimes called the *pooled formula*, is used to compare two groups when the four assumptions for the *t* test are met.

Second, when the variances are *unequal*, the *separate formula* is used. This takes into account the fact that the variances are not alike. It is a more conservative measure.

Third, when the two sets of scores are not independent (assumption 2), that is, there is correlation between the data taken from the two groups, adjustment must be made for that relationship. That formula often is called the *correlated t test* or the *t*-test for *paired comparisons*. Comparing a group of subjects on their pretest and post-test scores is an example of when this technique would be used. Because these are not two independent groups, but rather one group measured twice, the scores will most likely be correlated. Another example is when the two groups consist of matched pairs. If the pairs are carefully matched, their scores will correlate, and the standard *t* test would not be appropriate.

COMPUTER ANALYSIS

As an example of a *t* test, suppose we randomly assigned patients scheduled for a diagnostic hysteroscopy to an experimental or control group. The experimental group was taught how to achieve a state of mental and physical relaxation; the control group was not. The Multiple Affect Adjective Checklist (MAACL) was used to measure anxiety at the beginning of the procedure. Table 6-1 contains the fictitious data.

We see that the experimental group had a lower (5.8) mean anxiety level than the control group (11.1). Is the 5.3-point difference between the two groups a statistically significant difference?

Before attempting to answer that question, consider the power of the analysis.

TABLE 6-1
*MAACL Anxiety Scores for the Experimental
and Control Group*

	Group 1 Experimental	Group 2 Control
	X_1	X_2
	8	15
	5	13
	7	12
	9	8
	7	11
	6	14
	5	9
	3	10
	4	9
	4	10
Σ_s	*58*	*111*
	$n = 10 \quad \overline{X}_1 = 5.8$	$n = 10 \quad \overline{X}_2 = 11.1$

Generally, 10 subjects per group would not be enough to achieve an adequate (approximately 0.80) level of power. According to Cohen (1987), for a two-tailed *t* test with an expected moderate effect size (0.5), probability level of 0.05, and desired power of 0.80, 64 subjects would be required in each group for a total sample of 128. For a one-tailed *t* test with the same effect, power, and alpha levels, 100 subjects would be required, 50 in each group (Cohen, 1987).

Suppose, however, that we had done work in this area before and knew that the standard deviation of the MAACL anxiety score would be approximately 3.0. A difference of 5.3 points between the two groups would result in an effect size of $5.3/3 = 1.77$ standard deviation units. This results in a power greater than 0.995 (Cohen, 1987).

To test the difference between the two groups, we use the SPSS/PC package. Figure 6-1 contains the results.

① The command line identifies the independent variable as GROUP with two values, 1 and 2. The experimental group was entered as 1, and the control as 2. The variable on which the two groups are being compared is ANXIETY.

② There are 10 subjects in each group. The mean of the experimental group is 5.8, and the mean of the control group is 11.1. The associated standard deviations and standard errors are listed.

③ The *F* value tests for homogeneity of variance. It answers the question of whether the two standard deviations are equivalent. The *F* value is the ratio of the larger to the smaller variance. The degrees of freedom equal the number in the group minus one. The two-tailed probability is 0.585, which, because it is greater than 0.05, indicates

SPSS/PC+

① T-TEST /GROUPS GROUP (1,2) /VARIABLES ANXIETY.

Independent samples of GROUP

Group 1: GROUP EQ 1   Group 2: GROUP EQ 2

t-test for: ANXIETY

	Number of Cases	Mean	Standard Deviation	Standard Error
② Group 1	10	5.8000	1.932	.611
Group 2	10	11.1000	2.331	.737

③   ④   ⑤

F Value	2-Tail Prob.	Pooled Variance Estimate			Separate Variance Estimate		
		t Value	Degrees of Freedom	2-Tail Prob.	t Value	Degrees of Freedom	2-Tail Prob.
1.46	.585	-5.54	18	.000	-5.54	17.40	.000

FIGURE 6-1
t-test analysis produced by SPSS/PC+.

that the standard deviations of the two groups are equivalent. Another way to say this is that the standard deviation of group 1 (1.932) is not statistically significantly different from the standard deviation of group 2 (2.331). Thus, the assumption of homogeneity of variance has been met, and the appropriate *t* test to use is the pooled variance estimate.

④ Pooled variance estimate.

⑤ If the *F* value had been significant, the separate variance estimate would have been the appropriate *t* test to report. As you can see, the computer output contains both estimates, and you must decide which to use based on the homogeneity of variance test.

For our example we would report a *t* value of −5.54 with 18 degrees of freedom (total number of subjects minus 2) and a two-tailed probability of 0.000 (or less than 0.001). (For a one-tailed *t* test, you divide the two-tailed probability by 2.) We would say that subjects taught relaxation are significantly less anxious ($p < 0.001$) at the beginning of the hysteroscopy procedure than subjects who were not taught relaxation.

CALCULATING THE BASIC (POOLED) t TEST

The *t* test formula consists of dividing the difference between the two means by the standard error. The standard error serves as an estimate of the standard deviation in the population from which our subjects are drawn. It represents the "pooled" variance of both groups and is appropriate when the variances of the two groups are equal. An example of the calculation is provided in Table 6-2.

TABLE 6-2
Calculation of Pooled t Test

Group 1 Experimental		Group 2 Control	
X_1	X_1^2	X_2	X_2^2
8	64	15	225
5	25	13	169
7	49	12	144
9	81	8	64
7	49	11	121
6	36	14	196
5	25	9	81
3	9	10	100
4	16	9	81
4	16	10	100
58	370	111	1281

Group 1	Group 2

$$\overline{X} = 5.8 \qquad\qquad \overline{X} = 11.1$$

$$n = 10 \qquad\qquad n = 10$$

$$\text{sum of squares } (\Sigma \chi_1)^2 = 370 - \frac{(58)^2}{10} \qquad \text{sum of squares } (\Sigma \chi_2)^2 = 1281 - \frac{(111)^2}{10}$$

$$= 33.6 \qquad\qquad = 48.9$$

$$t = \frac{(\overline{X}_1 - \overline{X}_2)}{\sqrt{\left(\dfrac{\Sigma \chi_1^2 + \Sigma \chi_2^2}{n_1 + n_2 - 2}\right)\left(\dfrac{1}{n_1} + \dfrac{1}{n_2}\right)}}$$

$$t = \frac{5.8 - 11.1}{\sqrt{\left(\dfrac{33.6 + 48.9}{10 + 10 - 2}\right)\left(\dfrac{1}{10} + \dfrac{1}{10}\right)}}$$

$$t = -5.54$$

Using the table in Appendix C, we find that a *t* value of -5.54 with 18 *df* has a probability level of 0.001 for the two-tailed test and 0.0005 for the one-tailed test.

CALCULATING THE "SEPARATE" t TEST

If the variances for the two groups were not the same, we would use a more conservative formula, because it would be an error to "pool" different variances. The formula for this *t* test is:

$$t = \frac{\overline{X}_1 - \overline{X}_2}{\sqrt{\dfrac{s_1^2}{n_1} + \dfrac{s_2^2}{n_2}}}$$

where s_1^2 = variance for group 1
        s_2^2 = variance for group 2

CORRELATED OR PAIRED t TEST

If the two groups being compared are matched or paired on some basis, the scores are likely to be similar. The chance differences between the two groups will not be as large as when they are drawn independently. In the correlated t test, a correction is made that has the effect of increasing t, thus making it more likely to find a significant difference if one exists.

Suppose we had two measures on our subjects. Table 6-3 contains the raw data, and Figure 6-2 contains the computer analysis.

① The command line requests a paired t test for the two variables PRETEST and POSTTEST.

② On the pretest, the mean score was 17.1, and on the post-test, 9.8. Was there a significant decrease from pretest to post-test?

③ The difference between the two means is 7.3. There is a correlation of 0.846 between the means, indicating that people who score high on the pretest are likely to score high on the post-test, and people who scored low on the pretest are likely to score low on the post-test. That correlation is significant at the 0.002 level. Because there is correlation between the measures, the correlated or paired t is the appropriate test to use. The t value of 8.93 is significant at less than 0.001. Therefore, we would say that subjects' scores decreased significantly from pretest to post-test.

TABLE 6-3
Data for Correlated t Test

Subjects	Pretest	Post-test
1	20	13
2	15	8
3	18	10
4	12	7
5	14	8
6	17	9
7	19	14
8	10	6
9	22	11
10	24	12

①
                                       SPSS/PC+
T-TEST /PAIRS PRETEST WITH POSTTEST.

   Paired samples t-test: PRETEST
                            POSTTEST

   Variable   Number   Standard   Standard
                of Cases   Mean   Deviation   Error

② PRETEST   10   17.1000   4.408   1.394
   POSTTEST   10   9.8000   2.658   .841

③ (Difference) Standard   Standard | 2-Tail | t   Degrees of   2-Tail
       Mean   Deviation   Error | Corr. Prob. | Value   Freedom   Prob.

      7.3000   2.584   .817 | .846   .002 | 8.93   9   .000

FIGURE 6-2
Paired *t*-test analysis produced by SPSS/PC+.

For those interested in the calculation, the formula follows:

$$t = \frac{\overline{X}_1 - \overline{X}_2}{\sqrt{\dfrac{s_1^2}{n_1} + \dfrac{s_2^2}{n_2} - 2r\left(\dfrac{s_1}{\sqrt{n_1}}\right)\left(\dfrac{s_2}{\sqrt{n_2}}\right)}}$$

where s_1^2 = variance for group 1
        s_2^2 = variance for group 2
        s_1 = standard deviation for group 1
        s_2 = standard deviation for group 2

The correlated *t* test uses the pooled estimate of variance, so we do not have to decide whether to use a separate or pooled formula.

SUMMARY

The *t* test is a statistical method for comparing differences between two groups. The *t* statistic is similar to the *z* statistic. It uses an estimate of the population parameters and thereby is substituted for the *z* statistic when these parameters are unknown. The test requires interval or ratio measurement of the variable on which the groups are being compared. The test assumes that the variable is normally distributed in the populations from which the samples are drawn and that the samples have equivalent variances. The *t* test is particularly useful in experimental and quasiexperimental designs in which an experimental and control group are compared.

7

Differences Among Group Means: *One-Way Analysis of Variance*

Barbara Hazard Munro

OBJECTIVES FOR CHAPTER 7

After reading this chapter you should be able to do the following:

1. **Determine when analysis of variance is the appropriate statistical method to use.**

2. **Interpret a computer printout of a one-way analysis of variance.**

3. **Describe between, within, and total variance.**

4. **Explain the use of post-hoc tests.**

5. **Report the results of one-way analysis of variance in a summary table.**

Many times, a clinical research question involves a comparison of several groups on a particular measure. When the measure is represented by interval- or ratio-level data, we want to determine whether the groups vary from one another in their distribution of scores. In Chapter 6 we discuss the *t* test as a method for examining the difference between *two* groups. The basic *t* test compares two means in relation to the distribution of the differences between pairs of means drawn from a random sample. When

Barbara Hazard Munro and Ellis Batten Page: STATISTICAL METHODS FOR HEALTH CARE RESEARCH, SECOND EDITION. © 1993, 1986 by J. B. Lippincott Company.

we have more than two groups and are interested in the differences among the set of groups, we are dealing with different combinations of pairs of means. If we choose to analyze the differences by *t* test analysis, we would need to do a number of *t* tests. Suppose, for example, that we had four different groups—A, B, C, and D—that we wished to compare on a particular variable. If we were interested in the differences among the four groups, we would need to do a *t* test for each of the possible pairs that exist in the four groups. We would have A vs. B, A vs. C, A vs. D, B vs. C, B vs. D, and C vs. D. In all, we would have six separate comparisons, each requiring a separate analysis.

The problem with conducting such multiple group comparisons relates to the underlying concept of statistical analysis. Each test is based on the probability that the *null hypothesis is true*. Therefore, each time we conduct a test, we are running the risk of a Type I error. The probability level we set as the point at which we reject the null hypothesis also is the level of risk with which we are comfortable. If that level is 0.05, we are accepting the risk that 5 of 100 times our rejection of the null hypothesis will be in error.

However, when we calculate multiple *t* tests on independent samples that are being measured on the same variable, the rate of error increases exponentially by the number of tests conducted. For example with our four-group problem, the error rate increases to 18 of 100 times, a substantial increase in risk of incorrectly rejecting the null hypothesis.*

Instead of using a series of individual comparisons, we examine the differences among the groups through an analysis that considers the variation across all groups at once. This test is the Analysis of Variance (ANOVA).

The question answered by the ANOVA test is whether group means differ from each other. For example Forrester (1990) studied the effect of acquired immune deficiency syndrome (AIDS)-related risk factors on nurses' attitudes toward aggressiveness of nursing care. Through the use of vignettes, nurses were asked to rate their attitudes toward aggressiveness of nursing care for three types of patients: intravenous (IV) drug users, homosexual men, and individuals who neither used IV drugs nor were homosexual. Analysis of variance was used to compare the means of these three groups. The overall analysis was significant at the 0.0001 level. This result indicates differences among the groups but does not tell us which pairs of groups were different. To ascertain where the differences occurred, the investigator did a post-hoc (after the fact) test and determined that the means for the IV group (42.7) and for the homosexual group (41.9) were significantly higher than the mean for the group without an AIDS-related risk factor (38.5). The means for the IV and homosexual group did not differ significantly.

The calculation of the rate of Type I errors is determined by the following formula:

$$1 - (1 + \alpha)^t$$

where α = *the level of significance for the tests*

   t = *the number of test comparisons used*

   In our example the calculation would give us $1 - (1 - 0.05)^4 = 0.18.$

TYPE OF DATA REQUIRED

With ANOVA the independent variable(s) are at the nominal level. A one-way ANOVA means that there is only *one* independent variable (often called *factor*). That independent variable has two or more levels. Sex would be a variable with two levels, whereas race, religion, and so forth may have varying numbers of levels depending on how the variable is defined. Two-way ANOVA indicates two independent variables, and *n*-way ANOVA indicates that the number of independent variables is defined by *n*. The dependent variable should be interval or ratio level.

ASSUMPTIONS

Analysis of variance has been shown to be fairly "robust." This means that even if the assumptions are not rigidly adhered to, the results may still be close to the truth.

The assumptions for ANOVA are the same as those for the *t* test; that is, the dependent variable should be measured at the interval or ratio level, the groups should be mutually exclusive (independent of each other), the dependent variable should be normally distributed, and the groups should have equal variances (homogeneity of variance requirement).

THE STATISTICAL QUESTION IN ANALYSIS OF VARIANCE

The statistical question using ANOVA is based on the null hypothesis: the assumption that all groups are equal and drawn from the same population. Any difference comes from a random sampling difference.

SOURCE OF VARIANCE

According to the null hypothesis, all groups are from the same population, and each of their scores also comes from the same population of measures. Any variability of scores can be seen in two ways: First, the scores vary from each other in their own group; second, the groups vary from each other. The first variation is called *within-group variation*; the second variation is called *between-group variation*. Together the two types of variation add up to the *total variation*.

Students often are confused when we say that ANOVA tells us whether or not the means of groups differ significantly and then proceed to talk about analyzing variance. The *t* test was clearly a test of mean difference, because the difference between the two means was contained in the numerator of the *t* test formula. It is important to understand how analyzing the variability of groups on some measure can tell us whether their measures of central tendency (means) differ.

In analysis of variance the variance of each group is measured separately; all the subjects are then lumped together, and the variance of the total group is computed. If the variance of the total group (total variation) is about the same as the average of the variances of the separate groups (within-group variation), the *means* of the separate groups are not different. This is because if total variation is the sum of within-group variation and between-group variation and if within group variation and total variation are equal, there is no between-group variation. This will hopefully become more clear in the diagrams that follow. If, on the other hand, the variance of the total group is much larger than the average variation within the separate groups, a significant mean difference exists between at least two of the subgroups. In that case the within-group variation does not equal total variation. The difference between them must equal the between-group variation.

To visualize the difference in the types of variation, consider the three groups in the experiment described previously. Suppose that the three conditions yielded widely different scores, so different that there was no overlap between the three groups in terms of the outcome measure (Fig. 7-1). We could then represent our three groups in terms of their relationship to each other and in terms of a *total group*. Each group would then have its own mean and its own distribution around its mean. At the same time there would be a *grand mean*, which is a mean for all the groups combined. Now, as we can see from Figure 7-1, we can look at the variation *within* the groups as well as the variation *between* the groups. The combination of the within-group and between-group variation equals the *total* variation.

The ANOVA test examines the variation and tests whether the between-group

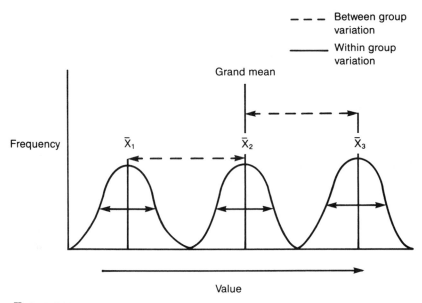

FIGURE 7-1

Between-group and within-group variation: the case of no overlap.

variation is greater than the within-group variation. When the between-group variance is greater (statistically greater) than the within-group variance, the means of the groups must be different. On the other hand when the within-group variance is approximately the same as the between-group variance, the groups' means are not importantly different. This relationship between the difference among group and the different types of variance is shown in Figure 7-2.

When the null hypothesis is true, the groups overlap to a large extent, and the within-group variation is greater than the between-group variation. When the null hypothesis is false, the groups show little overlapping, and the distance between groups is greater.

As we can infer from Figure 7-2, the group variation and the deviation between group means determine the likelihood that the null hypothesis is true. More explicitly,

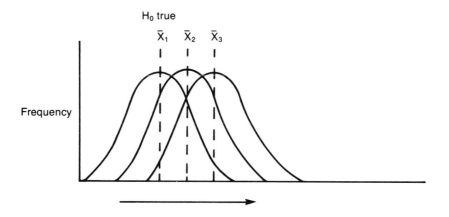

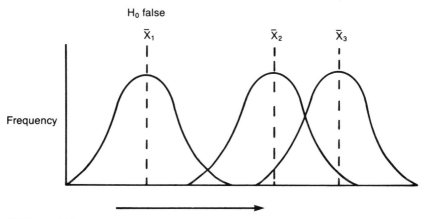

FIGURE 7-2
Relationship of variation to null hypothesis.

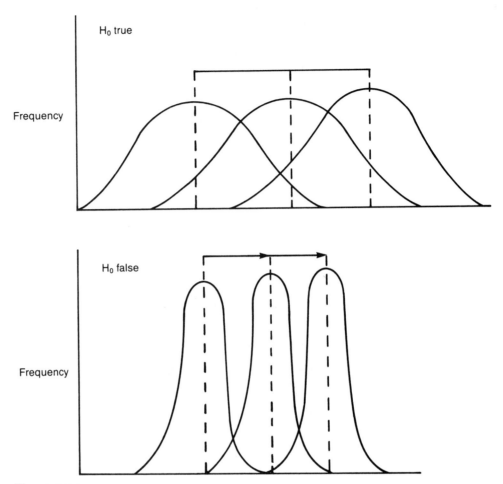

FIGURE 7-3
Effect of within-group variation on null hypothesis.

when the variation within a group or groups is great, the difference between the groups must be greater than when the distribution within groups is narrow to reject the null hypothesis (Fig. 7-3). In the same way when the group distributions are narrow (low within-group variance), relatively small between-group differences will be significant.

THE MEASURE OF VARIANCE: SUMS OF SQUARES

The concept of the kinds of variation we find when examining scores within groups has an intuitive and a statistical meaning. We have discussed the intuitive meaning as the extent to which the scores within a group vary from each other and the extent to which the groups vary from each other. The statistical concept of this variation involves a quantification of the amount of variation of scores around the mean. We have already defined and used this concept with the term *sum of squares*.

The *sum of squares* is the sum of the squared deviations of each of the scores around a respective mean. In analysis of variance the sum of squares is used to measure the total variation, between-group variation, and within-group variation. Table 7-1 contains an example of the calculation of the sums of squares using the formulas based on the deviations of the scores from their respective means. The data consist of three

TABLE 7-1
Calculation of Sum of Squares

	Group 1	Group 2	Group 3
	1	4	7
	2	5	8
	3	6	9
	—	—	—
$\overline{X}_s$	2	5	8

TOTAL SUM OF SQUARES

Raw Scores	Deviations From Grand Mean	Squared Deviation
1	$1 - 5 = -4$	16
2	$2 - 5 = -3$	9
3	$3 - 5 = -2$	4
4	$4 - 5 = -1$	1
5	$5 - 5 = 0$	0
6	$6 - 5 = 1$	1
7	$7 - 5 = 2$	4
8	$8 - 5 = 3$	9
9	$9 - 5 = 4$	16
Grand Mean $= 5$	Sum $= 0$	Sum $= 60$

Total sum of squares $= 60$.

WITHIN SUM OF SQUARES

Group 1		
Raw Scores	Deviations From Group Mean	Squared Deviations
1	$1 - 2 = -1$	1
2	$2 - 2 = 0$	0
3	$3 - 2 = 1$	1
$\overline{X} = 2$	Sum $= 0$	Sum $= 2$

(*continued*)

TABLE 7-1   (CONTINUED)

WITHIN SUM OF SQUARES   *(continued)*

Group 2

Raw Scores	Deviations From Group Mean	Squared Deviations
4	4 − 5 = −1	1
5	5 − 5 = 0	0
6	6 − 5 = 1	1
$\overline{X} = 5$	Sum = 0	Sum = 2

Group 3

7	7 − 8 = −1	1
8	8 − 8 = 0	0
9	9 − 8 = 1	1
$\overline{X} = 8$	Sum = 0	Sum = 2

Within sum of squares = 2 + 2 + 2 = 6.

BETWEEN SUM OF SQUARES

Deviations of Group Means From Grand Mean	Squared Deviations	Number in Group
Group 1 2 − 5 = −3	9	3
Group 2 5 − 5 = 0	0	3
Group 3 8 − 5 = 3	9	3

Between sum of squares = (3)(9) + 3(0) + 3(9) = 54.

SUMMARY TABLE

Source of Variance	SS	df	MS	F	p
Between group	54	2	27	27	0.01
Within group	6	6	1		
Total	60				

scores in each of three groups. The means for the three groups are 2, 5, and 8, respectively.

The Sum of Squares for Total Variation

The total sum of squares is equal to the sum of the squared deviations of each score in all groups from the grand mean. In our example the grand mean (mean of the nine scores) is 5. The sum of the deviations around the mean equals zero, and the sum of the squared deviations equals 60. This total sum of squares represents the basis of the null hypothesis that all the subjects belong to one population, which is described by the grand mean.

The Sum of Squares for Within-Group Variation

The within-group variation is the total of the variation that occurs in each subgroup. It is calculated by finding the sum of squares for each group separately and then summing the results. The sum of the squared deviations for each group is 2, and the sum across the three groups is 6.

The Sum of Squares for Between-Group Variation

The between-group variation examines how each of the groups varies from the grand mean. For this calculation we use group means as representative of the individual groups. The between-group variation examines the variation of the group means from the grand mean. As you can see in Table 7-1, the mean for group 1 is 3 less than the grand mean. The sum of the deviations around the grand mean is (as always) zero, and the squared deviations are 9, 0, and 9, respectively. Because the weight of the difference of any mean from the grand mean is influenced by the number of the scores in the group, we weight the squared deviations by the number in the group. The weighted squared deviations are then summed to provide the between sum of squares (54).

In summary these three sums of squares define the three different kinds of variation that exist when subjects are members of different groups and measured on a single variable. They include the *total variation* of each of the scores around the grand mean, the variation of scores *within* their respective groups, and the deviation *between* groups measured by the deviation of group means from the grand mean.

DISPLAYING THE RESULTS: THE SUMMARY OF ANALYSIS OF VARIANCE

The results of the calculations leading to the *F* ratio are summarized in table form that is standard for presenting ANOVA results. This presentation of the results is called the *summary of ANOVA* table.

In Table 7-1 *SS* stands for sum of squares, *df* for degrees of freedom, *MS* for mean square, *F* for the statistic generated, and *p* for the probability level.

Degrees of Freedom

The *df* for the between-group variance is equal to the number of groups minus one. In our example this is $3 - 1 = 2$. The *df* for the within-group variance is equal to the total number of subjects minus the number of groups, or $9 - 3 = 6$. The mean square is simply the sum of squares divided by its degrees of freedom. Thus, the between-group sum of squares, 54, divided by 2 results in a mean square of 27.

Testing the Difference Among Groups: The F Ratio

To determine whether the between-group difference is great enough to reject the null hypothesis, we compare it statistically to the within-group variance. The F represents the ratio of between to within variance and is calculated as the between mean square divided by the within mean square, or $27/1 = 27$. We interpret the F value by comparing it to the values obtained when the null hypothesis is true and the scores randomly selected from one population. To make the interpretation we use the table that presents the F distributions (Appendix D). We locate the critical values for comparison by using the *df* for the between and within mean squares.

In the example the between *df* was 2, and the within *df* was 6. We locate the between *df* on the row across the top of the table, and we locate the within *df* on the column on the left side of the table. With these points as coordinates, we locate two critical values for F.

The top value (in light print) is 5.14. This is the value required to reject the null hypothesis at a probability level of 0.05 (given a one-tailed test). The value below (in bold print) is 10.92, the value required to reject the null hypothesis at the 0.01 level.

The value of 27 is greater than the value required to reach an alpha of 0.01. Therefore, we can reject the null hypothesis at the 0.01 level. We say we have reached a probability level of "less than 0.01." In summary we obtained an F value of 27. We therefore rejected the null hypothesis that there were no differences between the groups, and we concluded that the groups were different. In other standard presentations of ANOVA summary tables, the within variance is sometimes called the *error variance* or *error term*. This terminology reflects the assumption of the analysis of variance: The within difference is sampling error or random difference.

In addition to the summary table, often it is helpful to include a table in your results section that shows the means and standard deviations for the scores of each group. One can then see which group scored higher and by how much. Without further analysis, however, we do not know which pairs of means differ significantly. A post-hoc analysis would allow us to compare group 1 with group 2, group 1 with group 3, and group 2 with group 3. Before discussing such contrasts in detail, however, we first present another example with a computer analysis of the data.

ONE-WAY ANALYSIS OF VARIANCE

We have one independent categorical variable with n levels and one continuous dependent variable. To demonstrate we will extend the example used in Chapter 6. In that example we compared an experimental group and a control group on their anxiety as measured by the Multiple Affect Adjective Checklist. The data on the experimental and control groups remain the same as in the previous example (see Table 6-1). Here we add a second experimental group (Table 7-2). We randomly assign women being prepared for a diagnostic hysteroscopy to one of three groups. All receive the usual care, but subjects in experimental I also are taught a relaxation technique; in experimental II a nurse spends additional time answering the patients' questions about the procedure; and the control group receives usual care only.

TABLE 7-2
Scores on the MAACL Anxiety Score Across Groups

Experimental I Relaxation	Experimental II Procedure Information	Control
8	8	15
5	9	13
7	7	12
9	9	8
7	10	11
6	6	14
5	10	9
3	12	10
4	7	9
4	11	10
$\overline{X} = 5.8$	$\overline{X} = 8.9$	$\overline{X} = 11.1$
$s = 1.93$	$s = 1.91$	$s = 2.33$

The question is whether the groups score differently on the anxiety measure. If the groups differ in their scores, the question is which groups are different from which other groups? That is, where is the difference?

COMPUTER ANALYSIS

To answer the research question, the data were submitted to analysis by the ONEWAY program in SPSS/PC+. This program handles one-way analysis of variance (one independent variable) and post-hoc tests necessary to compare pairs of means. Figure 7-4 contains the computer output.

① The command line requests a one-way analysis of variance. ANXIETY is the dependent variable, and GROUP is the independent variable. The groups are coded from one to three. The post-hoc test, Scheffé, is requested. Statistic 1 is the group descriptive statistics, and statistic 3 is the homogeneity of variance tests.

② The analysis of variance summary table is typical of what is reported in the literature. The components of variance are given first. These are explained in more detail in a subsequent section. "Between groups" indicates the difference between the three groups, "within groups" is the error term, and "total" is the total variance in the dependent variable.

Degrees of freedom, or df, are given first. Because there are three groups, $df = 2$ (number of groups minus one). Dividing the sum of squares by its associated degree of freedom gives the mean square value. For example for between groups, $141.8/2 = 70.9$. The F is the ratio of between to within variance, or $70.9/4.2741 = 16.5884$. This number is significant at the 0.0000 (or <0.0001) level.

SPSS/PC+ The Statistical Package for IBM PC

SPSS/PC+

(1) ONEWAY /VARIABLES ANXIETY BY GROUP (1,3) /RANGES SCHEFFE /STATISTICS 1 3.

- - - - - - - - - - O N E W A Y - - - - - - - - - - -

Variable   ANXIETY

By Variable   GROUP

(2)   Analysis of Variance

Source	D.F.	Sum of Squares	Mean Squares	F Ratio	F Prob.
Between Groups	2	141.8000	70.9000	16.5884	.0000
Within Groups	27	115.4000	4.2741		
Total	29	257.2000			

(3)

Group	Count	Mean	Standard Deviation	Standard Error	95 Pct Conf Int for Mean		
Grp 1	10	5.8000	1.9322	.6110	4.4178	To	7.1822
Grp 2	10	8.9000	1.9120	.6046	7.5323	To	10.2677
Grp 3	10	11.1000	2.3310	.7371	9.4325	To	12.7675
Total	30	8.6000	2.9781	.5437	7.4880	To	9.7120

Group	Minimum	Maximum
Grp 1	3.0000	9.0000
Grp 2	6.0000	12.0000
Grp 3	8.0000	15.0000
Total	3.0000	15.0000

(4) Tests for Homogeneity of Variances

Cochrans C = Max. Variance/Sum(Variances) = .4237, P = .696 (Approx.)
Bartlett-Box F =   .221 , P = .802
Maximum Variance / Minimum Variance   1.486

FIGURE 7-4

One-way analysis of variance produced by SPSS/PC +.

(5) (*) Denotes pairs of groups significantly different at the   .050 level

        Variable ANXIETY
        (Continued)

                                    G G G
                                    r r r
                                    p p p

        Mean   Group   1 2 3

         5.8000   Grp 1
         8.9000   Grp 2   *
        11.1000   Grp 3   *

    Homogeneous Subsets   (Subsets of groups, whose highest and lowest means
                             do not differ by more than the shortest
                             significant range for a subset of that size)

    SUBSET 1

    Group   Grp 1
    Mean   5.8000
    - - - - - - - - - -

    SUBSET 2

    Group   Grp 2   Grp 3
    Mean   8.9000   11.1000
    - - - - - - - - - - - - - - - - -

FIGURE 7-4 (CONTINUED)

(3) The group statistics, requested through STATISTICS 1, are given next. (Group 1 is experimental I, group 2 is experimental II, and group 3 is the control group.) There were 10 subjects in each group, and group means, standard deviations, and standard errors are listed. Based on the standard errors, 95% confidence intervals also are listed. For group 1 the 95% CI is 4.4178 to 7.1822. The minimum and maximum score for each group also are listed.

(4) The homogeneity of variance is a test of one of the major assumptions underlying the use of analysis of variance; that is, the variances in the groups should be equal. Actually, this should be inspected first because if the assumption is violated, the analysis would be inappropriate. We can see that the standard deviations for the three groups were 1.9322, 1.9120, and 2.3310. The tests indicate that the differences among these groups in terms of variance is not significant. For Cochrans and Bartlett-Box F probability levels are given. Maximum/minimum variance would be $(2.3310)^2/(1.9120)^2$ or 1.486. This figure can be looked up in Appendix D (the F distribution) with 9,9 df (number in each of groups minus one). Because 3.18 is the critical value at the 0.05 level, this number is not significant. Thus, the assumption is met, and the analysis is appropriate.

⑤ Because the overall F is significant, we now want to know which pairs of means are significantly different. The Scheffé procedure was requested. The asterisks indicate that group 1 differs significantly from groups 2 and 3, but groups 2 and 3 do not differ significantly from each other. Therefore, the group taught relaxation (experimental I), scored significantly lower on the measure of anxiety than the other two groups. Although the control group (group 3) scored the highest, the mean of 11.1 was not significantly higher than the mean of 8.9 for the procedure group (group 2).

MULTIPLE GROUP COMPARISONS

Two types of comparisons can be made among group means. The most commonly reported are post-hoc (after the fact) comparisons and a priori (planned) comparisons, based on hypotheses stated prior to the analysis.

Post-Hoc Tests

When a significant F test is obtained, we are able to reject the null hypothesis that all the groups are from the same population or that all the populations are equal; that is, we are able to state that there is a difference among the groups. However, when more than two groups are being compared, we cannot determine from the F test alone which of the groups differ from each other. In other words a significant F test does not mean that every group in the analysis is different from every other group. Many patterns of difference are possible. Some of the groups may be similar, forming a cluster that is different from another select group, or depending on the number of groups being compared, there may be wide deviation between each pair of the groups.

To determine where the significant differences lie, further analysis is required. Therefore, we are confronted with the task of comparing group means. However, if we decide to use the standard t test, we are confronted with the possibility of an increased rate of Type I errors. To prevent this a number of secondary analyses following the computation of the F ratio are available to pinpoint the source of the difference.

A variety of techniques exists. For example SPSS/PC+ has seven available. A discussion of each is beyond the scope of this book, but the aim of all is to decrease the likelihood of making a Type I error when making multiple comparisons. The Scheffé test is reported frequently. The formula is based on the usual formula for the calculation of a t test or F ratio. The critical value used for determining whether the resulting F statistic is significant is different. In other words the F associated with comparing the two means is the same as if they had been compared in the usual ANOVA, but the critical value is changed based on the number of comparisons. The new critical value is simply the usual value multiplied by the number of groups being compared minus one. In our example the critical value at the 0.05 level with 2 and 6 degrees of freedom was 5.14. Multiplying that by 2 (the number of groups minus one) results in a critical value of 10.28. Thus, the critical value is twice as stringent when making all possible comparisons among three groups than it was for the overall analysis. The Scheffé test is quite stringent, but it can be used with groups of equal and unequal size. For more detail on post-hoc tests following analysis of variance, we suggest the article by Holm and Christman (1985).

Planned Comparisons

Planned comparisons, or a priori contrasts, are based on hypotheses stated before data are collected. As previously mentioned when you hypothesize ahead of time, you are able to use more powerful statistical tests. One way to do this is through the development of prespecified contrasts that are orthogonal to each other. *Orthogonal* means that the hypothesis tests are unrelated to each other; that is, knowing one result tells you nothing about the other. For an overview of planned comparisons vs. omnibus tests, you can refer to a *Nursing Research* "Methodology Corner" by Wu and Slakter (1990).

Here we demonstrate how orthogonal contrasts can be developed and analyzed in SPSS/PC + . To have comparisons that are independent, only $n - 1$ comparisons can be made; that is, if there were three groups (experimental 1, experimental 2, and control), there could only be two orthogonal contrasts. In our example we might want to know if the experimental groups differed from the control group and if the experimental groups differed from each other. Table 7-3 contains the vectors necessary to code such a contrast. On vector $X1$ subjects in both experimental groups receive a -1, and the control group subjects receive 2. This contrast tests the difference between the mean anxiety score for all the experimental subjects and the mean for the control group subjects. The second contrast is given in vector $X2$. The first experimental group is compared with the second.

To ensure that hypothesized contrasts are orthogonal, three tests must be applied:

There must be only $n - 1$ contrasts.
The sum of each vector must equal zero. In the example the sum of $X1$ is $-1 + (-1) + 2 = 0$, and the sum of $X2$ is $1 + (-1) + 0 = 0$.
The sum of the cross-products must equal zero. In the example $(-1 \times 1) + (-1 \times -1) + (2 \times 0) = 0$.

TABLE 7-3
Orthogonal Coding

Groups	Vectors	
	X1	X2
Experimental 1	−1	1
Experimental 2	−1	−1
Control	2	0

TABLE 7-4
Contrasts

	Pairs of Vectors					
Groups	X1	X2	Y1	Y2	Z1	Z2
1	2	0	−1	1	−1	1
2	−1	1	2	0	0	−1
3	−1	−1	−1	−1	1	0

```
          SPSS/PC+ The Statistical Package for IBM PC
```

① `ONEWAY /VARIABLES ANXIETY BY GROUP (1,3) /CONTRAST -1 -1 2`
`/CONTRAST 1 -1 0.`

```
              - - - - - - - - - O N E W A Y - - - - - - - - - -
```

Variable ANXIETY

By Variable GROUP

Analysis of Variance

Source	D.F.	Sum of Squares	Mean Squares	F Ratio	F Prob.
Between Groups	2	141.8000	70.9000	16.5884	.0000
Within Groups	27	115.4000	4.2741		
Total	29	257.2000			

```
              - - - - - - - - - O N E W A Y - - - - - - - - - -
```

Variable ANXIETY
By Variable GROUP

Contrast Coefficient Matrix

	Grp 1	Grp 2	Grp 3
Contrast 1	-1.0	-1.0	2.0
Contrast 2	1.0	-1.0	.0

```
              - - - - - - - - - O N E W A Y - - - - - - - - - -
```

②

	Value	S. Error	Pooled Variance Estimate T Value	D.F.	T Prob.
Contrast 1	7.5000	1.6014	4.683	27.0	.000
Contrast 2	-3.1000	.9246	-3.353	27.0	.002

FIGURE 7-5
One-way analysis of variance with specified contrasts produced by SPSS/PC+.

In Table 7-4 there are some other examples of possible contrasts, given three groups. Are they all orthogonal? The vectors $X1$ and $X2$ reflect an orthogonal contrast, as do the vectors $Y1$ and $Y2$. Vectors $Z1$ and $Z2$ do not reflect an orthogonal contrast; group 1 is compared to group 2 and to group 3. The sum of the cross-products does not equal zero $(-1 \times 1) + (0 \times -1) + (1 \times 0) = -1$.

We now demonstrate the use of the contrasts specified in Table 7-3 in a computer analysis of these data. See Figure 7-5 for the computer output.

① A one-way analysis of variance is requested with ANXIETY as the dependent variable and GROUP as the independent variable. Remember that group 1 is experimental I, the group taught relaxation; group 2 is experimental II, the group that received information about the procedure; and group 3, the control group, received no experimental intervention. Two contrasts are requested. In the first groups 1 and 2 are contrasted with group 3, and in the second, groups 1 and 2 are compared. The analysis of variance table is the same as in Figure 7-4.

② Contrast 1 is significant at the 0.000 level; that is, the two experimental groups differed significantly from the control group. Looking at the group means in Table 7-2, we can see that the two experimental groups scored significantly *lower* on anxiety than the control group.

Contrast 2 is significant at the 0.002 level; that is, experimental group I scored significantly *lower* on anxiety than experimental group II.

CALCULATION OF SUMS OF SQUARES USING COMPUTATIONAL FORMULAS

Although the use of the formulas based on the deviations of scores from their means demonstrates most clearly how the variance is partitioned in an analysis of variance, two formulas are equivalent and easier to calculate. For those who would like to work with those formulas, Table 7-5 contains the hand calculations.

SUMMARY

One-way analysis of variance is used to compare the means of two or more groups. When the overall F is significant and more than two groups are being compared, post-hoc tests are necessary to determine which pairs of means differ from each other. Additionally, a priori contrasts may be specified and tested.

TABLE 7-5
Data for Calculation of One-Way ANOVA

Experimental I Relaxation		Experimental II Procedure Information		Control	
X_1	X_1^2	X_2	X_2^2	X_3	X_3^2
8	64	8	64	15	225
5	25	9	81	13	169
7	49	7	49	12	144
9	81	9	81	8	64
7	49	10	100	11	121
6	36	6	36	14	196
5	25	10	100	9	81
3	9	12	144	10	100
4	16	7	49	9	81
4	16	11	121	10	100
Σ_s 58	370	89	825	111	1281
$\overline{X}_1 = 5.8$		$\overline{X}_2 = 8.9$		$\overline{X}_3 = 11.1$	

HOMOGENEITY OF VARIANCE

$$\text{Variance} = \frac{\Sigma X^2 - \dfrac{(\Sigma X)^2}{n}}{n - 1}$$

$$\text{Experimental group I} = \frac{370 - \dfrac{(58)^2}{10}}{10 - 1} = 3.73$$

$$\text{Experimental group II} = 3.66$$

$$\text{Control group} = 5.43$$

$$F = \frac{\text{largest group variance}}{\text{smallest group variance}}$$

$$F_{9,9} = \frac{5.43}{3.66} = 1.4836 \qquad \text{not significant}$$

Total Sum of Squares

$$SS_{\text{tot}} = \Sigma X_{\text{tot}}^2 - \frac{(\Sigma X_{\text{tot}})^2}{n_{\text{tot}}}$$

$$\Sigma X_{\text{tot}}^2 = \Sigma X_1^2 + \Sigma X_2^2 + \Sigma X_3^2 = 370 + 825 + 1281 = 2476$$

$$\Sigma X_{\text{tot}} = 58 + 89 + 111 = 258$$

$$n_{\text{tot}} = 10 + 10 + 10 = 30$$

$$SS_{\text{tot}} = 2476 - \frac{(258)^2}{30} = 257.2$$

(*continued*)

TABLE 7-5　(CONTINUED)
Data for Calculation of One-Way ANOVA

Between Sum of Squares

$$SS_b = \left[\frac{(\Sigma X_1)^2}{n_1} + \frac{(\Sigma X_2)^2}{n_2} + \frac{(\Sigma X_3)^2}{n_3} + \cdots \frac{(\Sigma X_k)^2}{n_k} \right] - \frac{(\Sigma X_{tot})^2}{n_{tot}}$$

$$SS_b = \left[\frac{(58)^2}{10} + \frac{(89)^2}{10} + \frac{(111)^2}{10} \right] - \frac{(258)^2}{30} = 141.8$$

Within Sum of Squares

$$SS_w = \Sigma_{x_1}^2 + \Sigma_{x_2}^2 + \Sigma_{x_3}^2$$

$$\Sigma_{x_1}^2 = \Sigma X_1^2 - \frac{(\Sigma X_1)^2}{n_1}$$

$$= 370 - \frac{(58)^2}{10}$$

$$= 33.6$$

$$\Sigma_{x_2}^2 = \Sigma X_2^2 - \frac{(\Sigma X_2)^2}{n_2}$$

$$= 825 - \frac{(89)^2}{10}$$

$$= 32.9$$

$$\Sigma_{x_3}^2 = \Sigma X_3^2 - \frac{(\Sigma X_3)^2}{n_3}$$

$$= 1281 - \frac{(111)^2}{10}$$

$$= 48.9$$

$$SS_w = 33.6 + 32.9 + 48.9 = 115.4$$

8

Differences Among Group Means: *Multifactorial Analysis of Variance*

Barbara Hazard Munro

OBJECTIVES FOR CHAPTER 8

After reading this chapter you should be able to do the following:

1. Discuss the advantages of testing for interactions.

2. Interpret computer output from a two-way analysis of variance.

3. Determine when it is appropriate to use a multivariate analysis of variance (MANOVA).

TWO-WAY ANALYSIS OF VARIANCE

We have discussed the use of analysis of variance (ANOVA) with one categorical independent variable (with two or more levels) and one continuous dependent variable. In this chapter we discuss the use of ANOVA with more than one independent variable. We then extend the discussion into an analysis that includes more than one dependent variable. Such an analysis usually is referred to as multivariate analysis of variance (MANOVA) and allows the researcher to look for relationships among dependent, as well as independent, variables.

There are great advantages in having more than one independent variable in an ANOVA. One advantage is economy: Many hypotheses can be

Barbara Hazard Munro and Ellis Batten Page: STATISTICAL METHODS FOR HEALTH CARE RESEARCH, SECOND EDITION. © 1993, 1986 by J. B. Lippincott Company.

tested for almost the same cost. The other is the ability to test for *interactions*. Although it is interesting and valuable to learn whether a particular approach works better than another, it may be even more important to find out whether the effect of an approach varies depending on the group of subjects. Testing for an interaction allows us to answer the question of whether or not the results of a given treatment vary depending on the groups or conditions in which it is applied.

Table 8-1 illustrates this with a contrived example, first published in *Clinical Nurse Specialist* (Munro, 1990). This is an example of a 2 × 2 design, often called a 2 × 2 factorial design. Each of the two independent variables (or factors) has two levels. The first between-subject factor is information, with two groups, one that received information (yes) and one that did not receive information (no). The second factor (independent variable) is information style, with two groups (information seekers and information avoiders). If we analyzed each independent variable separately, we would not derive the information that is provided by studying the interaction effect in the two-way analysis of variance. If we compared those who received information with those who did not, there would be no difference between the groups, because the mean of each group (column means) is 75. Similarly, if we compared information seekers with information avoiders, we would find no difference (row means). Looking at the cells in the table, however, we can see that those whose information style fit with the information provided did much better (means of 100) than those whose style did not fit (means of 50). The test of the interaction is the statistical comparison of the diagonal means, 100 vs. 50.

In the example provided three research questions (or hypotheses) can be addressed:

1. Is there a significant difference between those who receive information and those who do not?
2. Is there a significant difference between those who seek information and those who avoid it?

TABLE 8-1
Example of an Interaction (Numbers Represent Group Means)

	Information		Row Means
	Yes	*No*	
Information Style			
Information-seeker	100	50	75
Information-avoider	50	100	75
Column means	75	75	
Diagonals: Seek/yes and Avoid/no	Mean = 100		
Seek/no and Avoid/yes	Mean = 50		

(From Munro, B. H. [1990]. Testing for interactions: The analysis of variance model. Clinical Nurse Specialist, 4(3), 128–129.)

TABLE 8-2
Two-Way Analysis of Variance of Aggressiveness of Nursing Care by Medical Diagnosis and DNR Status (N = 600)

	F-Value	*p*
Main Effects	28.56	<.001
Medical Diagnosis *(AIDS v. Non-AIDS)*	18.70	<.001
DNR Status *(DNR order v. No DNR order)*	38.42	<.001
Interaction Effects (*df* = 3,596)	0.47	.495

(From Forrester, D. A. [1990]. AIDS-related risk factors medical diagnosis, do-not-resuscitate orders and aggressiveness of nursing care. Nursing Research, 39(6), *350–354.)*

3. Is there a significant interaction between information provided and the information-seeking style of the subject?

Testing of the interaction provides information about whether or not effects are altered by other factors. This allows us to investigate differences among groups of subjects in relation to an outcome measure.

Forrester (1990) used a two-way ANOVA to test the hypothesis that there was no interaction between medical diagnosis and do not resuscitate (DNR) orders in relation to nurses' attitudes toward aggressiveness of care. As you can see in Table 8-2, the hypothesis was supported ($F = 0.47, p = 0.495$). There were significant main effects. Nurses' scores on aggressiveness of care were significantly higher for AIDS patients than for non-AIDS (oat cell carcinoma) patients ($F = 18.70, p < 0.001$), and the aggressiveness scores were significantly lower for patients with a DNR order than for patients with no DNR order ($F = 38.42, p < 0.001$).

EXAMPLE OF A COMPUTER PRINTOUT OF A TWO-WAY ANALYSIS OF VARIANCE

Table 8-3 contains fictitious data to provide another example of a two-way ANOVA. As can be seen, there are two independent variables, treatment and sex, and each has two levels. Overall, those who had treatment A had a mean score of 5.5; those who had treatment B had a mean of 5.4 (column means). Males had a mean of 5.2, and females had a mean of 5.7 (row means). These represent the two main effects. Looking at the cell means, we see that males exposed to treatment B and females exposed to treatment A, had higher means (8.0 and 8.6) than males exposed to treatment A (2.4) and females exposed to treatment B (2.8). One could say that males do better with treatment B, and females do better with treatment A. Determining whether this is a significant difference

TABLE 8-3
Data for Two-Way ANOVA (Outcome = X)

Sex	Treatment		Row Means
	A	B	
Males	1	8	
	3	9	
	4	10	
	2	6	
	2	7	
Means	2.4	8.0	5.2
Females	10	4	
	9	2	
	9	3	
	7	4	
	8	1	
Means	8.6	2.8	5.7
Column Means	5.5	5.4	

is a test of the interaction between treatment and sex. Figure 8-1 contains the computer analysis of these data produced by SPSS/PC+.

① The command line requests the ANOVA procedure. The dependent variable is X, and RX and SEX are the independent variables. STATISTICS 3 causes cell means and counts to be displayed. Unfortunately, tests for homogeneity of variance are not included in the ANOVA program. To test that assumption, the ONEWAY program must be used. In this example two one-way analyses are conducted, with each independent variable (RX and SEX) taken separately. The homogeneity of variance tests are then checked to determine if the assumption has been met. In this example those results are nonsignificant (i.e., the assumption is met).

② The mean in the total group is 5.45. The means are provided for the treatment groups (A and B) and males and females, and then the cell means are listed. The numbers in parentheses indicate the number of subjects.

③ Neither of the two main effects is significant. The sum of squares for the treatment effect is 0.050. Dividing that by its degrees of freedom results in the mean square. Dividing the mean square, 0.050, by the residual mean square, 1.7, results in an F value of 0.029, which with 1,16 degrees of freedom has a probability level of 0.866.

The interaction of RX and SEX is significant, however, at the 0.000 level. Comparing the means, we see that males in group A and females in group B scored significantly lower than males in group B and females in group A.

The degrees of freedom for the main effects equal the number of groups minus 1. Because we have two groups in each independent variable, the degrees of freedom for each main effect is 1. The degrees of freedom for the interaction is the product of the degrees of freedom for each variable in the interaction. In our example it is RX × SEX or 1 × 1 = 1. The total degrees of freedom equal the number of subjects minus 1.

COMPUTATION OF TWO-WAY ANALYSIS OF VARIANCE

The data for computation of a two-way ANOVA are outlined in Table 8-4 for those who wish to work the hand calculations.

MULTIVARIATE ANALYSIS OF VARIANCE

Many times we are interested in more than one outcome. For example Maikler (1991) studied the effects of a skin refrigerant or anesthetic and age on the pain responses of infants receiving immunizations. Infants were randomly assigned to receive the skin refrigerant or compressed air and were categorized into two age groups (younger than or older than 16 weeks). The outcome measures included facial expression, cry, and body movements. Rather than conduct separate analyses for each outcome measure (which would have increased the chance of a Type I error), the investigator used a MANOVA to "consider all measures of facial expression, cry, and body movements simultaneously." The infants who received the skin refrigerant startled less and took longer to cry than those in the control group. The duration of pain expression was longer in the younger infants.

Another example is a study of the outcomes of developmentally supportive nursing care for very low-birth-weight infants (Becker, Grunwald, Moorman, & Stuhr, 1991). A MANOVA was used to compare two groups of infants (before and after a staff education program) on seven outcome measures. Infants in the staff education group "had more optimal respiratory and feeding status, lower levels of morbidity, shorter hospitalization, and improved behavioral organization."

Although MANOVA techniques were developed in the 1930s and 1940s, not until the computer software became readily available were they reported in the social science literature. Today, MANOVA can be performed on a personal computer. Because in health professions, we are usually interested in more than one outcome, MANOVA is a very important technique and is being reported with increasing frequency in research publications. An in-depth presentation of the technique is beyond the scope of this book, and readers are referred to Bray and Maxwell (1985) for a more comprehensive presentation.

Advantages of MANOVA

Health-care outcomes measures, including physiological, psychological, and sociological, often are correlated. MANOVA includes the inter-relation among the outcome measures, whereas separate ANOVAs (one for each dependent variable) do not. Good-

SPSS/PC+

(1) ANOVA /VARIABLES X BY RX (1,2) SEX (1,2) /STATISTICS 3.

* * * C E L L   M E A N S * * *

```
              X            SCORE ON OUTCOME MEASURE
           BY RX           TREATMENT GROUP
              SEX
```

(2) TOTAL POPULATION

```
        5.45
     (    20)
```

RX

```
          A             B

        5.50          5.40
     (    10)    (     10)
```

SEX

```
       MALE        FEMALE

        5.20          5.70
     (    10)    (     10)
```

```
           SEX
                   MALE        FEMALE
      RX
             A      2.40          8.60
                 (     5)    (      5)

             B      8.00          2.80
                 (     5)    (      5)
```

FIGURE 8-1

Two-way ANOVA produced by SPSS/PC+.

win (1984) cites three general advantages of a multivariate, rather than several univariate analyses, to test hypotheses: (1) to keep alpha at a known level; (2) to increase power; and (3) for ease in computation and interpretation. Conducting one overall analysis protects against Type I errors. An alternative would be to use a Bonferroni correction, but that would still ignore any relationship among the dependent variables. MANOVA is more powerful than separate ANOVAs, and the interpretation of the results may be improved by considering the outcome measures simultaneously (Bray & Maxwell, 1985, pp. 10–12). If the outcome measures are not correlated, however, there is no advantage to conducting a MANOVA.

```
* * *   A N A L Y S I S   O F   V A R I A N C E   * * *

         X           SCORE ON OUTCOME MEASURE
    BY   RX          TREATMENT GROUP
         SEX
```

③ Source of Variation	Sum of Squares	DF	Mean Square	F	Signif of F
Main Effects	1.300	2	.650	.382	.688
RX	.050	1	.050	.029	.866
SEX	1.250	1	1.250	.735	.404
2-way Interactions	162.450	1	162.450	95.559	.000
RX SEX	162.450	1	162.450	95.559	.000
Explained	163.750	3	54.583	32.108	.000
Residual	27.200	16	1.700		
Total	190.950	19	10.050		

```
   20 Cases were processed.
    0 Cases (   .0 PCT) were missing.
```

FIGURE 8-1 (CONTINUED)

Assumptions of MANOVA

For ANOVA the assumptions include random sample, normal distribution, and equal variances across the groups on the dependent variable. When this is extended to MANOVA, not only should the univariate assumptions hold, but the dependent variable should have a "multivariate normal distribution with the same variance covariance matrix in each group" (Norusis, 1990b, p. B-64). To meet the assumption of multivariate normal distribution, each dependent variable must have a normal distribution, but this does not ensure that the overall measure of the dependent variables taken together will be normally distributed. Thus, the multivariate assumption needs to be tested. The requirement that each group will have the same variance–covariance matrix means that the homogeneity of variance assumption is met for each dependent variable and that the correlation between any two dependent variables must be the same in all groups (Bray & Maxwell, 1985, pp. 32–33).

Statistical Power

It is difficult to ascertain the power when planning a MANOVA study, due to the number of parameters to be estimated. Increasing the number of dependent variables requires an increase in sample size to maintain a given level of power. For example for two groups with an alpha of 0.05, power of 0.80, and moderate effect size, 64 subjects in each

(text continues on page 139)

TABLE 8-4
Computation of Two-Way Analysis of Variance

DATA FOR COMPUTATION OF A TWO-WAY ANOVA

Sex	Treatment A X	Treatment A X^2	Treatment B X	Treatment B X^2	Row Totals X	Row Totals X^2
Males	1	1	8	64		
	3	9	9	81		
	4	16	10	100		
	2	4	6	36		
	2	4	7	49		
Subtotal	*12*	*34*	*40*	*330*	52	364
Females	10	100	4	16		
	9	81	2	4		
	9	81	3	9		
	7	49	4	16		
	8	64	1	1		
Subtotal	*43*	*375*	*14*	*46*	57	421
Column Totals	*55*	*409*	*54*	*376*	*109*	*Overall Total 785*

HOMOGENEITY OF VARIANCE

$$\text{Variance} = \frac{\Sigma X^2 - \dfrac{(\Sigma X)^2}{n}}{n-1},$$

degrees of freedom = number in group -1

Variances for the Four Groups	**Degrees of Freedom**
Rx A, Males 1.3	4
Rx B, Males 2.5	4
Rx A, Females 1.3	4
Rx B, Females 1.7	4

$$F \text{ ratio} = \frac{\text{largest variance}}{\text{smallest variance}}$$

$$F = \frac{2.5}{1.3}$$

$F = 1.9$ with 4,4 degrees of freedom, not significant

(*continued*)

TABLE 8-4   (CONTINUED)
Computation of Two-Way Analysis of Variance

SUM OF SQUARES

Total Sum of Squares

$$\Sigma X_{tot}^2 - \frac{(\Sigma X_{tot})^2}{n_{tot}}$$

$$785 - \frac{(109)^2}{20} = 785 - 594.05 = 190.95$$

Between Groups Sum of Squares.

Since we have two groups (treatment and sex), we will calculate *two* between groups sums of squares. The formula is

$$\Sigma \frac{(\Sigma X_g)^2}{n_g} - \frac{(\Sigma X_{tot})^2}{n_{tot}}$$

$$\text{Treatment group } SS = \frac{(55)^2}{10} + \frac{(54)^2}{10} - \frac{(109)^2}{20}$$

$$= 302.5 + 291.6 - 594.05$$

$$= 0.05$$

$$\text{Sex group } SS = \frac{(52)^2}{10} + \frac{(57)^2}{10} - \frac{(109)^2}{20}$$

$$= 270.4 + 324.9 - 594.05$$

$$= 1.25$$

Interaction Sum of Squares.

The *first* step is to calculate the sum of squares for each individual cell. The formula is

$$\text{Subgroups } SS = \Sigma \frac{(\Sigma X_{sg})^2}{n_{sg}} - \frac{(\Sigma X_{tot})^2}{n_{tot}}$$

$$= \frac{(12)^2}{5} + \frac{(40)^2}{5} + \frac{(43)^2}{5} + \frac{(14)^2}{5} - \frac{(109)^2}{20}$$

$$= 28.8 + 320 + 396.8 + 39.2 - 594.05$$

$$= 163.75$$

The *second* step is to calculate the interaction sum of squares using the following formula:

$$\text{Interaction } SS = \text{Subgroup } SS - \text{Between } SS$$

$$\text{Interaction } SS = 163.75 - (.05 + 1.25)$$

$$= 163.75 - 1.3$$

$$= 162.45$$

(continued)

TABLE 8-4 (CONTINUED)
Computation of Two-Way Analysis of Variance

SUM OF SQUARES

Total Sum of Squares

Within SS = Total SS − (Between SS + *Interaction*)

Within SS = 190.95 − (.05 + 1.25 + 162.45)

$$= 190.95 − 163.75$$

$$= 27.2$$

Degrees of Freedom

The following formulas are used:

Total between SS = number of subgroups − 1

Factor (independent variable) SS = $k − 1$

Interaction SS = df for first group × df for second group

Within SS = number in sample − number of groups in first variable × number of groups in second variable

Total SS = number in sample − 1

In our example, we have the following *df*:

	df
Total between groups	4 − 1 = 3
Treatment	2 − 1 = 1
Sex	2 − 1 = 1
Interaction	1 × 1 = 1
Within groups	20 − (2 × 2) = 16
Total	20 − 1 = 19

SUMMARY TABLE FOR TWO-WAY ANALYSIS OF VARIANCE

Source of Variance	*SS*	*df*	*MS*	*F*	*p*
Between group	163.75	3	54.78	32.108	<.01
Treatment	.05	1	.05	.029	ns
Sex	1.25	1	1.25	.735	ns
Treatment × sex	162.45	1	162.45	95.559	<.01
Within groups	27.20	16	1.70		
Total	*190.95*	*19*			

group are required when there is one dependent variable. With two dependent variables, 80 subjects are required in each group (Lauter, Lauter, & Schmidtke, 1978).

Results of MANOVA

The first step in assessing the results is to look at the overall MANOVA. This is similar to looking at the F in the ANOVA. It tells whether there is an overall significant result. If there is, it indicates that there is a difference in at least one of the dependent variables. While there is only one outcome measure for ANOVA, F, there are four outcome measures for MANOVA:

1. Wilks' lambda
2. Pillai-Bartlett trace
3. Roy's greatest characteristic root
4. Hotelling-Lawley trace

Wilks' lambda is explained in the sections on canonical correlation and discriminant analysis. It represents the product of the unexplained variances, that is, the error variance. Thus, a small value indicates significance.

Pillai-Bartlett trace represents the sum of the explained variances; therefore, a large value indicates significance.

Roy's greatest characteristic root is based on the first discriminant variate (see the section on discriminant function analysis).

Hotelling-Lawley trace is the sum of the ratio of the between and within sums of squares for each of the discriminant variates.

Any of these statistics might be used to test the overall multivariate hypothesis. According to Bray and Maxwell (1985, p. 28), choosing the appropriate test involves a complex consideration of robustness and statistical power, but Wilks' lambda is historically the most widely used, and Pillai-Bartlett trace has been found to be the most robust.

If the overall MANOVA is significant, one wants to determine where the differences lie. Do the groups differ on all the dependent variables or only one? Generally, investigators have conducted univariate analyses following a multivariate significant result; that is, they conduct an ANOVA for each dependent variable. The danger of Type I error is thought of as being "protected" by the overall significant MANOVA. This has been referred to as the least significant difference test or the protected F (Bray & Maxwell, 1985, p. 40). This approach has been criticized, however, because it does not control for the number of comparisons made and does not adequately analyze the multivariate nature of the analysis. According to Bray and Maxwell (1985, p. 45) the most general method of analyzing a significant MANOVA is to use Roy-Bose simultaneous confidence intervals. "This is a completely multivariate approach in which any linear combination of the classification or criterion variables can be investigated" (p. 53). This approach is not available in SPSS/PC+, and our computer example will use the univariate analysis following the significant multivariate result.

Computer Output of a MANOVA Analysis

To demonstrate a MANOVA analysis, we return to the example used earlier in this chapter (see Table 8-3). There we have a two-way ANOVA (TREATMENT and SEX) with one dependent variable, X. Suppose we measured the same subjects on an additional outcome measure, Y. Table 8-5 contains the additional data. Here we see that the mean for treatment A was higher than the mean for treatment B (column means), and males scored higher than females (row means). We add the second outcome measure to the database and produce a MANOVA, which is given in Figure 8-2. Although the numbers of subjects are too small for such a complex analysis, we hope that this example will help clarify the main points and enable the interested reader to replicate the analysis.

①　The MANOVA procedure lists two dependent variables, X and Y, and two independent variables, RX and SEX. OMEANS requests the observed means for the overall groups (SEX and RX). The PRINT line requests the means of the cells and the homogeneity of variance test.

②　First the cell means for variable X are given (compare with Table 8-3), and then the means for variable Y are given (compare with Table 8-5).

③　Box's M is a measure of the multivariate test for homogeneity of variance. With a p of 0.889, the assumption has been met. It should be noted, however, that Box's M, although widely used, is very sensitive to departures from normality (Olson, 1974). It is essential that the data be submitted to preliminary checks for meeting the underlying assumptions, for outliers, and so forth before the analysis is conducted.

(*text continues on page 144*)

TABLE 8-5
Data for Two-Way MANOVA (Outcome = Y)

	Treatment		
Sex	A	B	Row Means
Males	10	5	
	6	4	
	8	6	
	9	4	
	7	5	
Means	8	4.8	6.4
Females	6	1	
	3	2	
	4	2	
	5	4	
	7	3	
Means	5	2.4	3.7
Column Means	6.5	3.6	

SPSS/PC+

(1) MANOVA X Y BY RX (1,2) SEX (1,2)
    /OMEANS=VARIABLES (X Y) TABLES (SEX RX)
    /PRINT=CELLINFO (MEANS) HOMOGENEITY (BOXM)
    /DESIGN.

        20 cases accepted.
         0 cases rejected because of out-of-range factor values.
         0 cases rejected because of missing data.
         4 non-empty cells.

         1 design will be processed.

(2) - - - - - - - - - -
Cell Means and Standard Deviations
Variable .. X   SCORE ON OUTCOME MEASURE
     FACTOR   CODE   Mean Std. Dev.   N

   RX   A
    SEX   MALE   2.400   1.140   5
    SEX   FEMALE   8.600   1.140   5

 * * ANALYSIS OF VARIANCE -- DESIGN   1 * *

 Cell Means and Standard Deviations   (CONT.)
 Variable .. X   SCORE ON OUTCOME MEASURE
     FACTOR   CODE   Mean Std. Dev.   N

   RX   B
    SEX   MALE   8.000   1.581   5
    SEX   FEMALE   2.800   1.304   5
 For entire sample   5.450   3.170   20

 - - - - - - - - - -
 Variable .. Y   SCORE ON Y
     FACTOR   CODE   Mean Std. Dev.   N

   RX   A
    SEX   MALE   8.000   1.581   5
    SEX   FEMALE   5.000   1.581   5
   RX   B
    SEX   MALE   4.800   .837   5
    SEX   FEMALE   2.400   1.140   5
 For entire sample   5.050   2.373   20

 * * ANALYSIS OF VARIANCE -- DESIGN   1 * *

(3) Multivariate test for Homogeneity of Dispersion matrices

   Boxs M =   5.60215
   F WITH (9,2933) DF =   .48007, P =   .889 (Approx.)
   Chi-Square with 9 DF =   4.33777, P =   .888 (Approx.)

FIGURE 8-2
Multivariate analysis of variance produced by SPSS/PC+. (*continued*)

```
(4) - - - - - - - - -
    * * ANALYSIS  OF  VARIANCE -- DESIGN   1 * *

    Combined Observed Means for SEX
    Variable .. X
              SEX
              MALE          WGT.     5.20000
                            UNWGT.   5.20000
           FEMALE           WGT.     5.70000
                            UNWGT.   5.70000

    - - - - - - - - - - -
    Variable .. Y
              SEX
              MALE          WGT.     6.40000
                            UNWGT.   6.40000
           FEMALE           WGT.     3.70000
                            UNWGT.   3.70000


    * * ANALYSIS  OF  VARIANCE -- DESIGN   1 * *

    Combined Observed Means for RX
    Variable .. X
              RX
              A             WGT.     5.50000
                            UNWGT.   5.50000
              B             WGT.     5.40000
                            UNWGT.   5.40000

    - - - - - - - - - - -
    Variable .. Y
              RX
              A             WGT.     6.50000
                            UNWGT.   6.50000
              B             WGT.     3.60000
                            UNWGT.   3.60000

    * * ANALYSIS  OF  VARIANCE -- DESIGN   1 * *

(5) EFFECT .. RX BY SEX
    Multivariate Tests of Significance (S = 1, M = 0, N = 6 1/2)

    Test Name       Value   Approx. F Hypoth. DF   Error DF  Sig. of F

    Pillais        .85680   44.87421      2.00       15.00     .000
    Hotellings    5.98323   44.87421      2.00       15.00     .000
    Wilks          .14320   44.87421      2.00       15.00     .000
    Roys           .85680

    - - - - - - - - - - -
    Univariate F-tests with (1,16) D. F.

    Variable   Hypoth. SS   Error SS Hypoth. MS    Error MS         F  Sig. of F

    X          162.45000    27.20000  162.45000     1.70000  95.55882      .000
    Y             .45000    28.00000     .45000      1.75000    .25714      .619

    * * ANALYSIS  OF  VARIANCE -- DESIGN   1 * *
```

FIGURE 8-2 (CONTINUED)

⑥ EFFECT .. SEX
Multivariate Tests of Significance (S = 1, M = 0, N = 6 1/2)

Test Name	Value	Approx. F	Hypoth. DF	Error DF	Sig. of F
Pillais	.56772	9.84984	2.00	15.00	.002
Hotellings	1.31331	9.84984	2.00	15.00	.002
Wilks	.43228	9.84984	2.00	15.00	.002
Roys	.56772				

- - - - - - - - - -
Univariate F-tests with (1,16) D. F.

Variable	Hypoth. SS	Error SS	Hypoth. MS	Error MS	F	Sig. of F
X	1.25000	27.20000	1.25000	1.70000	.73529	.404
Y	36.45000	28.00000	36.45000	1.75000	20.82857	.000

* * ANALYSIS OF VARIANCE -- DESIGN 1 * *

⑦ EFFECT .. RX
Multivariate Tests of Significance (S = 1, M = 0, N = 6 1/2)

Test Name	Value	Approx. F	Hypoth. DF	Error DF	Sig. of F
Pillais	.60429	11.45309	2.00	15.00	.001
Hotellings	1.52708	11.45309	2.00	15.00	.001
Wilks	.39571	11.45309	2.00	15.00	.001
Roys	.60429				

- - - - - - - - - -
Univariate F-tests with (1,16) D. F.

Variable	Hypoth. SS	Error SS	Hypoth. MS	Error MS	F	Sig. of F
X	.05000	27.20000	.05000	1.70000	.02941	.866
Y	42.05000	28.00000	42.05000	1.75000	24.02857	.000

* * ANALYSIS OF VARIANCE -- DESIGN 1 * *

⑧ EFFECT .. CONSTANT
Multivariate Tests of Significance (S = 1, M = 0, N = 6 1/2)

Test Name	Value	Approx. F	Hypoth. DF	Error DF	Sig. of F
Pillais	.97788	331.55139	2.00	15.00	.000
Hotellings	44.20685	331.55139	2.00	15.00	.000
Wilks	.02212	331.55139	2.00	15.00	.000
Roys	.97788				

- - - - - - - - - -
Univariate F-tests with (1,16) D. F.

Variable	Hypoth. SS	Error SS	Hypoth. MS	Error MS	F	Sig. of F
X	594.05000	27.20000	594.05000	1.70000	349.44118	.000
Y	510.05000	28.00000	510.05000	1.75000	291.45714	.000

FIGURE 8-2 (CONTINUED)

④ The combined means are presented. First, the means for males and females on variable X and then on variable Y are listed. Then, the combined means for the second major variable are presented. The means for treatments A and B are listed for each of the two outcome measures.

⑤ The multivariate tests of the interaction are given first. The four tests are listed, and they are significant at the 0.000 level. The univariate test is then given. Here we see that there is a significant interaction on the X variable ($p = 0.000$) but not on the Y variable ($p = 0.619$).

As noted previously, this interaction is based on the fact that on the dependent variable X, males do best with treatment B, and females do best with treatment A.

⑥ The multivariate tests of the main effect, SEX, are given next. They are significant at the 0.002 level. Looking at the univariate test, we see that the difference occurs for the Y but not the X variable. Looking at the combined means for variable Y, we see that the males scored significantly higher (mean = 6.4) than the females (mean = 3.7).

⑦ The multivariate tests of the other main effect, RX, also are significant ($p = 0.001$). Here treatment groups differ significantly on Y ($p = 0.000$) but not on X ($p = 0.866$). Looking at the combined means for variable Y, we see that subjects scored higher on A (mean = 6.5) than on B (mean = 3.6).

⑧ The test of the constant is the test of the overall analysis, including main effects and interaction effects. The multivariate tests are significant, and there are significant effects for both dependent variables. There is a significant interaction effect for the X variable and significant main effects for the Y variable.

SUMMARY

Analysis of variance is a powerful, robust test that allows us to test for relationships between categorical independent variables and a continuous (measured at the interval or ratio level) dependent variable. Testing for interactions between the independent variables is particularly useful when we want to determine whether or not the effects of some intervention will be the same for all types of people or conditions. ANOVA may be extended to the use of more than one dependent variable in a given analysis. This analysis is usually referred to as MANOVA and allows the researcher to look for relationships among dependent, as well as many independent, variables.

9

Analysis of Covariance

*Barbara
Hazard Munro*

OBJECTIVES FOR CHAPTER 9

After reading this chapter you should be able to do the following:

1. **Determine when analysis of covariance is the appropriate technique to use.**
2. **Explain the relationship between analysis of variance and regression.**
3. **Discuss the assumptions, interpretations, and limitations of analysis of covariance.**

In the preceding chapters the statistical methods of analysis of variance (ANOVA)—one-way and complex—were described as techniques to investigate differences among group means. Those tests were used when more than two groups were involved or when we were interested in the effects of several categorical (independent) variables on a "continuous" (dependent) measure.

In this chapter we present another ANOVA technique: the analysis of covariance (ANCOVA). This technique combines the ANOVA with regression to measure the differences among group means. The advantages that ANCOVA holds over other techniques are the ability to reduce the error variance in the outcome measure and the ability to measure group differences after allowing for other differences between subjects. The error variance is reduced by controlling for variation in the dependent measure that comes from separate measurable variables that influence all the groups being compared. Such a separate variable is considered to be neither "independent" nor "dependent" in the ANOVA. However, it

Barbara Hazard Munro and Ellis Batten Page: STATISTICAL METHODS FOR HEALTH CARE RESEARCH, SECOND EDITION. © 1993, 1986 by J. B. Lippincott Company.

contributes to the variation and reduces the magnitude of the differences among groups. In ANCOVA the variation from this variable is measured and extracted from the within (or error) variation. The effect is the reduction of error variance and therefore an increase in the power of the analysis. Recall that power is the *likelihood of correctly rejecting the null hypothesis*. With ANCOVA the control of the extraneous variation will provide a more accurate estimate of the real difference among groups.

STATISTICAL QUESTIONS FOR ANCOVA

In general ANCOVA answers the same research question that ANOVA addresses: Do the experimental groups differ to a greater degree than we would expect by chance alone? However, with ANOVA two sets of variables were involved in the analysis: the independent variables and the dependent variable. With ANCOVA a third type of variable is included: the *covariate*.

For example Gulick and Bugg (1992) compared multidimensional health patterning in three groups of people with multiple sclerosis. They used ANCOVA "to control for age at diagnosis since a more rapid disease progression has been reported when persons are older at time of diagnosis" (p. 178). They found that older age at diagnosis was related to decreased functioning in activities of daily living in several areas. If they had not included age as a covariate, they would have been unable to explain the variability due to age; it would have been relegated to the "error" term. Thus, their analysis was more powerful in that the error term was reduced, and they were able to validate previous research that indicated that age is an important variable when studying multiple sclerosis.

Such an approach is typical of the original purpose for using ANCOVA. Since then, the technique has been used in other ways as well. Frequently, it has been used to "equate" groups. In quasiexperimental designs individuals have not been randomly assigned to groups, and intact groups are often used. A typical example is using already established classes in a school to test different teaching methods. Because the subjects are not randomly assigned, there may be initial differences among groups. In classroom situations the major concern would be that the groups might differ in intelligence. In a hospital situation one might be concerned that patients in one unit were sicker than those in another unit. If the groups are found to be different, ANCOVA is often used to "equate" them; that is, in the classroom example IQ would be the covariate, and the effect of intelligence would be "removed" before the means of the groups on the dependent variable were compared. In the hospital example degree of illness might be used as a covariate.

In a related example Moore (1983) studied the effect of prepared childbirth on marital satisfaction. This is a very interesting example because if the investigator had not used ANCOVA, her results would have been misleading. She had two groups of couples: One was prepared for childbirth through Lamaze classes, and the other received hospital classes. Subjects were measured on marital satisfaction during pregnancy and after the birth of the child. The theory was that because Lamaze is a shared experience with a common goal, the Lamaze group should have higher marital satisfaction than the hospital class group. This was a nonexperimental design in that the investigator did not randomly assign subjects to the groups; assignment was by self-selection. Because group equality could not be assumed, Moore measured marital satisfaction before the childbearing experience, as well as at two later times. The groups were not equivalent on marital satisfaction prior to their childbearing experience. The Lamaze group had significantly higher marital satisfaction than the hospital class group before any of them had attended childbirth classes. To control for that initial difference, Moore used the first measure of marital satisfaction as a covariate. The outcome measures of marital satisfaction were "adjusted" for the initial group differences. The adjusted postpartum scores showed no significant differences between the two groups. The unadjusted scores were significantly different; that is, without ANCOVA the results would have indicated that Lamaze couples had higher marital satisfaction when that was simply due to initial group differences.

ANCOVA also has been used when random assignment has not "worked." Especially with small samples, an investigator may find that even after random assignment, the groups differ on some important variable. ANCOVA might then be used to equate the groups statistically.

Although ANCOVA has been widely used for such statistical "equalization" of groups, it is not a cure-all and should be used with caution. Some authors condemn its use for anything but the intent to remove another source of variation from the dependent variable. They do not believe that it should be used to equate groups. To use ANCOVA with dissimilar groups, one would have to be able to assert that the groups were essentially equivalent except for the variable(s) being used as covariate(s). This equivalence is virtually impossible to know for certain.

TYPE OF DATA REQUIRED

As with ANOVA we have one or more categorical variables as independent variables, and the dependent variable is measured at the interval or ratio level. In addition the covariate should be at the interval or ratio level. This is discussed in further detail in the following section.

ASSUMPTIONS

To ensure a valid interpretation of ANCOVA results, several assumptions should be met. These assumptions are based on requirements necessary for the validity of the regression and the ANOVA components of the test. The first four assumptions are those associated with ANOVA:

1. The groups should be mutually exclusive.
2. The variances of the groups should be equivalent (homogeneity of variance).
3. Interval or ratio level data should be used for the dependent variable.
4. The dependent variable should be normally distributed.

In addition,

5. The covariate should be measured at the interval or ratio level. If a variable is at the nominal level, it cannot be used as a covariate. (However, a nominal variable may be included as an additional independent variable in ANOVA, rather than as a covariate.)
6. The covariate and the dependent variable must show a linear relationship. When this assumption is violated, the analysis will have little benefit, because there will be little reduction in error variance. The test is most effective when that relationship lies above $r = 0.30$. The stronger the relationship, the more effective the ANCOVA analysis will be; that is, the more the two variables are related, the greater is the reduction in the error variance by controlling for the covariate. In cases in which the relationship between the covariate and dependent variable is not linear, one appropriate test would be the complex ANOVA, with the levels of the covariate as another independent variable. Another possibility would be mathematical transformation of the variables to achieve a linear relationship. The transformed variables could then be used in ANCOVA.

Consider an example that demonstrates a violation of this assumption. Suppose that we wished to study the effects of two different teaching methods on student performance. Suppose also that the investigator wished to control for the effects of anxiety. Previous research implies that there is a U-shaped relationship between anxiety and performance; that is, performance seems to be enhanced by moderate levels of anxiety. However, at high and low levels, performance is hampered. This relation is depicted graphically in Figure 9-1. Therefore, ANCOVA analysis with level

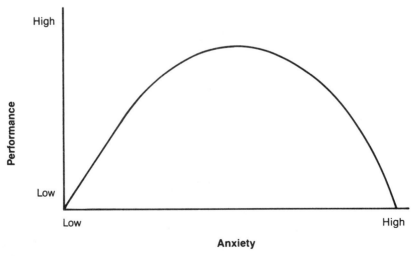

FIGURE 9-1
Possible relationship between performance and anxiety.

of anxiety as a covariate would violate the assumption of a linear correlation between the covariate and the outcome variable.

One appropriate analysis in this case would be a complex ANOVA with three levels of anxiety as one main effect variable and types of teaching as a second main effect. Another approach would be to use curvilinear regression analysis, in which case the anxiety scores could be treated as continuous, rather than categorical, data. For further information on curvilinear regression, see Pedhazur (1982, Chapter 11).

7. The direction and strength of the relationship between the covariate and dependent variable must be similar in each group. We call this requirement *homogeneity of regression across groups*. When this assumption is violated, the chance of a Type I error is increased. This assumption can be expressed in another way: The independent variable should not have an effect on *the relationship between the covariate and the dependent variable*. Another way to say this is that the covariate has the same effect on the dependent variable in all the groups.

Finally, in the graph in Figure 9-2 we see that when there is homogeneity of regression, the regression lines will be parallel. In the example the lines are not parallel, indicating that the interventions affected the covariate-dependent relationship differentially. In Figure 9-2 IQ is the covariate (varying from low to high) and the score on the final examination is the outcome measure. There are two groups, one taught by the lecture method and one by programmed instruction (PI). The covariate, IQ, does not have the same relationship with the dependent variable in these two groups. In the programmed instruction (PI) group, students with higher IQs score lower on the final examination (a negative correlation). In the lecture group the opposite is true. Students with higher IQs score higher on the final.

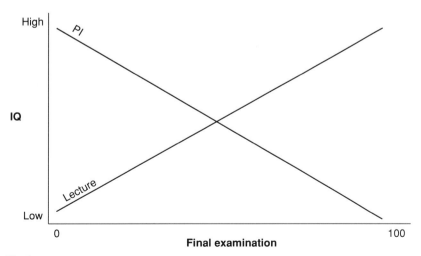

FIGURE 9-2
Lack of homogeneity of regression across two groups.

RELATIONSHIP OF ANOVA AND REGRESSION TO ANCOVA

To understand the rationale behind the mathematical operations involved in ANCOVA, it is necessary to understand the concept of *residual*. This notion is well explained in Kerlinger and Pedhazur (1973), and the following explanation relies heavily on their work.

In Chapter 11 we explain that squaring the correlation coefficient results in a quantity, r^2, known as a *coefficient of determination*. This coefficient is often used as a measure of the meaningfulness of r, because it is a measure of the variance shared by the two variables. To calculate the proportion of variance that is *not shared* by the two variables, we would subtract r^2 from 1. For example if the correlation between two variables is 0.50, then $r^2 = 0.25$, and $1 - r^2 = 0.75$. We could then state that 25% of the variance was shared by the two variables, and 75% was not shared. This 75% is called the *variance of the residual*. The residual variance is not due to the relationship between the two variables. In regression analysis we talk about the regression sum of squares and the residual sum of squares. With ANOVA the within sum of squares, or error term, is analogous to the residual sum of squares. Thus, the residual variance is the variation not explained by the variables in the study. With ANCOVA we use the residuals to determine whether groups differ *after* the effect of some other variable has been removed.

EXAMPLE OF A COMPUTER PRINTOUT

First, let us suppose that we wanted to test two nursing interventions designed to improve posthospital adjustment (1 and 2). There are two medical units in our hospital, so we randomly assign intervention 1 to one unit and intervention 2 to the other. The posthospital adjustment scale measures physical, psychological, and social adjustment and has a potential range of scores of 1 to 20. Table 9-1 contains the fictitious results from this study. The means of the two groups are similar, 8.5 and 8. Applying the pooled *t* test to these data results in a *t* value of -0.273, which is nonsignificant. We could therefore conclude that there is no difference between interventions 1 and 2 in relation to posthospital adjustment.

However, suppose that the two units are not really equivalent: The unit assigned the 1 intervention has much sicker patients than the other unit. Degree of illness would be expected to be related to posthospital adjustment. We rate all the subjects on their degree of illness (on a scale ranging from 0 to 10, with 10 being the sickest) and present the additional data in Table 9-2. Now we see that the patients exposed to treatment 1 had a much higher mean illness score (8) than the patients exposed to treatment 2 (3.5). To adjust for this difference between the groups, we use ANCOVA with one independent variable, treatment group; one covariate, illness score; and one dependent variable, posthospital adjustment score. Figure 9-3 contains the computer analysis of these data. While the ANOVA procedure in SPSS can be used to produce an analysis of covariance, it does not allow us to test the assumption that the regression lines are equivalent. The MANOVA program does enable us to test this important assumption.

(*text continues on page 154*)

TABLE 9-1
Comparison of the Effect of Two Nursing Interventions on Posthospital Adjustment

	TREATMENT GROUPS	
	1	**2**
	Adjustment Scores	*Adjustment Scores*
	3	10
	5	7
	14	7
	8	3
	7	3
	10	12
	6	14
	15	9
	13	4
	4	11
	—	—
	85	80
$\overline{X}s$	8.5	8.0

TABLE 9-2
Comparison of Illness Scores for Two Units

	TREATMENT GROUPS		
	1		**2**	
Illness Scale	*Adjustment Score*	*Illness Scale*	*Adjustment Score*
10	3	3	10
9	5	4	7
6	14	4	7
8	8	6	3
8	7	5	3
7	10	2	12
9	6	1	14
6	15	3	9
7	13	5	4
10	4	2	11
—	—	—	—
80	85	35	80
$\overline{X}s$ 8.0	8.5	3.5	8.0

SPSS/PC+

(1) MANOVA ADJUST BY GROUP (1,2) WITH ILLNESS
(2)   /PMEANS
  /DESIGN
(3)   /ANALYSIS=ADJUST
  /DESIGN=ILLNESS GROUP GROUP BY ILLNESS
(4)   /DESIGN=ILLNESS WITHIN GROUP GROUP.
        20 cases accepted.
         0 cases rejected because of out-of-range factor values.
         0 cases rejected because of missing data.
         2 non-empty cells.

        3 designs will be processed.
- - - - - - - - -
         CELL NUMBER
         1   2
Variable
  GROUP   1   2

(5) * * ANALYSIS OF VARIANCE -- DESIGN 1 * *

Tests of Significance for ADJUST using UNIQUE sums of squares

Source of Variation	SS	DF	MS	F	Sig of F
WITHIN CELLS	15.79	17	.93		
REGRESSION	284.71	1	284.71	306.44	.000
CONSTANT	646.31	1	646.31	695.65	.000
GROUP	218.12	1	218.12	234.77	.000

- - - - - - - - - -
Regression analysis for WITHIN CELLS error term
Dependent variable .. ADJUST   ADJUSTMENT SCORE

COVARIATE	B	Beta	Std. Err.	t-Value	Sig. of t
ILLNESS	-2.58824	-.97337	.148	-17.506	.000

COVARIATE	Lower -95% CL- Upper	
ILLNESS	-2.900	-2.276

* * ANALYSIS OF VARIANCE -- DESIGN 1 * *

Adjusted and Observed Means
Variable .. ADJUST   ADJUSTMENT SCORE

CELL	Obs. Mean	Adj. Mean
1	8.500	14.324
2	8.000	2.176

FIGURE 9-3

Analysis of covariance produced by SPSS/PC+.

(6) * * ANALYSIS OF VARIANCE -- DESIGN   2 * *
  Order of Variables for Analysis

    Variates   Covariates

    ADJUST

    1 Dependent Variable
    0 Covariates

* * ANALYSIS OF VARIANCE -- DESIGN   2 * *

Tests of Significance for ADJUST using UNIQUE sums of squares
Source of Variation   SS   DF   MS   F Sig of F

WITHIN+RESIDUAL   14.10   16   .88
CONSTANT   567.20   1   567.20   643.63   .000
ILLNESS   286.31   1   286.31   324.89   .000
GROUP   53.30   1   53.30   60.49   .000
GROUP BY ILLNESS   1.69   1   1.69   1.92   .185

Adjusted and Observed Means
Variable .. ADJUST   ADJUSTMENT SCORE
   CELL   Obs. Mean   Adj. Mean

      1   8.500   8.500
      2   8.000   8.000

(7) * * ANALYSIS OF VARIANCE -- DESIGN   3 * *
  Order of Variables for Analysis

    Variates   Covariates

    ADJUST

    1 Dependent Variable
    0 Covariates

* * ANALYSIS OF VARIANCE -- DESIGN   3 * *

Tests of Significance for ADJUST using UNIQUE sums of squares
Source of Variation   SS   DF   MS   F Sig of F

WITHIN+RESIDUAL   14.10   16   .88
CONSTANT   567.20   1   567.20   643.63   .000
ILLNESS WITHIN GROUP   286.40   2   143.20   162.50   .000
GROUP   53.30   1   53.30   60.49   .000
- - - - - - - - - -
Adjusted and Observed Means
Variable .. ADJUST   ADJUSTMENT SCORE
   CELL   Obs. Mean   Adj. Mean

      1   8.500   8.500
      2   8.000   8.000

FIGURE 9-3 (CONTINUED)

① The MANOVA command indicates that ADJUST (adjustment score) is the dependent variable; GROUP, with two levels (1 and 2) is the independent variable; and ILLNESS is the covariate. The adjusted means (PMEANS) are requested. There are three design commands, and ADJUST is the dependent variable in all of them (ANALYSIS = ADJUST).

② The first design statement is the default and produces the analysis described in the MANOVA command (i.e., an analysis of covariance with GROUP as the independent variable and ILLNESS as the covariate).

③ The second design statement tests the assumption of homogeneity of regression. If the interaction term is significant, the assumption has *not* been met, and the regular analysis of covariance would be inappropriate.

④ The third design statement is the appropriate analysis if the assumption has not been met.

To summarize these three design statements, if the interaction (requested in the second design statement) is *not significant*, the results of the first design statement should be reported. If the interaction is *significant*, the results from the third design statement should be reported.

⑤ This contains the analysis of covariance.

⑥ This shows the test of the homogeneity of regression.

⑦ The within-group analysis is shown here, that is, the regression line is fit for each group.

Let's look first at ⑥, because this contains the test that will determine the appropriate analysis (⑤ or ⑦). To adjust for a covariate, the difference between the score of an individual on the covariate and the grand mean of the covariate is weighted by a *common* regression coefficient (b). Use of such a common regression coefficient is based on the assumption that there is no interaction between the covariate and the independent variable. If such an interaction exists, ANCOVA should *not* be used. Alternate approaches were discussed under the assumptions for ANCOVA.

The main interest in this analysis is whether there is an interaction between the independent variable (GROUP) and the covariate (ILLNESS). We see that there is a significant relationship between the covariate and the dependent variable ($F = 324.89$, $p = 0.000$) and between the independent variable and the dependent variable ($F = 60.49$, $p = 0.000$). There is *no significant interaction* between the independent variable and the covariate ($F = 1.92$, $p = 0.185$). Thus, the assumption is met, and design 1 is appropriate.

In ⑤ we see a significant regression effect ($F = 695.65$, $p = 0.000$). That is the effect of the covariate, illness, so level of illness is significantly related to adjustment. Additionally, there is a significant group effect ($F = 234.77$, $p = 0.000$). To interpret the group effect, we look at the group means. Adjusted and observed means are listed immediately after the section that contains the b and beta weights (used in the calculation of the adjusted means).

Although the original means were almost equal, adjusting for the differences measured by the illness scale changes the means dramatically. We see that the adjusted mean for group 1 (14.324) is significantly higher than the adjusted mean for group 2 (2.176). The use of ANCOVA allowed us to compare our two nursing interventions as though they were applied to groups who were equivalent in terms of level of illness.

SUMMARY

ANCOVA is an extension of ANOVA that allows us to remove additional sources of variation from the error term, thus enhancing the power of our analysis. This technique is not a cure-all for difficulties with unequal groups and should be used only after careful consideration has been given to meeting the underlying assumptions. It is especially important to check for homogeneity of regression, because if that assumption is violated, ANCOVA can lead to improper interpretation of results.

10 Repeated Measures Analysis of Variance

Barbara Hazard Munro

OBJECTIVES FOR CHAPTER 10

After reading this chapter you should be able to do the following:

1. **Describe the two major ways in which repeated measures ANOVA is used.**
2. **Explain the assumption of compound symmetry.**
3. **Interpret a repeated measures ANOVA computer printout.**
4. **Discuss difficulties that may arise with the use of this technique.**

Repeated measures analysis of variance (ANOVA) is an approach that helps us deal with individual differences. These differences usually are part of the error term. Because they increase the error term, they decrease the likelihood of finding a significant result. While individual differences reflect actual differences among individuals, they also reflect the individual's particular state when the instrument was administered (e.g., tired, bored, angry), environmental factors (e.g., noise, heat, cold), and response styles (e.g., unwillingness to check extreme value). With repeated measures ANOVA we may be able to measure, and thus control, some of this variation.

There are two main types of repeated measures designs (also called within-subjects designs). One type involves taking repeated measures of the same variable(s) over time on a group or groups of subjects. For example if we were studying hypertension, we would probably want more than one blood pressure reading on our subjects.

The other main type of repeated measures design involves exposing the same subjects to all levels of the treatment. Suppose we wanted to see

Barbara Hazard Munro and Ellis Batten Page: STATISTICAL METHODS FOR HEALTH CARE RESEARCH, SECOND EDITION. © 1993, 1986 by J. B. Lippincott Company.

whether therapeutic touch or meditation reduced pain any more than the standard treatment. We could randomly assign individuals experiencing pain to one of the following three conditions: touch, meditation, or control.

However, if our subjects varied widely in the amount of pain they reported, the within-subject variability would be very large. Because the F statistic is based on the ratio of between-group variance to within-group variance, there would have to be a very large between-group difference to attain a significant result; that is, the large variability among the subjects could obscure any real differences between the groups. This would be especially true if the groups were small. One way to remove these individual differences would be to assign each subject to all treatments. Each subject would be exposed to touch, meditation, and regular treatment. Thus, each subject would serve as his or her own control, and the within or error variance would be decreased. This would result in a more powerful test and would decrease the number of subjects needed for the study.

TYPE OF DATA REQUIRED

The requirements are the same as those for the usual ANOVA. The independent variable(s) are categorical, and the dependent variable is measured at the interval or ratio level.

ASSUMPTIONS

The basic assumptions for the t test and ANOVA also are necessary here. The dependent variable should be normally distributed, and the homogeneity of variance requirement should be met.

There is one major difference, however. With ANOVA the observations are independent of each other. This is achieved by randomly assigning subjects to mutually exclusive groups. With repeated measures, however, there is correlation between the measures because they are from the same people. It is necessary, therefore, to meet another assumption. This is called the assumption of *compound symmetry*.

There are two parts to this assumption. The first part is the assumption that the correlations across the measurements are the same. Suppose you measured a variable three times. You could then calculate the correlation between the first measure and the second, between the first and the third, and between the second and the third. All three of these correlations should be about the same, or $r_{12} = r_{13} = r_{23}$.

The second part of the assumption is that the variances should be equal across measurements. With three measurements the variance of 1 = variance of 2 = variance of 3. The assumption of compound symmetry is critical. The general robustness of the ANOVA model does not withstand much violation of this assumption.

REPEATED MEASURES OVER TIME

The simplest example of such an analysis is presented in Chapter 6, in which is discussed the use of the correlated *t* test to compare the means of a pretest and a post-test administered to the same people. Because the same people took both tests, their scores should be correlated. The correlated *t* test removes this relationship and thus increases the power of the comparison of the two means. We can extend this concept to situations in which there are more than one group and to situations in which subjects are measured several times on the same variable.

Suppose that instead of one group measured pretreatment and post-treatment, we had a true experimental design with subjects assigned randomly to an experimental group and to a control group. If we measured these subjects pre-experiment and postexperiment, we could no longer use the correlated *t* test. We would now have two groups that were measured twice. This is called a *mixed design* because we have between- and within-subjects measures. First, we have two different groups: the experimental and the control group. These two groups constitute the between-group measure. Comparing these groups answers the question of whether the experimental condition had an effect on the outcome. The second part of the design, or the within-group component, concerns the fact that each group is measured twice on the same variable. The question answered here is whether there is a difference between the pretest and post-test measures. Because there are two independent variables, we also would have an interaction effect (i.e., is there an interaction between study group and time?).

Another example is presented in Figure 10-1. We want to study the effectiveness of various treatment modalities on hypertension, and we want to examine the effects over time. We randomly assign individuals with hypertension to one of three groups: drug

| | **Treatment group** | | | |
	Drug therapy (DT) $n = 10$	Relaxation therapy (RT) $n = 10$	Control (C) $n = 10$	Row $\bar{X}_s$
1 week	$\bar{X}_{DT}$, 1 week	$\bar{X}_{RT}$, 1 week	$\bar{X}_C$, 1 week	$\bar{X}$ 1 week
1 month	$\bar{X}_{DT}$, 1 month	$\bar{X}_{RT}$, 1 month	$\bar{X}_C$, 1 month	$\bar{X}$ 1 month
3 months	$\bar{X}_{DT}$, 3 months	$\bar{X}_{RT}$, 3 months	$\bar{X}_C$, 3 months	$\bar{X}$ 3 months
6 months	$\bar{X}_{DT}$, 6 months	$\bar{X}_{RT}$, 6 months	$\bar{X}_C$, 6 months	$\bar{X}$ 6 months
Column $\bar{X}_s$	$\bar{X}_{DT}$	$\bar{X}_{RT}$	$\bar{X}_C$	

(Time, labeled vertically on the left side of the rows)

FIGURE 10-1
A mixed design.

therapy, relaxation therapy, or control. Each subject is in only one group. All subjects' blood pressure is measured at the following intervals: 1 week, 1 month, 3 months, and 6 months.

If we were to use regular one-way ANOVA to analyze these data, we would have to calculate four ANOVAs, one for each time the blood pressure was measured. The individual differences would be part of the error term.

If we use repeated measures ANOVA, we have two independent variables (rather than one independent variable measured against four different measures of the same variable). One independent variable is treatment group, with three levels. The other independent variable is time, with four levels. With the repeated measures approach, we can answer three main questions:

1. Do the three groups have significantly different blood pressures after treatment? All blood pressure recordings would be included here; that is, the time component is ignored, and the question is answered by comparing the three column means, $\overline{X}DT$, $\overline{X}RT$, and $\overline{X}C$ (see Fig. 10-1). If the overall F is significant, post-hoc tests would be used to find differences between pairs of scores.
2. Are there significant differences in blood pressure across the four time periods? Treatment group is ignored here, and the mean blood pressure is calculated for each of the time periods. In our example the row means would be compared.
3. Is there an interaction between treatment type and time? Twelve means would be compared to answer this question (three levels of first independent variable times four levels of second). In Figure 10-1 those means are shown in the cells. This would tell us whether different approaches worked better at one point than another.

In a study of the treatment of pressure ulcers (Munro, Brown, & Heitman, 1989), 40 male patients with stage II or III ulcers were randomly assigned to the Clinitron bed or to a standard hospital bed (control condition). Patients in the control condition were treated with usual nursing measures, such as sheepskin or gel pads placed beneath ulcer areas, positioning, and massage. Ulcer size was measured on the 3rd, 8th, and 15th days after treatment began. See Table 10-1 for the results. There was a significant group by time interaction. Using Table 10-1 try to determine why the interaction was significant. (The size of the ulcers in the control group became *larger* with time, whereas the ulcers in the experimental group were *smaller*.)

TABLE 10-1
Ulcer Size (mm²): Group Means Over Time

Day	Control	Experimental
3rd	1704	1970
8th	1708	1659
15th	2051	1158

EXAMPLE OF COMPUTER ANALYSIS

Table 10-2 contains the data for the analysis. It is based on the example given in Figure 10-1. Diastolic blood pressure is the dependent variable. For the drug therapy group, we see that the group means decreased from 105.8 at the end of the first week to 90.2 at the sixth month. The means for the relaxation therapy group also decreased with time, but six months later the control group means increased from 105.4 at week 1 to 111.8. The computer printout is shown in Figure 10-2.

① MANOVA is used for the analysis. WEEK1, MONTH1, MONTH3, and MONTH6 are the repeated measures (i.e, the four levels of the within-subjects factor). They are the diastolic blood pressures recorded four times on the same subjects. GROUP is the between-subjects factor, with three levels. In this example the three groups were coded 1 for drug therapy, 2 for relaxation therapy, and 3 for control. The WSFACTORS indicates that there are four repeated measures, which the researcher has named TIME. The PRINT command requests the means and standard deviations for the groups at each time period, the averaged and multivariate tests of significance, and tests of the underlying assumptions (HOMOGENEITY, BARTLETT, BOXM).

② Compare the cell means with those listed in Table 10-2.

③ The Bartlett-Box univariate homogeneity of variance tests are listed for each of the repeated measures. This tests whether the three groups have equal variances at each of the time periods. Since the p values range from 0.716 to 0.975, we know that the groups do not differ significantly in terms of variance. Next, Box's M is given as the test to determine if the variance–covariance matrices are equal across all levels of the between-subjects factor. Again, the p value of greater than 0.05 indicates that the assumption has been met.

④ First, the between-subjects effect is given. For GROUP, $F = 5.00$, and $p = 0.014$. There is an overall difference among our three groups. Post-hoc tests will be necessary to determine where the differences lie.

⑤ Next, tests of the assumptions underlying the repeated measures are presented. The most important is meeting the criterion for compound symmetry. This assumption is often violated, leading to improper interpretation of results. According to Finn and Mattsson (1978), "In practice, behavioral data rarely meet the assumption of compound symmetry" (p. 83). They also state, "It is a critical assumption in the univariate analysis of repeated measures data, and it is one that is not required by the corresponding *multivariate* analysis" (p. 82).

By "multivariate" Finn and Mattsson (1978) are referring to the use of more than one dependent variable in an analysis. In our example time is the second independent variable. Thus, we have two independent variables, and the dependent variable is diastolic blood pressure. With a multivariate approach, the analysis would be treated as including only one independent variable: treatment group. It would also include four dependent variables. These would be the four measures of diastolic pressure. This sounds like the separate ANOVAs that could be used. However, the analysis does not take each ANOVA separately, but rather examines the relationships among the levels of the dependent variable, as well as the relationship between the independent variable and

(*text continues on page 164*)

TABLE 10-2
Data for Mixed Design Repeated Measures of Analysis

Group		Week 1	Month 1	Month 3	Month 6
Drug Therapy		90	88	84	80
		94	90	90	86
		100	96	90	86
		106	100	96	90
		110	106	100	100
		114	110	106	96
		120	110	106	100
		112	106	96	90
		108	104	90	86
		104	100	94	88
	$\overline{X}_s$	105.8	101.0	95.2	90.2
Relaxation Therapy		92	90	86	84
		94	92	90	90
		100	96	90	86
		106	100	96	88
		110	106	100	94
		114	112	108	98
		118	114	110	100
		114	114	112	110
		106	100	90	84
		108	100	92	86
	$\overline{X}_s$	106.2	102.4	97.4	92.0
Control		92	94	98	100
		94	96	96	100
		98	100	102	104
		104	104	106	108
		108	110	112	114
		118	120	118	120
		120	120	118	118
		110	112	116	120
		104	110	116	118
		106	112	114	116
	$\overline{X}_s$	105.4	107.8	109.6	111.8

SPSS/PC+

(1) MANOVA WEEK1 MONTH1 MONTH3 MONTH6 BY GROUP (1,3)
    /WSFACTORS=TIME(4)
    /PRINT=CELLINFO(MEANS) SIGNIF(AVERF) HOMOGENEITY (BARTLETT BOXM).

        30 cases accepted.
         0 cases rejected because of out-of-range factor values.
         0 cases rejected because of missing data.
         3 non-empty cells.

         1 design will be processed.

    * * ANALYSIS   OF   VARIANCE -- DESIGN   1 * *

(2) Cell Means and Standard Deviations
     Variable .. WEEK1

FACTOR	CODE	Mean	Std. Dev.	N
GROUP	DRUG	105.800	9.163	10
GROUP	RELAXATION	106.200	8.613	10
GROUP	CONTROL	105.400	9.240	10
For entire sample		105.800	8.700	30

- - - - - - - - -
     Variable .. MONTH1

FACTOR	CODE	Mean	Std. Dev.	N
GROUP	DRUG	101.000	7.732	10
GROUP	RELAXATION	102.400	8.784	10
GROUP	CONTROL	107.800	9.114	10
For entire sample		103.733	8.785	30

    * * ANALYSIS   OF   VARIANCE -- DESIGN   1 * *

    Cell Means and Standard Deviations   (CONT.)
    Variable .. MONTH3

FACTOR	CODE	Mean	Std. Dev.	N
GROUP	DRUG	95.200	7.193	10
GROUP	RELAXATION	97.400	9.524	10
GROUP	CONTROL	109.600	8.422	10
For entire sample		100.733	10.379	30

- - - - - - - - - - -
    Variable .. MONTH6

FACTOR	CODE	Mean	Std. Dev.	N
GROUP	DRUG	90.200	6.563	10
GROUP	RELAXATION	92.000	8.485	10
GROUP	CONTROL	111.800	8.080	10
For entire sample		98.000	12.451	30

FIGURE 10-2

Repeated measures over time produced by SPSS/PC+. (*continued*)

```
* * ANALYSIS  OF  VARIANCE -- DESIGN  1 * *

Cell Means and Standard Deviations  (CONT.)
Univariate Homogeneity of Variance Tests
```

③ `Variable .. WEEK1`

```
        Bartlett-Box F(2,1640) =              .02490, P =  .975
```

```
Variable .. MONTH1
```

```
        Bartlett-Box F(2,1640) =              .12400, P =  .883
```

```
Variable .. MONTH3
```

```
        Bartlett-Box F(2,1640) =              .33352, P =  .716
```

```
* * ANALYSIS  OF  VARIANCE -- DESIGN  1 * *

Univariate Homogeneity of Variance Tests (CONT.)

Variable .. MONTH6
```

```
        Bartlett-Box F(2,1640) =              .30301, P =  .739
```

```
* * ANALYSIS  OF  VARIANCE -- DESIGN  1 * *

Multivariate test for Homogeneity of Dispersion matrices


Boxs M =                          31.92928
F WITH (20,2616) DF =              1.24526, P =   .206 (Approx.)
Chi-Square with 20 DF =          25.14924, P =   .196 (Approx.)


- - - - - - - - - -

* * ANALYSIS  OF  VARIANCE -- DESIGN  1 * *
```

④ `Tests of Between-Subjects Effects.`

```
Tests of Significance for T1 using UNIQUE sums of squares
Source of Variation         SS        DF        MS        F    Sig of F

WITHIN CELLS           7129.00       27    264.04
CONSTANT            1250112.53        1  1250112.5   4734.61      .000
GROUP                  2642.47        2   1321.23      5.00      .014
```

FIGURE 10-2 (CONTINUED)

each dependent variable. This multivariate approach is more robust and can therefore handle the failure to meet the compound symmetry requirement. According to Finn and Mattsson (1978), "The multivariate approach to the analysis of repeated measures is not only less restrictive, but usually more realistic. Especially in longitudinal data, we expect the correlations will not be uniform. If, however, the assumptions of the univariate model are met, the univariate analysis should be used, because it is more powerful and requires fewer subjects" (p. 80).

```
* * ANALYSIS  OF  VARIANCE -- DESIGN   1 * *
```

(5) Tests involving 'TIME' Within-Subject Effect.


```
Mauchly sphericity test, W =        .15158
Chi-square approx. =             48.52906 with 5 D. F.
Significance =                      .000

Greenhouse-Geisser Epsilon =        .47476
Huynh-Feldt Epsilon =               .53082
Lower-bound Epsilon =               .33333
```

AVERAGED Tests of Significance that follow multivariate tests are equivalent to univariate or split-plot or mixed-model approach to repeated measures. Epsilons may be used to adjust d.f. for the AVERAGED results.

```
* * ANALYSIS  OF  VARIANCE -- DESIGN   1 * *
```

(6) EFFECT .. GROUP BY TIME
Multivariate Tests of Significance (S = 2, M = 0, N = 11 1/2)

Test Name	Value	Approx. F	Hypoth. DF	Error DF	Sig. of F
Pillais	.84021	6.27860	6.00	52.00	.000
Hotellings	3.89930	15.59719	6.00	48.00	.000
Wilks	.19660	10.46112	6.00	50.00	.000
Roys	.79384				

```
* * ANALYSIS  OF  VARIANCE -- DESIGN   1 * *
```

(7) EFFECT .. TIME
Multivariate Tests of Significance (S = 1, M = 1/2, N = 11 1/2)

Test Name	Value	Approx. F	Hypoth. DF	Error DF	Sig. of F
Pillais	.69713	19.18158	3.00	25.00	.000
Hotellings	2.30179	19.18158	3.00	25.00	.000
Wilks	.30287	19.18158	3.00	25.00	.000
Roys	.69713				

```
- - - - - - - - - -
* * ANALYSIS  OF  VARIANCE -- DESIGN   1 * *
```

(8) Tests involving 'TIME' Within-Subject Effect.

AVERAGED Tests of Significance for MEAS.1 using UNIQUE sums of squares

Source of Variation	SS	DF	MS	F	Sig of F
WITHIN CELLS	586.20	81	7.24		
TIME	1050.93	3	350.31	48.41	.000
GROUP BY TIME	1694.87	6	282.48	39.03	.000

FIGURE 10-2 (CONTINUED)

Mauchly's test of sphericity is used to test the assumptions underlying the univariate approach. As can be seen, this test is significant ($p = 0.000$), indicating that the assumption has not been met. The univariate approach is not appropriate in this case.

⑥ and ⑦ The multivariate tests are given first. Because the assumptions were not met for the univariate model, the multivariate results would be appropriate to report. The GROUP BY TIME interaction with 6 *df* is significant at the 0.000 level. (See the section on MANOVA in Chapter 8 for a description of the four multivariate tests.) The TIME effect with 3 *df* (four time periods minus one) also is significant ($p = 0.000$). Post-hoc tests are necessary to determine where the differences lie.

⑧ Although Finn and Mattsson (1978) strongly advocate the use of the multivariate approach when the assumption of compound symmetry is not met, other approaches may be taken. Rather than use the multivariate approach, adjustments can be made to the *df* in the univariate approach to decrease the likelihood of a Type I error. This is done through the use of an "epsilon" correction. Epsilon is multiplied by the *df* in the numerator and the denominator, and the new *df* is used to test *F*. The Greenhouse-Geisser epsilon is conservative; Huynh-Feldt epsilon is an improved, more robust test; and SPSS also produces the lowest possible correction factor (lower-bound epsilon).

In our example the *df* for TIME is 3 (number of repeated measures minus 1) and 81 (*df* associated with the error or WITHIN CELLS term). Multiplying them by Huynh-Feldt epsilon (0.53082), we derive the following *df*s: 1.59, 42.97. The *df*s are smaller, thus requiring a larger *F* for significance. Even with the more conservative *df*s, however, TIME with an *F* of 48.41 is still significant at less than 0.01 (see Appendix D). Similarly, the *df*s for GROUP BY TIME are 6 and 81, and with the Huynh-Feldt epsilon correction they become 3.18 and 42.97. The *F* value of 39.03 is still significant at less than 0.01. Thus, in this example the multivariate and the corrected univariate results are equivalent. As is

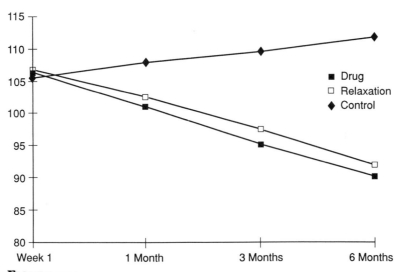

FIGURE 10-3
Graph of interaction.

TABLE 10-3
Table of Means for Effect of Treatment

Time	Drug	Relaxation	Control
1 Week	105.8	106.2	105.4
1 Month	101.0	102.4	107.8
3 Months	95.2	97.4	109.6
6 Months	90.2	92.0	111.8

pointed out in Chapter 8, a significant interaction is examined first because it affects the interpretation of the main effects. Figure 10-3 contains a graph of the interaction. Here we see that in the two treatment groups, drug and relaxation therapy, the means for diastolic pressure decreased with time, but in the control group the means increased. To examine the main effects, additional analyses are required. First, we can use separate one-way ANOVAs to compare the three groups at each of the four time periods. We summarize the results here rather than showing all the computer printouts. See Table 10-3 for a summary of the group means. The three groups did not differ significantly at the pretest ($p = 0.980$) or at the 1-month measure ($p = 0.192$); however, they did differ at the 3- ($p = 0.001$) and 6-month ($p = 0.000$) measures. Scheffé tests indicated that at each of these time periods, the control group scored significantly higher than the treatment groups. The treatment groups did not differ significantly from each other.

The second main effect, time, can be examined by using paired t tests to compare the four time periods. Table 10-4 contains the means for all subjects at each time period. The pretest was significantly higher than any of the other three time periods. Month 1 was significantly higher than months 3 and 6, and month 3 was significantly higher than month 6.

SUBJECTS EXPOSED TO ALL TREATMENT LEVELS

An example is given in Figure 10-4. Ten subjects are exposed to four different methods of pain control. The dependent variable is a rating by the patient of his or her perceived level of pain. This rating is taken four times, once after each treatment. Note that each

TABLE 10-4
Table of Means for Effect of Time

Time	Means
1 Week	105.8
1 Month	103.7
3 Months	100.7
6 Months	98.0

Treatments

Subjects	Drug therapy	Laughter therapy	Therapeutic touch	Distraction
1	6	5	8	9
2	7	8	10	9
3	4	4	6	7
4	1	2	4	5
5	3	2	3	3
6	5	6	8	7
7	2	3	7	6
8	4	3	8	7
9	0	1	4	6
10	5	4	7	5
Col $\overline{X}_S$	3.7	3.8	6.5	6.4

FIGURE 10-4
Within-subjects design.

cell contains only one score. Subject 1's rating of perceived pain after exposure to drug therapy (6) is the only score in the upper left cell. Because there is only one score in each cell, there is no variability within the cells of this design.

The total variation consists of *between-subjects variation* and *within-subjects variation*. Between-subjects variation consists of the differences among the 10 subjects in this design. Testing the significance of that amount of variation would tell us whether the row means differed significantly from each other. We are not interested in this because it tells us only whether the subjects differed from each other. We want to know whether there were differences among the treatments. By calculating the between-people variation, however, we are able to remove that source of variation from the error term. If the variability among subjects is large, the error term would be substantially reduced.

The second main source of variation is the within-subject variation. This measures how much each subject's scores varied across the treatment levels. We are interested in this. Do the subjects have lower ratings of pain with some treatments than with others? There are two components to this within-people variation. One is due to the effect of treatment, and the other is due to uncontrolled factors that influence how a subject rates his or her pain at any time.

Example of Computer Analysis of Within-Subjects Design

Figure 10-5 contains the computer output produced by analysis of the data in Figure 10-4.

① MANOVA is used, and there are four measures, one for each treatment: DRUG, LAUGHTER, TT (therapeutic touch), and DISTRACT (distraction) (i.e., there is one within-subjects factor with four levels). The investigator has labeled the within-subjects factor RX (treatment). The PRINT command requests cell means and standard deviations, averaged and multivariate significance tests, and tests of the assumptions.

② This contains the means, standard deviations, and number in each cell.

③ Because the Mauchly sphericity test is not significant ($p = 0.466$), the assump-

```
                            SPSS/PC+

① MANOVA DRUG LAUGHTER TT DISTRACT
     /WSFACTORS=RX(4)
     /PRINT=CELLINFO (MEANS) SIGNIF (AVERF) HOMOGENEITY (BARTLETT BOXM).

       10 cases accepted.
        0 cases rejected because of out-of-range factor values.
        0 cases rejected because of missing data.
        1 non-empty cells.

        1 design will be processed.


  * * ANALYSIS  OF  VARIANCE -- DESIGN  1 * *

② Cell Means and Standard Deviations
     Variable .. DRUG
                                   Mean   Std. Dev.         N

     For entire sample            3.700     2.214          10

     - - - - - - - - -
     Variable .. LAUGHTER
                                   Mean   Std. Dev.         N

     For entire sample            3.800     2.098          10

     - - - - - - - - - -
     Variable .. TT
                                   Mean   Std. Dev.         N

     For entire sample            6.500     2.224          10


  * * ANALYSIS  OF  VARIANCE -- DESIGN  1 * *

     Cell Means and Standard Deviations   (CONT.)
     Variable .. DISTRACT
                                   Mean   Std. Dev.         N

     For entire sample            6.400     1.838          10
```

FIGURE 10-5

Within-subjects analysis produced by SPSS/PC+. (*continued*)

```
* * ANALYSIS  OF  VARIANCE -- DESIGN   1 * *

Tests involving 'RX' Within-Subject Effect.
```

(3)
```
Mauchly sphericity test, W =          .55103
Chi-square approx. =              4.60218 with 5 D. F.
Significance =                        .466

Greenhouse-Geisser Epsilon =          .70904
Huynh-Feldt Epsilon =                 .93465
Lower-bound Epsilon =                 .33333
```

```
AVERAGED Tests of Significance that follow multivariate tests are equivalent to
univariate or split-plot or mixed-model approach to repeated measures.
Epsilons may be used to adjust d.f. for the AVERAGED results.

* * ANALYSIS  OF  VARIANCE -- DESIGN   1 * *
```

(4)
```
EFFECT .. RX
Multivariate Tests of Significance (S = 1, M = 1/2, N = 2 1/2)

Test Name        Value    Approx. F Hypoth. DF   Error DF  Sig. of F

Pillais         .86680   15.18456      3.00       7.00       .002
Hotellings     6.50767   15.18456      3.00       7.00       .002
Wilks           .13320   15.18456      3.00       7.00       .002
Roys            .86680

- - - - - - - - - -
* * ANALYSIS  OF  VARIANCE -- DESIGN   1 * *
```

(5)
```
Tests involving 'RX' Within-Subject Effect.

AVERAGED Tests of Significance for MEAS.1 using UNIQUE sums of squares
Source of Variation          SS       DF       MS        F   Sig of F

WITHIN CELLS              26.00       27      .96
RX                       73.00        3    24.33     25.27     .000

- - - - - - - - - -
```

FIGURE 10-5 (CONTINUED)

tion of compound symmetry has been met, and the averaged ((5)), rather than the multivariate ((4)), test is appropriate (and more powerful).

(4) These are multivariate tests of significance.

(5) The averaged tests indicate that there is a significant overall difference among the four treatment groups (p = 0.000). Follow-up tests are necessary to determine where the differences lie.

Paired t tests can compare each pair of means. Table 10-5 contains the means. As would be expected from looking at the means, paired t tests demonstrate that the drug and laughter therapy group means were significantly lower than the means for therapeutic touch and distraction. Thus, we would report that drug therapy and laughter therapy are related to significantly lower reports of pain than therapeutic touch and distraction.

TABLE 10-5
Table of Means for Within-Subjects Design

Group	Mean
Drug therapy	3.7
Laughter therapy	3.8
Therapeutic touch	6.5
Distraction	6.4

An example of a within-subjects design in which subjects are used as their own control is a study of the measurement of specific gravity in infants' urine (Lybrand, Medoff-Cooper, & Munro, 1990). The urine was collected by two different methods from each baby and measured at three different times. The results are displayed in Table 10-6. The two methods of collection were from a collecting bag and aspiration from the diaper. The specific gravity was measured after the infant voided, 1 hour after voiding, and 2 hours after voiding. Thus, we have a design with two within-subjects measures. One is the method of collection with two levels, bag and diaper, and the other is time, with three measurements. There were no significant differences for either of the two effects. Thus, whether the urine is measured from the collecting bag or from the diaper, the resulting specific gravity measure is the same, and the measure does not change if it is measured 1 or 2 hours after the infant has voided.

PROBLEMS WITH USE OF REPEATED MEASURES

Norusis (1990b) summarizes the problems as "the carry-over effect, the latent effect, and the order or learning effect." When subjects are exposed to more than one treatment, we need to consider that previous treatments may still be having an effect. In

TABLE 10-6
*Mean Specific Gravity Measurements Using
Two Methods of Urine Collection*

	Specific Gravity	
	Bag	Diaper
First measurement	1.0058	1.0059
One hour after voiding	1.0058	1.0061
Two hours after voiding	1.0060	1.0060

(From Lybrand, M., Medoff-Cooper, B., & Munro, B. H. [1990]. Periodic comparisons of specific gravity using urine from a diaper and collecting bag. MCN American Journal of Maternal Child Nursing, 1[4], 238.)

drug trials, for example, time is allowed for one drug to "wash out" before a second drug is tested. Adequate time should be allowed to prevent carry-over effects. Pilot testing can be used to determine whether carry-over is a problem.

The latency effect is more subtle and involves an interaction with a previous treatment. Would exposure to one treatment have an enhancing or depressing effect on a subsequent treatment?

Repeated exposure to measures may result in an increase in the outcome measure that is related to the subject learning about the measure, rather than a real change. Because subjects are measured repeatedly, such things as sensitization to the instruments may cause difficulties. Scores on an anxiety scale may vary due to repeated exposure to the scale, rather than to real changes in anxiety. Even physiological measures may reflect this. For example vital signs may increase with a new situation, then decrease with repeated measures. Practice with previous tests may increase scores on later tests. Subjects may be bored by repeated measures and be careless with later tests.

If such sequence effects are relatively small, repeated measures designs can be used. Randomizing the order in which the subjects are exposed to the treatments tends to spread the sequence effects over all the treatment levels and prevents them from being a confounding influence on only certain levels (Winer, 1971).

SUMMARY

Repeated measures ANOVA is a particularly interesting technique because we tend to take repeated measures on our patients, and it often makes sense to do so with our research subjects as well. There are stringent requirements for this analysis, however. If the requirements cannot be met and we have enough subjects, it is possible to use a multivariate approach or the epsilon correction.

11

Correlation

Barbara Hazard Munro

OBJECTIVES FOR CHAPTER 11

After reading this chapter you should be able to do the following:

1. **Explain when to use correlational techniques to answer research questions or test hypotheses.**

2. **Be able to read a computer printout reporting correlations.**

3. **Report a correlation coefficient in terms of its statistical significance and meaningfulness.**

4. **Understand measures of relationship other than the Pearson Product Moment Correlation Coefficient.**

5. **Know when it is appropriate to use multiple correlation, partial correlation, and semipartial correlation.**

Correlational techniques are used to study relationships. They may be used in exploratory studies in which one intent is to determine whether relationships exist and in hypothesis-testing studies in which we test a hypothesis about a particular relationship.

Lee (1991) conducted a descriptive study to explore the relationship of hardiness and current life events to perceived health in rural adults. One question she addressed was, "What relationship exists between the personality characteristic of hardiness and self-perception of health?" The correlation between hardiness and perceived health was -0.37, with a p value <0.001. What does that tell you about the relationship between these two variables? What does the negative sign indicate? What does a value of 0.37 mean? What does the p value indicate? One aim of this chapter is to help you answer such questions.

To interpret correlation coefficients, you must know how the variables are measured. A negative sign indicates that individuals who score high on one of these variables tend to score low on the other. Does this mean that

Barbara Hazard Munro and Ellis Batten Page: STATISTICAL METHODS FOR HEALTH CARE RESEARCH, SECOND EDITION. © 1993, 1986 by J. B. Lippincott Company.

those with high hardiness scores have lower perceived health? Not in this case, because the variable "hardiness" was scored in such a way that a high score indicated low hardiness. Thus, subjects in this study who rated themselves higher on hardiness also tended to rate themselves higher on health status. To judge the strength of the relationship, one must consider the actual number of the correlation coefficient (0.37) and the associated p value (<0.001). We discuss a measure of the "meaningfulness" of the coefficient and the effect of the number of subjects on the p value in subsequent sections of this chapter.

It was hypothesized that perceived stress was related to trait anger and four anger expression modes (anger-in, anger-out, anger-discuss, and anger symptoms) (Thomas & Williams, 1991). See Table 11-1 for the correlations reported for males in the study.

The hypothesis was supported because all of the anger variables correlated significantly with stress. Anger-discuss is a positive way of dealing with anger and had a negative correlation with stress. Although all the correlations are significant, two are less than 0.20, which means they each account for less than 4% of the shared variance between the two variables. With 720 subjects, even fairly small correlations have p values of less than 0.05.

The term *correlation* is used in everyday language. We hear people state that something is correlated with something else. In this chapter we are speaking about a relation that can be measured mathematically; we can calculate a number representing how strong a relation is. However, a correlation, which shows that two variables are related, does *not* mean that one variable *caused* the other. It is a mistake to infer causation from correlation alone. For example more people die in hospitals than anyplace else. Does that mean that hospitals cause deaths? There is a relation between the number of police cars at an accident and the amount of damage done to the vehicles and people involved. Do police cars cause the damage? Therefore, although a relationship may exist, other factors also may be affecting the variables under study.

TABLE 11-1
Correlations Between Stress and Anger

Anger Variable	Correlation	p value
Anger symptoms	0.44	<0.0001
Trait anger	0.35	<0.0001
Anger-out	0.32	<0.0001
Anger-discuss	−0.16	<0.05
Anger-in	0.14	<0.05

(Adapted from Thomas, S. P., & Williams, R. L. [1991]. Perceived stress, trait anger, modes of anger expression, and health status of college men and women. Nursing Research, 40[5], 303–307.)

TYPE OF DATA REQUIRED

The Pearson Product Moment Correlation Coefficient (r) is the most usual method by which the relation between two variables is quantified and is the focus of this chapter. A brief description of other formulas, most of which have been derived from the Pearson r, are given. To calculate r, there must be at least two measures on each subject. It is often assumed that both of these measures must be at the interval level. In most cases, however, valid results also may be obtained with ordinal data. Moreover, we can code categorical variables for use with r and with regression equations. Mathematically, it is possible to use any level of data when calculating r, but factors other than the level of the data must be considered when deciding whether a correlation coefficient is appropriate.

ASSUMPTIONS

Although we can calculate correlations with data at all levels, certain assumptions must be made if we are to generalize beyond the sample statistic, that is, if we are to make inferences about the population itself.

First, the sample must be representative of the population to which the inference will be made.

Second, the variables that are being correlated, say X and Y, must each have a normal distribution; that is, the distribution of their scores must approximate the normal curve.

Third, for every value of X the distribution of Y scores must have approximately equal variability. This is called the *assumption of homoscedasticity*.

Fourth, the relationship between X and Y must be linear; that is, when the two scores for each individual are graphed, they should tend to form a straight line. The points will not all fall on this line, but they should be scattered closely around it. The technique for graphing the relationship between two variables is demonstrated in the next section of this chapter. In Figure 11-1, **A** and **B** demonstrate linear relationships, and **D** shows a curvilinear relationship. A technique for measuring curvilinear relationships is presented later in this chapter.

CORRELATION COEFFICIENT

The correlation coefficient r allows us to state mathematically the relationship that exists between two variables. The correlation coefficient may range for $+1.00$ through 0.00 to -1.00. A $+1.00$ indicates a perfect positive relationship, 0.00 indicates no relationship, and -1.00 indicates a perfect negative relationship.

The correlation coefficient also tells us the *type* of relationship that exists, that is, whether the relationship is *positive* or *negative*. The relationship between job satisfaction and job turnover has been shown to be negative (we say that an *inverse* relationship

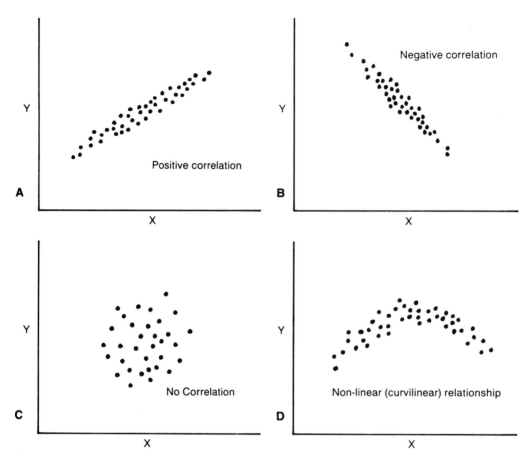

FIGURE 11-1
Linear and nonlinear relationships.

exists between them). These terms mean that as one variable increases, the other decreases. People with higher job satisfaction have lower rates of job turnover and vice versa. Similarly, those with higher college grades have lower dropout rates. There is a positive relationship between graduate requirement examination (GRE) scores and graduate grades; that is, those with higher GRE scores usually have higher grades.

If you were to look at scores on two variables, as in Table 11-2, you might observe that those who scored high on one measure tended to score high on the other, and those who did poorly on one measure did poorly on the other. (It is common to use X to designate the independent variable and Y for the dependent variable.) In this example, however, it is not necessary to think of one as independent and the other as dependent. The two sets of scores might represent a quiz and an examination given to students in some class, with no notion of one causing the other.

In addition to "eyeballing" these figures, you might graph the data to see what they

TABLE 11-2
Subjects' Scores on Two Measures

Subjects	X	Y
1	2	1
2	5	6
3	7	9
4	3	2
5	10	8
6	1	3
7	9	10
8	4	3
9	8	9
10	6	7

look like. Such a graph is called a *scatter diagram* (Fig. 11-2). To draw such a graph, you plot the pair of scores for each subject. For subject 1 the X score was 2, so you move to 2 on the horizontal scale where the X scores are plotted. The Y score was one, so you move straight up from the 2 on the horizontal axis to the spot opposite the 1 on the vertical axis where the Y scores are plotted. The dot that represents subject 1's scores is labeled in the graph. All other scores are plotted in the same way. In this example the scores

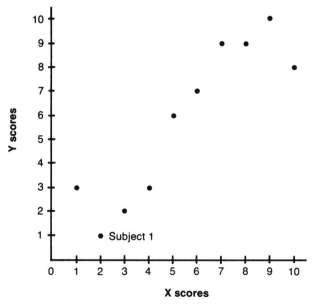

FIGURE 11-2
Graph of scores from Table 11-2.

extend diagonally from the lower left to the upper right corner of the graph. Such a configuration indicates a positive relationship between the two scores: low scores on X tend to go with low scores on Y, and vice versa. If there were a negative relationship, high scores on one variable with low scores on the other, the dots on the graph would go from the upper left to the lower right. When no relationship exists, the dots are scattered into a central cluster, like a target (see Fig. 11-1**C**). Although the graph indicates a positive relationship between the two variables, it does not tell us how strong the relationship is. To make such a determination, we need to calculate a correlation coefficient, r.

Computer Analysis

Adapting the variables used in the Thomas and Williams (1991) study, suppose we measured 20 students on their anger symptoms and their perceived stress. Scores on anger range from 0 to 15, with 0 indicating no anger and 15 the most anger. Scores on perceived stress range from 0 to 20, with 0 indicating no stress. The fictitious data are contained in Table 11-3. The computer output is shown in Figure 11-3.

TABLE 11-3
Data for Computer Analysis

Subjects	Scores on Variables	
	Anger	Perceived Stress
1	0	2
2	7	9
3	8	11
4	6	7
5	8	7
6	9	20
7	7	10
8	2	2
9	15	18
10	9	12
11	13	16
12	3	5
13	8	11
14	6	5
15	10	18
16	7	10
17	6	6
18	7	9
19	11	10
20	5	4

SPSS/PC+

① CORRELATIONS /VARIABLES ANGER WITH STRESS /OPTIONS 5.

Correlations: STRESS

② ANGER   .8396
                   (20)
                   P= .000

③ (Coefficient / (Cases) / 1-tailed Significance)

FIGURE 11-3
Correlation coefficient produced by SPSS/PC+.

① The command line requests a correlation between the variables ANGER and STRESS. OPTIONS 5 requests the actual *p* value, rather than *s indicating <0.05, <0.01, and so forth. By default, a one-tailed test of significance is provided. If you were exploring relationships rather than testing hypothesized relationships, you would request a two-tailed test through OPTIONS 3.

② The correlation between stress and anger is 0.8396. There were 20 subjects in the analysis, and the *p* value equals 0.000 (or is less than 0.001).

③ This gives you the order of the numbers provided; that is, the coefficient is given first, then the number of cases, and then the significance.

The results indicate a significant positive relationship between stress and anger. Before demonstrating the hand calculations associated with this analysis, we use *z*-scores, as explained in Chapter 3, to clarify what is being measured by this technique.

Relationships Measured With Correlation Coefficients

When using the formula with *z*-scores, *r* is the average of the cross-products of the *z*-scores ($r = [\Sigma zXzY]/n$). (Hopefully, this will be clear when we have taken you through this process.) Later in this chapter the "computational" formula for *r* is introduced. It is commonly used and easier to calculate than the *z*-score formula, but it is not as simple conceptually.

A perfect positive relationship, +1.00, is demonstrated in Table 11-4. The five subjects took a quiz, *X*, on which the scores ranged from 6 to 10 and an examination, *Y*, on which the scores ranged from 82 to 98. You can see that the subjects have the same *rank* on both measures. Subject 1 had the lowest score on both tests, and subject 2 had the next lowest scores on both, and so forth.

Because the means and standard deviations (*s*) of the two tests are different, we cannot directly compare the scores from the two tests. We can, however, transform the scores to *z*-scores with a mean of zero and a standard deviation of 1. In Chapter 3 the formula for converting a score to a *z*-score was given as

$$z = \frac{X - \overline{X}}{s}$$

TABLE 11-4
A Perfect Positive Relationship Between Two Variables

Subjects	X	Y	zX	zY	zXzY
1	6	82	−1.42	−1.42	2.0
2	7	86	−0.71	−0.71	0.5
3	8	90	0.00	0.00	0.0
4	9	94	0.71	0.71	0.5
5	10	98	1.42	1.42	2.0

$$\bar{X} = 8, s = 1.41 \qquad \bar{Y} = 90, s = 5.66 \qquad \Sigma zXzY = 5.00$$

$$r = \frac{\Sigma zXzY}{n} = \frac{5.00}{5} = 1$$

in which   X = individual's score

$\bar{X}$ = mean

s = standard deviation.

In Table 11-4, the z-scores for the X variable are listed under zX, and the z-scores for the Y variable are under zY. We can now compare the z-scores for X and Y and see that each subject received matching z-scores for the two tests. This is a perfect positive correlation.

The correlation is the mean of the cross-product of the z-scores for each subject. This is a measure of how much each pair of scores varies together. The cross-products are labeled as zXzY in the table. For subject 2 the cross-product is calculated as −0.071 × −0.071 and is 0.50. To take the average of the cross-products, add them and divide by the number of cross-products. Thus, the formula for r is ($\Sigma zXzY$)/n. The sum of the cross-products ($\Sigma zXzY$) is 5; dividing that by 5 (the number of cross-products) results in an r equal to 1. The scores are plotted in Figure 11-4. When the dots are joined they form a straight line, which indicates a perfect relationship.

To demonstrate a perfect negative correlation, reverse the scores on the Y variable (Table 11-5). Subject 1 still gets the lowest score on X but now also gets the highest score on Y. Carrying out the same procedure, the sum of the cross-products is −5; thus, r = −5/5, or −1, a perfect negative correlation. Figure 11-5 shows the graph of these scores.

In Table 11-6 the Y scores are scrambled in such a way that there is no relationship between the X and Y scores. These scores are plotted in Figure 11-6.

Strength of Correlation Coefficient

How large should r be for it to be useful? As is often the case, the answer is, "it depends." Alternate forms of a test should be measuring the same thing, so the correlation between them should be high. With tests (such as GREs), results of which are used in

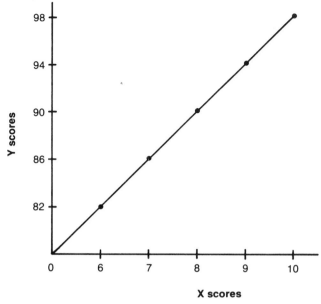

FIGURE 11-4
Graph of scores from Table 11-4.

important decision making, the correlations between two forms of the same test must be very high, approximately 0.95. However, when studying the relationships among various aspects of human behavior, we may be happy with a correlation of 0.50. Some "descriptors" that can be attached to rs of varying strengths are listed below. The *direction* of the relationship does not affect the *strength* of the relationship. A correlation of -0.90 is just as high, or just as "strong," as an r of $+0.90$. The following categories include $+$ and $-$ rs:

0.00–0.25	little if any
0.26–0.49	low
0.50–0.69	moderate
0.70–0.89	high
0.90–1.00	very high

Significance of the Correlation

If you want to generalize the r that you calculate from the sample to the correlation of these two variables in the population, you must determine the level of probability of r, that is, the probability that this r occurred by chance alone. You may use either a one- or two-tailed test for significance, depending on whether you hypothesized about the relationship. When you use statistical programs for the computer, the exact probability of r may be retrieved. When you calculate r by hand, you can consult a table such as that in Appendix E. The level of statistical significance is greatly affected by the size of the

TABLE 11-5
A Perfect Negative Correlation Between Two Variables

Subjects	X	Y	zX	zY	zXzY
1	6	98	−1.42	1.42	−2.0
2	7	94	−0.71	0.71	−0.5
3	8	90	0.00	0.00	0.0
4	9	86	0.71	−0.71	−0.5
5	10	82	1.42	−1.42	−2.0

$\overline{X} = 8, s = 1.41 \qquad \overline{Y} = 90, s = 5.66 \qquad \Sigma zXzY = -5.00$

$$r = \frac{\Sigma zXzY}{n} = \frac{-5.00}{5} = -1.00$$

sample, n. It makes sense that if r is based on a sample of 1000, there is a much greater likelihood that it represents the r of the population than if r was based on a sample of 10. With a two-tailed test and a sample of 100, an r of 0.20 is statistically significant at the 0.05 level, but with a sample of 10, the correlation must be 0.632 or larger to be significant. With large samples rs that are described as demonstrating "little if any" relationship are statistically significant. To reiterate, the statistical significance implies that the r did not occur by chance; the relationship actually is greater than zero. However, a "highly

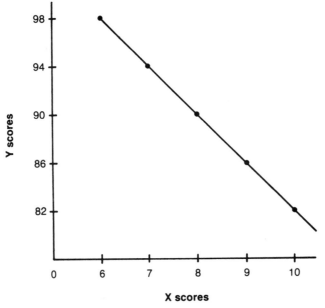

FIGURE 11-5
Graph of scores in Table 11-5.

TABLE 11-6
A Demonstration of No Relationship Between Two Variables

Subjects	X	Y	zX	zY	zXzY
1	6	94	−1.42	0.71	−1.0
2	7	82	−0.71	−1.42	1.0
3	8	90	0.00	0.00	0.0
4	9	98	0.71	1.42	1.0
5	10	86	1.42	−0.71	−1.0

$\bar{X} = 8, s = 1.41$ $\bar{Y} = 90, s = 5.66$ $\Sigma zXzY = 0.00$

$$r = \frac{\Sigma zXzY}{n} = \frac{0.00}{5} = 0.00$$

significant" correlation may in fact be quite small. For this reason many people also speak about the *meaningfulness* of r.

Meaningfulness of the Correlation Coefficient

The coefficient of determination, r^2, often is used as a measure of the "meaningfulness" of r. This is a measure of the amount of variance the two variables share. The circle containing X represents all the variability or variance of X, and the other circle

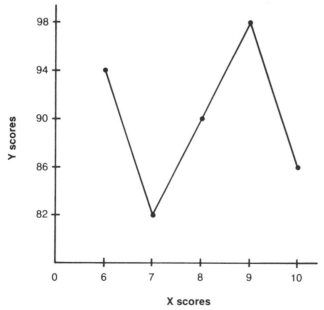

FIGURE 11-6
Graph of scores in Table 11-6.

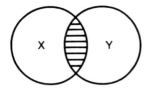

represents the total variance for Y. The overlapping area indicates their shared variance. This area can be determined by squaring the correlation coefficient r. To determine the meaningfulness of an r of 0.20, square the coefficient: $r^2 = (0.20)^2 = 0.04$, or 4%. You can then say that the variance shared between these two variables equals 4%. When reporting this, researchers usually say that the independent variable, X, accounts for 4% of the variance of the dependent variable. Obviously, this is not very much, because another 96% of variance is unaccounted for. To account for approximately half of the variance, you would need an r of 0.70 (because $0.70^2 = 0.49$, or 49%).

Confidence Intervals

We constructed confidence intervals around mean scores and stated that 95% (or 99%) of the confidence intervals would include the population mean. We also may construct confidence intervals around r. This is another way of determining the meaning of the r you calculate. We demonstrate the construction of these intervals after demonstrating the calculation of r by the most commonly used formula.

CALCULATIONS

Pearson Product Moment Correlation

The following formula is mathematically equivalent to the z-score formula that we have already demonstrated. This formula looks more complicated than the z-score formula but is actually easier to calculate because all the scores are not subtracted from their respective means.

$$r = \frac{\Sigma XY - \frac{(\Sigma X)(\Sigma Y)}{n}}{\sqrt{\left(\Sigma X^2 - \frac{(\Sigma X)^2}{n}\right)\left(\Sigma Y^2 - \frac{(\Sigma Y)^2}{n}\right)}}$$

The calculation of r is demonstrated in Table 11-7 using the data from the computer analysis (see Table 11-3).

To determine the statistical significance of the correlation, use the table in Appendix E. The value for r must equal or exceed the tabled value for it to be significant at a given level. The df for r is $n - 2$, that is, the number of subjects minus two. In our example we had 20 subjects, so the $df = 18$. For a one-tailed test an r of 0.8396 with 18 df, exceeds the tabled value of 0.561 for the 0.005 level. (Note that for a given tabled value, the significance level is twice as high for a two-tailed as for a one-tailed test.)

TABLE 11-7
Calculation of the Pearson Product Moment Correlation Coefficient

Subjects	Anger X	Perceived Stress Y	X^2	Y^2	XY
1	0	2	0	4	0
2	7	9	49	81	63
3	8	11	64	121	88
4	6	7	36	49	42
5	8	7	64	49	56
6	9	20	81	400	180
7	7	10	49	100	70
8	2	2	4	4	4
9	15	18	225	324	270
10	9	12	81	144	108
11	13	16	169	256	208
12	3	5	9	25	15
13	8	11	64	121	88
14	6	5	36	25	30
15	10	18	100	324	180
16	7	10	49	100	70
17	6	6	36	36	36
18	7	9	49	81	63
19	11	10	121	100	110
20	5	4	25	16	20
	147	192	1311	2360	1701

$$r = \frac{\Sigma XY - \dfrac{(\Sigma X)(\Sigma Y)}{n}}{\sqrt{\left(\Sigma X^2 - \dfrac{(\Sigma X)^2}{n}\right)\left(\Sigma Y^2 - \dfrac{(\Sigma Y)^2}{n}\right)}}$$

$$r = \frac{1701 - \dfrac{(147)(192)}{20}}{\sqrt{\left(1311 - \dfrac{(147)^2}{20}\right)\left(2360 - \dfrac{(192)^2}{20}\right)}}$$

$$r = \frac{289.8}{\sqrt{(230.55)(516.80)}}$$

$$r = \frac{289.8}{345.18}$$

$$r = 0.8396$$

$n = 20$

$\Sigma X = 147$

$\Sigma Y = 192$

$\Sigma X^2 = 1311$

$\Sigma Y^2 = 2360$

$\Sigma XY = 1701$

Transforming r Values

Methods for testing differences between means and developing confidence intervals are based on the characteristics of the normal curve. When a distribution is asymmetric, these methods are not appropriate. When the value of r in the population exceeds approximately 0.25, the sampling distribution becomes skewed and becomes more skewed as the value of r increases (Thorndike, 1988, p. 616). Thus, before rs in different samples can be compared and before confidence intervals can be constructed, the r values must be transformed to values for which distribution will be symmetric. This transformation is known as Fisher's z. Appendix F contains a table that can be used to transform r values into z_r values.

When comparing r values from two different groups, you would transform the r values to z_r values, and then apply the t-test (or ANOVA) to the z_r values to determine whether they were statistically different. You would also transform r values to z_rs before attempting to average them. We will demonstrate the use of Fisher's z values in constructing confidence intervals.

Confidence Intervals

To set up the confidence interval around a given r, r must first be transformed into a *Fisher's z_r* using the table in Appendix F. For example assume that we had 103 subjects and an r of 0.9.

The first step is to convert r to z_r. In Appendix F note that an r of 0.9 equals a z_r of 1.472.

The second step is to determine the standard error. The formula for the standard error is $1/\sqrt{n - 3}$. In this example that is $1/\sqrt{103 - 3} = 0.1$.

The third step is to determine the confidence interval to choose. The 95% and 99% levels are commonly used. The formulas follow:

a. 95% $= z_r \pm (1.96)$ (standard error)
b. 99% $= z_r \pm (2.58)$ (standard error)

For our example they become the following:

a. 95% $= 1.472 \pm (1.96)(0.1) = 1.276$ and 1.668
b. 99% $= 1.472 \pm (2.58)(0.1) = 1.214$ and 1.730

The fourth step is to transform the z_rs back to rs using Appendix F. When using the table, you will see that not every possible z_r is listed. Select the one closest to the number you calculated.

a. 95%: z_rs $= 1.276$ and 1.668; after transformation back to rs, they become 0.855 and 0.930, respectively.
b. 99%: z_rs $= 1.214$ and 1.730; after transformation back to rs, they become 0.840 and 0.940, respectively.

The fifth step is to set up the confidence intervals.
Note that the confidence intervals are not symmetric around the r value.

Level	Bound for r
a. 95%	0.855–0.930
b. 99%	0.840–0.940

Brief Description of Other Measures of Relationship

There are measures other than the Pearson *r* for measuring relationships. An overview is given here, but computational formulas are not presented. Three "short-cut" versions of *r* are *phi*, point-biserial, and *Spearman rho*.

Short-Cut Versions of r

There tends to be some confusion about short-cut versions of *r*; many researchers assume that they are different from Pearson's *r* and that applying *r* and one of these formulas to a set of data would result in different results. Actually, these measures usually give the same result as *r*. The only advantage of using them is when doing hand calculations. They are really short-cut versions of *r* that can be used with specific types of data.

Phi

When both variables being correlated are *dichotomous*, that is, each has only two levels, a short-cut version of *r* can be used. Examples of dichotomous variables include sex (male and female), a yes or no response choice, and pass or fail. If using the computer to analyze your data, you can use *r* and will get exactly the same result as if you had used phi. See Chapter 5 for a more complete description of phi.

Point-Biserial and Spearman Rho

When you want to correlate one dichotomous variable with one continuous variable, you can use the point-biserial formula. When you have two sets of ranks, you can use the Spearman rho formula. You might ask two groups to rank a list of stressors from most stressful to least stressful. You could compare the rankings of the two groups by using the Spearman rho formula. Spearman rho is often referred to as a *nonparametric* test, as though it were distribution-free, which is not true. It is better thought of as a short-cut version of *r*.

Nonparametric Measures

Kendall's Tau

This measure is a nonparametric measure and is not a short-cut formula for *r*. It was developed as an alternate procedure for Spearman rho. It is sometimes used when measuring the relation between two ranked (ordinal) variables. Kendall's tau might be an alternative if your data seriously violated the assumptions underlying r. It can be calculated using most of the major computer packages, such as SAS or SPSS.

Contingency Coefficient

One nonparametric technique can be used to measure the relationship between two nominal level variables. The variables need not be dichotomous variables but may have multiple levels. For example this technique could be used to determine the relationship between race and political affiliation.

To calculate this coefficient you must use the chi-square statistic, which is discussed in Chapter 5.

Estimating r

Two formulas are not short-cut versions of r, but instead estimate results that might be obtained using r. Nunnally (1978) recommends that, in general, these techniques should *not* be used. Because they are sometimes reported in the literature and often mentioned in statistics texts, they are outlined here.

Biserial

This technique can be used when one variable is dichotomized and the other is continuous. *Dichotomized* means that the variable has been made dichotomous, cut into two levels from a variable that would have been naturally continuous. For example scores could be divided into high and low, creating a dichotomized variable. A biserial correlation might be used with a scale on which people rated items with agree or disagree (a dichotomized variable) that a continuous variable, such as age; you want to know what the correlation would be if you changed the dichotomized variable into a continuous variable (perhaps by adding response categories). If you calculated the biserial correlation between the dichotomized variable (agree or disagree) and the continuous variable (age), you would have an estimate of what r would be if the dichotomized variable were changed to a continuous one. Nunnally (1978) argues against such a use, stating that the resulting coefficient is usually artificially high.

Tetrachoric

This coefficient estimates r from the relationship between two dichotomized variables. If there are serious problems with estimating r from one dichotomized variable (biserial), there are obviously even more difficulties with estimating r from two dichotomized variables.

"Universal" Measure

We have been discussing the relationship between two variables that have a linear relationship. When we graph these relationships, they suggest a straight line across the graph. Although the relationship may be positive or negative, it is the same across all the scores. An example of a nonlinear relationship can be seen in Figure 11-1D. In this case low scores on the X variable are related to low scores on the Y variable, but high scores on X also are related to low scores on Y. Such a relationship is called *curvilinear*. An example might be the possible relationship between anxiety and test scores. In this graph those with moderate anxiety could perform the best on tests. Those with very low or very high anxiety perform poorly. There is a real advantage to having data plotted to determine whether a nonlinear relationship exists, because r cannot be used to test such a relationship.

Eta

Eta, sometimes called the *correlation ratio*, can be used to measure a nonlinear relationship. The range of values for eta is from 0 to $+1$. It can be used with all variables, whether nominal or continuous. Eta is closely related to r and has been called a "universal" relationship because it can be used "regardless of the form of the relationship" (Nunnally, 1978, p. 147). When it is used with two continuous variables that have a linear relationship, it reduces to r.

PARTIAL CORRELATION

When discussing research design, we confront the notion of "control." How do we "control" variance that will distract or mislead us? There are several ways. If we are concerned about the impact of a variable, such as age, we might use random assignment of subjects to groups as a method of control, we might select only one age group, or we might match subjects by age before assigning them to groups. There also are statistical measures of control: We can record the age of the subjects and use that as a variable in the study. One method of statistical control is *partial correlation*.

This technique also allows us to describe the relationship between two variables (or more, if you go to multiple partial correlation) after statistically controlling for the influence of some third variable. When studying research design you learned that the relationship between two variables may be unclear because of the confounding influence of another variable. For example if you calculate the correlation between mental age and height in children 1 to 10 years of age, you will find a high correlation. Does that mean that height causes intelligence? Of course the key factor is age, not height. Once you control for age, the relationship between height and mental age becomes trivial.

One study was conducted to determine whether the number of hours studied was related to grades; the researchers found a negative correlation. Does this mean that studying less results in higher grades? No. Once they controlled for intelligence, the researchers found a significant positive relation between grades and hours of study. (Although that study indicates that "smarter" people study fewer hours, more recent evidence suggests that in most cases brighter students study more.)

Partial correlations may be written as $r_{12.3}$. This indicates that you are measuring the correlation between variables 1 and 2 with the effect of variable 3 removed from *both* the variables being correlated. Consider the example of college grades (variable 1) with hours of study (variable 2) and intelligence (variable 3). If we used partial correlation to study this relationship, the correlation between intelligence and grades (r_{13}) is removed, and the correlation between intelligence and hours of study (r_{23}) also is removed. The confounding influence of intelligence is thus removed statistically, and the relationship between the two variables, grades and hours of study, can be measured accurately. Partial correlation also may be written as $ry_{1.2}$, which would indicate the correlation of an independent variable 1, with a dependent variable, y, with the effect of variable 2 removed from the independent and the dependent variables.

SEMIPARTIAL CORRELATION

This is the correlation of two variables with the effect of a third variable removed from only *one* of the variables being correlated. It is closely tied to multiple correlation, as is discussed in the next section. Semipartial correlation may be written as $r_{1(2.3)}$ or $ry_{(1.2)}$. The first way would indicate the correlation between variables 1 and 2 with the effect of variable 3 removed from 2 alone; the second way would indicate the correlation between the dependent variable, y, and an independent variable, 1, with the effect of variable 2 removed from 1 alone. The following diagram explains further.

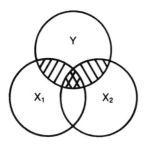

The circles represent the amount of variance of each of the variables. Remember that the variance shared by two variables is measured by r^2. If we take variable X_1 into account first, the variance accounted for in Y equals the variance contributed by X_1 (r_{y1}^2), plus the unique variance accounted for by X_2. That unique variance is the variance shared between Y and X_2 after the effect of X_1 on X_2 has been removed (or after the cross-hatched area has been subtracted). The squared semipartial correlation between X_2 and Y is the unique variance contributed by X_2 ($r_{y(2.1)}^2$). Therefore, in this case R^2 (the squared multiple correlation, which is explained more fully in the following section) = the r^2 between X_1 and Y + the semipartial correlation squared between X^2 and Y, or $R^2 = r_{y1}^2 + r_{y(2.1)}^2$.

MULTIPLE CORRELATION

We have been discussing correlation as measuring the relationship between two variables. This concept can be extended to one in which the relationship is measured between one variable and a combination of other variables. When discussing r, we were talking about one independent variable (X) and one dependent variable (Y). In multiple correlation (R), we are talking about more than one independent variable (X_1, X_2, X_3, and so on) and one dependent variable (Y). It is also possible to have more than one dependent variable (Y_1, Y_2, Y_3, and so on); this is called *canonical correlation* and is discussed in Chapter 12.

The multiple correlation, R, can go from 0 to 1. There are no negative Rs because the method of least squares is used to calculate R, and squaring numbers eliminates negatives. R^2 is the amount of variance accounted for in the dependent variable by the combination of independent variables. When reporting multiple correlations, R^2, rather than R, is often presented.

As we demonstrated in the discussion of semipartial correlation, the calculation of the squared multiple correlation, R^2, may require more than simply adding up the squared correlation of each independent variable with the dependent variable. This is because if there were no correlation between the independent variables, the correlations might be as follows:

	X_1	X_2	Y
X_1	1.00	0.00	0.40
X_2	0.00	1.00	0.30

This could be depicted as:

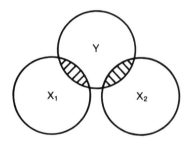

In this case there is no overlap between variables X_1 and X_2. They are not correlated; thus, each accounts for a different portion of the variance in Y. We could add up their squared correlation (r^2s) with Y (($0.40)^2$s $+ (0.30)^2$) and determine that $R^2 = 0.25$.

Usually in behavioral research, however, the independent variables are correlated among themselves as depicted in the following:

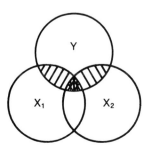

In this case there is correlation between X_1 and X_2, and if you add up the squared correlation of X_1 with Y and the squared correlation of X_2 with Y, you would add in the cross-hatched area twice. The variance accounted for in Y is actually all that is explained by one of the variables plus the *additional* variance explained by the second variable. The additional variance is measured by the squared semipartial correlation of the second variable with the dependent variable. If X_1 is counted first, it accounts for all of its shared variance with Y, and X_2 adds the variance that it alone contributes (its shared variance with Y minus the cross-hatched area). The first variable gets "credit" for the first piece of variance accounted for, even though it shares some of that with X_2. The order of entry of variables into a multiple correlation may be important when understanding the relationships being studied. This is discussed in more detail in Chapter 12. Multiple correlation is a technique for measuring the relationship between a dependent variable and a weighted combination of independent variables.

The following example comes from the Munro (1985) study of the predictors of success in graduate nursing education.

	Essay Score	*GREV*	*Master's GPA*
Essay	1.000	0.246	0.278
GRE-Verbal	0.246	1.000	0.216

The preadmission essay has a correlation of 0.278 with the final master's grade point average; that is, it accounts for almost 8% of the variance in grade point average (GPA) ($[0.278]^2 = 0.077$). The essay is also correlated with the GRE-verbal score ($r = 0.246$). The GRE-verbal accounts for approximately 5% of the variance in GPA ($[0.216]^2 = 0.047$), but part of the variance is shared with essay. When the multiple correlation is calculated, it shows that the essay accounts for 7.7% of the variance, and GRE-verbal adds another 2.3% of unique variance. $R^2 = 0.10$, or 10%, which is more than either of the variables could have accounted for alone. Because the essay was counted first, GRE-verbal was only credited with its squared semipartial correlation with master's GPA, rather than with its squared correlation with GPA $(0.216)^2$. The contribution of the essay to the explained variance was significant, but the 2.3% added by the GRE-verbal was not a significant addition ($p = 0.069$).

SUMMARY

Correlation is a procedure for quantifying the relationship between two or more variables. It measures the strength and indicates the direction of the relationship. Multiple correlation measures the relationship between one variable and a weighted composite of the other variables. Partial correlation is a statistical method for describing the relationship between two variables, with the effect of another confounding variable removed. In semipartial correlation, the influence of a third variable is removed from only one of the variables being correlated.

12 | Regression

Barbara Hazard Munro

OBJECTIVES FOR CHAPTER 12

After reading this chapter you should be able to do the following:

1. **Know when it is appropriate to use regression techniques.**

2. **Understand the statistics generated by the regression procedure.**

3. **Set up and solve a prediction equation.**

4. **Explain the difference between testing the significance of R^2 and the significance of a b-weight.**

5. **Code categorical variables.**

6. **Discuss methods for selecting variables for entry into a regression equation.**

7. **Understand the statistics generated by a canonical correlation.**

8. **Interpret the results section of research studies that report these techniques.**

We are constantly interested in predicting one thing based on another. We want to predict the weather to plan our weekend. We want to predict how well a student will do in nursing practice. We want to predict how long a patient may remain ill. Countless predictions are necessary for us simply to move through life.

A brilliant statistical invention is regression, which permits us to make predictions from some known evidence about some unknown future events. Only about a century old, regression is the basis of many statistical methods, and, in this book, there is nothing more important to understand.

Regression makes use of the correlation between variables and the notion of a straight line to develop a prediction equation. Once a relationship

Barbara Hazard Munro and Ellis Batten Page: STATISTICAL METHODS FOR HEALTH CARE RESEARCH, SECOND EDITION. © 1993, 1986 by J. B. Lippincott Company.

has been established between two variables, it is possible to develop an equation that will allow you to predict the score of one of the variables, given the score of the other. In the case of a multiple correlation, regression is used to establish a prediction equation in which the independent variables are each assigned a weight based on their relationship to the dependent variable. For example in a study of clinical predictors of intravenous (IV) site symptoms, multiple regression was used to develop a preliminary model of factors related to those symptoms. Dibble, Bostrom-Ezrati, and Rizzuto (1991) studied more than 500 patients at four institutions. Seven variables explained 18% of the variance in the number of IV site symptoms.

Regression is a useful technique that allows us to *predict* outcomes and *explain* the interrelationships among variables. The type of data required and the underlying assumptions are the same for regression as for correlation (see Chapter 11). Information about testing assumptions is provided later in this chapter in the discussion of the testing of residuals.

SIMPLE LINEAR REGRESSION

We begin by explaining *simple* regression. A correlation between two variables is used to develop a prediction equation. The techniques described in this chapter are for predictions based on a *linear* relationship between variables. If the relationship is curvilinear, other techniques, such as trend analysis, must be used.

If the correlation between two variables were perfect ($+1$ or -1), we would be able to make a perfect prediction about the score on one variable, given the score on the other variable. Of course we never get perfect correlations, so we are never able to make perfect predictions. The higher the correlation, the more accurate the prediction. If there were no correlation between two variables, knowing the score of one would not help in estimating the score on the other. When you have no information to aid you in predicting a score, your best guess for any subject would be the mean, because that is the center of the data.

To be able to make predictions, the relationship between two variables, the independent (X) and the dependent (Y), must be measured. If there is a correlation, a regression equation can be developed that will allow prediction of Y, given X. For example in the study previously mentioned, Dibble, Bostrom-Ezrati, and Rizzuto (1991) wanted to predict the number of IV site symptoms (Y') based on predictors (Xs), which included such things as duration of IV, osmolarity of solution, addition of potassium chloride, and so forth. They measured their subjects on all of the variables they believed to be related to the outcome measure, did preliminary analyses to determine which variables were correlated with their outcome measure, and then regressed the number of symptoms on those predictors. From this they were able to determine the relative relationship of the predictor variables to the outcome measure and to develop a prediction equation that would enable them to determine who would be more prone to developing these symptoms. The accuracy of that prediction is based on the strength of the correlations between the predictors and the outcome measure. Although 18% of the variation in symptoms was explained ($p = 0.0001$), 82% of the variation was not explained by this model.

Understanding Regression Through the Use of Standard Scores

In previous chapters standard scores (z-scores) are used to explain the concepts of standard deviation and correlation. Remember that once scores have been converted to z-scores, they have a mean of 0 and a standard deviation of 1 (Fig. 12-1). Direct comparisons between sets of z-scores can be made, because they are measured on the same scale. Given z-scores, the formula for a prediction (regression) equation is simple. It is $Y' = rX$, where Y' is the predicted score, and X is the "known" or predictor variable. Given a perfect positive correlation, Y' would equal X. For example someone with a z-score of $+2$ on X would also score $+2$ on Y.

$$Y' = (1)(2)$$

In Chapter 11 it is shown that with a perfect positive correlation ($r = +1$), everyone receives exactly the same z-score on Y as on X. It is shown that with a perfect negative correlation ($r = -1$), each subject receives exactly the opposite z-score on Y as on X. For example someone with a -3 on X would get a $+3$ on Y'.

$$Y' = (-1)(-3) = +3$$

As previously mentioned if there is *no* correlation between the variables, *no* prediction can be made, and our "best guess" for Y' is the mean. Using the formula for Y', with $r = 0$ and $X = +3$, we calculate Y' as $(0)(3) = 0$. Zero is, of course, the mean of a z-score distribution. These extreme cases, perfect correlations and zero correlations, however, are most uncommon in the world of research! Therefore, consider what happens with more reasonable correlations. Suppose an individual, Jill, scored $+2$ on X. Given the following rs, what Y score would you predict for Jill? Work these equations before reading on.

$$r = -0.20$$
$$r = 0.60$$
$$r = 0.20$$
$$r = -0.60$$

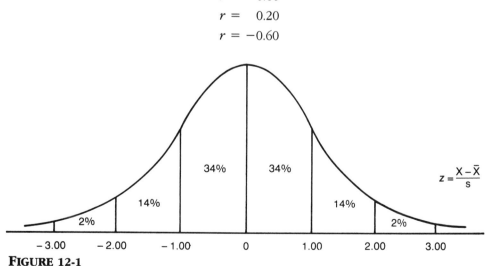

FIGURE 12-1
Normal curve with standardized scores.

For $r = -0.20$, our equation would be $Y' = (-0.20)(2)$ or -0.40. The other answers are, respectively, 1.20, 0.40, and -1.20. If you predicted each Y score correctly, you have mastered this simplest type of prediction, for which you have only the standard scores and the correlation coefficient.

Regression literally means a falling back toward the mean. With perfect correlations, there is no falling back; the predicted score is the same as the predictor. With less than perfect correlations, there is some error in the measurement, and we would expect that in the case of an individual who received an extremely high score, chance may have been working in her favor; therefore, on a second measure, her score would be somewhat less—it would have fallen back toward the mean. In the same way an individual with an extremely low score perhaps had all the fates against her and on a second measure would do better, thus moving her score closer to the mean.

Each prediction regresses toward the mean, depending on the strength of the correlation. If there is no correlation ($r = 0$), Y' equals zero (the mean). As the correlation rises toward 1, Y' moves proportionately outward from the mean, toward the position of the X predictor. The correlation coefficient tells us exactly what percentage of this distance Y' moves. Figure 12-2 shows predictions based on an r of 0.50. Note on the figure that all the predicted scores (Y's) are halfway between the mean and the X-score. This is because the correlation is 0.5. (If the correlation had been 0.7, the Y'-scores would have moved 0.7 times the distance between the mean and X.) If the X-score is above the mean, the predicted score will be lower than the X-score and closer to the mean. With an r of 0.5 and an X-score of $+2$, Y' would equal $(0.5)(2) = 1$. With a correlation of 0.5, an individual who was 2 standard deviations above the mean would be predicted to be 1 standard deviation above the mean on Y.

If the X-score is below the mean, the predicted score is higher and closer to the mean. An X-score of -3 would result in a predicted score of $(0.5)(-3) = -1.5$. Remember that these are predictions based on a correlation of 0.5, so you would not be able to predict perfectly an individual's score. The person's actual score will differ from the predicted score. This discrepancy between predicted and actual scores reflects the error in the prediction and is discussed more fully in the next section of this chapter. Because most measures will not be in z-scores, we now present the more general regression equation.

Prediction Equation

The regression equation is the equation for a straight line and is written as:

$$Y' = a + bX$$

Y' is the predicted score.

Given data on X and Y from a sample of subjects called the *regression sample, a* and b can be calculated. With these two measures Y can be predicted, given X. The letter a is called the *intercept constant* and is the value of Y when $X = 0$. It is the point at which the regression line intercepts the Y axis. The letter b is called the *regression coefficient* and is the rate of change in Y with a unit change in X. It is a measure of the slope of the regression line.

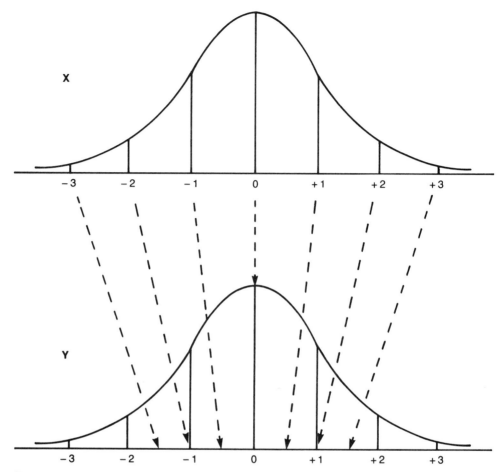

FIGURE 12-2
Predicting from X to Y, with $r = 0.50$.

An example is given in Figure 12-3. The intercept constant, a, is equal to 3; you can see that is the value of Y when $X = 0$. It is the point at which the regression line connects with the Y axis. The regression coefficient, b, is equal to 0.5. This means that the value of Y goes up 0.5 of a point for every 1-point change in X. When $X = 0$, $Y = 3$, and when X goes up to 1, Y goes up to 3.5. As you will see when we are calculating a and b, a is based on the means of the two variables, and b is based on the correlation between them.

The regression line is the "line of best fit" and is formed by a technique called the *method of least squares*. The concept of least squares is presented in Chapter 2 with a discussion of characteristics of the mean. Because the mean is (in one sense) the center of the data, the sum of the deviations of the scores around the mean, $\Sigma(X - \overline{X})$, adds up to 0. Also, if you square these deviations and add them, that number will be smaller than the sum of the squared deviations around any other measure of central tendency. In the

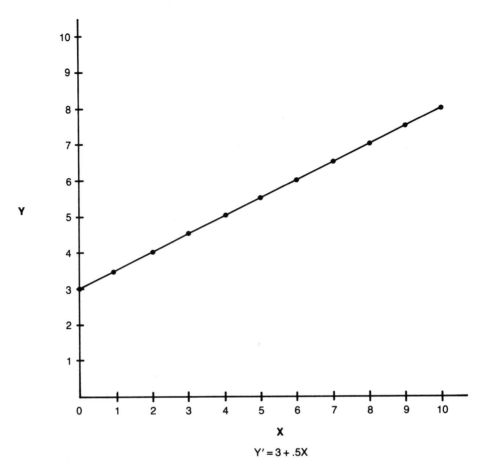

$$Y' = 3 + .5X$$

FIGURE 12-3
The regression line.

same way the regression line passes through the exact center of the data in the scatter diagram. Therefore, it is the "line of best fit." There are deviations around the regression line, just as there are deviations around the mean. The regression line represents the predicted scores (Y's), but because a prediction is not perfect, the actual scores (Ys) would deviate somewhat from the predicted scores. Because the regression line passes through the center of the pairs of scores, if you add up the deviations from the regression line ($Y - Y'$), they will equal 0. Also, if you square those deviations and add them, the sum of the squared deviations around the regression line is smaller than the sum of the squared deviations around any other line drawn through the scatter diagram.

If Dibble, Bostrom-Ezrati, and Rizzuto (1991) applied their prediction equation to the patients in their sample, they would find that the clients' *actual* number of symptoms (Y) would vary from their *predicted* (Y') number. Because the correlations between the predictors and the outcome measure were not perfect, there is error in the prediction. Even using the sample on which the prediction equation was calculated, there will be differences between Y and (Y'). $Y - Y'$ would equal the deviations from the predicted scores just as $X - \bar{X}$ equals the deviations around the mean. The regression equation minimizes the squared differences of the predicted score from the actual score.

Given a regression equation of $Y' = 4 + 0.2X$ and three individuals with scores on X of 5, 10, and 20, respectively, the predicted scores for the three would be calculated as follows:

$$a + \quad bX \quad = Y'$$

1. $4 + (0.2)\ (5) = 5$

2. $4 + (0.2)(10) = 6$

3. $4 + (0.2)(20) = 8$

Confidence Intervals

Because there is error in predictions, we need to know how accurate a prediction is. The standard error of estimate can be used to construct confidence intervals around predicted scores. The standard error of estimate is the standard deviation of the errors of prediction. We use that in the same way that we use the standard errors of the mean and the correlation coefficient to construct confidence intervals. Given a predicted score, we can then say that 95% or 99% of the confidence intervals will capture the actual score. (See Chapters 3 and 4 for a more complete description of confidence intervals.) The calculation of these intervals is presented after the calculation of a regression equation.

MULTIPLE REGRESSION

Multiple regression is possible when there is a measurable multiple correlation between a group of predictor variables and one dependent variable. The prediction equation is:

$$Y' = a + b_1X_1 + b_2X_2 + b_3X_3 + \ldots b_kX_k$$

There is still one intercept constant, a, but each independent variable (e.g., X_1, X_2, X_3) has a separate b-weight. Given a prediction equation of:

$$Y' = 2 + 0.5X_1 + 0.2X_2 + 0.4X_3$$

and three individuals with the following scores:

X_1	X_2	X_3
1. 8	4	7
2. 12	3	5
3. 10	6	9

their predicted scores would be calculated as:

---

1. $2 + (0.5)(8) + (0.2)(4) + (0.4)(7) = 9.6$
2. $2 + (0.5)(12) + (0.2)(3) + (0.4)(5) = 10.6$
3. $2 + (0.5)(10) + (0.2)(6) + (0.4)(9) = 11.8$

If adding extra variables increases the amount of variance accounted for in the dependent variable, that will also increase the accuracy of our prediction. Multiple regression simply extends the multiple correlation into the computation of the regression equation.

SIGNIFICANCE TESTING

When doing a simple linear regression, the correlation between the two variables is tested for significance, and r^2 represents meaningfulness. With multiple correlation we are interested not only in the significance of the overall R and the amount of variance accounted for (R^2), but also in the significance of each of the independent variables. Just because R^2 is significant does not mean that all the independent variables are contributing significantly to the explained variance. In multiple regression the multiple correlation is tested for significance and each of the b-weights also is tested for significance. Testing the b-weight tells us whether the independent variable associated with it is contributing significantly to the variance accounted for in the dependent variable.

The F-distribution is used for testing the significance of the R^2s, and either the F- or t-distribution is used to test the significance of the bs. See Appendix D for the F-distribution. When using the computer packaged programs, the Fs or ts and associated probabilities are printed out. The F-distribution is used for demonstration here.

The calculation of F is presented later in this chapter. When testing for the significance of R^2s, the degrees of freedom are calculated as $k/(n - k - 1)$. In other words there are two dfs; a numerator, k; and a denominator, $n - k - 1$. The k stands for the number of independent variables, and n stands for the number of subjects. When testing the significance of a b-weight, the df is $1/(n - k - 1)$.

We start with examples of testing the Fs associated with R^2s for significance. If we had two independent variables and a sample size of 63, the df would be $2/(63 - 2 - 1)$, or $2/60$. In Appendix D the dfs for the numerator are listed across the top of the page. The numerator also is known as the greater mean square. The dfs for the denominator are listed down the left side of the page. The denominator also is called the *lesser mean square*. In our example there are 2 dfs in the numerator and 60 dfs in the denominator. The tabled values for $2/60$ df, which must be equaled or exceeded, are 3.15 at the 0.05 level and 4.98 at the 0.01 level. Note that the 0.05 level is in light print, and the 0.01 level is in dark print. An F of 4.50 would be significant at the 0.05 level but not at the 0.01 level. Two additional examples follow:

F	k	n	df	p
4.05	3	129	3/125	<0.01
2.00	6	207	6/200	ns

To test the b-weights the procedure is the same except that the numerator of the df is always 1. Some examples for testing b-weights follow:

F	k	n	df	p
5.25	2	68	1/65	<0.05
8.00	3	154	1/150	<0.01

COMPUTER ANALYSIS

Simple Linear Regression

Two computer analyses are presented—first, a simple linear regression and then a multiple regression. The simple linear regression contains the same data used to calculate a correlation in Chapter 11 (see Table 11-3). These data also are used in the demonstration of the calculation of a simple linear regression. See Figure 12-4 for the computer printout generated by SPSS/PC+.

① The command line requests a regression procedure in which there are two variables, ANGER and STRESS. The dependent variable is STRESS. The method is ENTER, which means that all independent variables are entered together. In this example there is only one independent variable, ANGER.

② In Chapter 11 we find the correlation between ANGER and STRESS to be 0.8396 (see Fig. 11-3). Although the printout lists multiple R (the multiple correlation), because there is only one independent variable, the multiple R is the same as the correlation between the two variables, 0.83957. R square is the multiple R squared, or $0.83957^2 = 0.70487$. The adjusted R square corrects for the number of variables and number of subjects. It is a more conservative estimate of the statistic. More detail on this adjustment is provided in the last section of this chapter. The standard error is a measure of the difference between predicted and actual scores and can be used to construct confidence intervals.

③ In the analysis of variance (ANOVA) table, instead of between and within sum of squares, as reported in typical ANOVA tables, we see regression and residual sum of squares. The regression sum of squares is the portion of the total variance in the dependent variable that is explained through the analysis and therefore is analogous to the between sum of squares in ANOVA. The residual sum of squares is the unexplained or error variance and is analogous to within sum of squares in ANOVA.

SPSS/PC+

(1) REGRESSION /VARIABLES ANGER STRESS /DEPENDENT STRESS/METHOD ENTER.

```
* * * *   M U L T I P L E   R E G R E S S I O N   * * * *

Listwise Deletion of Missing Data

Equation Number 1    Dependent Variable..   STRESS

Block Number  1.  Method:  Enter

       * * * *   M U L T I P L E   R E G R E S S I O N   * * * *

Equation Number 1    Dependent Variable..   STRESS

Variable(s) Entered on Step Number
   1..    ANGER
```

(2)
```
Multiple R              .83957
R Square                .70487
Adjusted R Square       .68847
Standard Error         2.91093
```

(3) Analysis of Variance
```
                   DF      Sum of Squares      Mean Square
Regression          1           364.27690        364.27690
Residual           18           152.52310          8.47351

F =      42.99011      Signif F =  .0000
```

```
       * * * *   M U L T I P L E   R E G R E S S I O N   * * * *

Equation Number 1    Dependent Variable..   STRESS

----------------- Variables in the Equation ------------------
```

(4)
Variable	B	SE B	Beta	T	Sig T
ANGER	1.256994	.191712	.839565	6.557	.0000
(Constant)	.361093	1.552156		.233	.8187

```
End Block Number   1   All requested variables entered.
```

FIGURE 12-4
Simple linear regression produced by SPSS/PC+.

There is 1 *df* associated with the regression sum of squares because there is one independent variable. The *df* associated with the residual sum of squares is calculated as $n - k - 1$, where n = the number of subjects, and k = the number of independent variables. In our example this becomes $20 - 1 - 1 = 18$. Dividing each sum of squares by its respective *df* results in the mean square values. Dividing the regression sum of squares by the residual sum of squares gives the value for F (364.27690/8.47351 = 42.99011). That value of F with 1,18 *df* is significant at 0.0000 (or < 0.0001).

(4) Variables in the equation list each independent variable with its associated *b*

value, standard error of *b*, beta, *t* value, and significance of *t*. The constant or *a* value also is given. The prediction equation based on this table is:

$$\text{Predicted score for stress } (Y') = 0.361093 + 1.256994 \text{ (ANGER)}$$

Beta is the standardized regression coefficient. Because the *b*-weight reflects the actual measure with its associated mean and standard deviation, it is not directly interpretable. Beta reflects the weight associated with standardized scores (*z*-scores) on the variables. It is a partial correlation coefficient, a measure of the relationship between an independent and dependent variable with the influence of the other independent variables held constant. In this example with only one independent variable, it is simply the measure of the correlation between the two variables, 0.839565. With only one independent variable the measure of the variance accounted for in the overall regression (F) equals the variance accounted for by the independent variable. Because $F = t^2$, we see that F for the overall regression is 42.99, and F for the independent variable is $6.557^2 = 42.99$.

Multiple Regression

To extend the example from simple to multiple regression, we add an additional variable, HOPE. (Although 20 subjects is an inadequate number for two independent variables, we use this example to keep the demonstration of actual calculations as simple as possible.) For the actual data used see Table 12-1. Figure 12-5 contains the computer printout.

① The command line requests a REGRESSION with three variables, ANGER, STRESS, and HOPE. The DEPENDENT variable is STRESS, and all variables are entered together (ENTER).

② The independent variables entered into the equation are HOPE and ANGER. The multiple R is 0.87424, reflecting the contribution of both HOPE and ANGER. R square indicates that 76% of the variance in STRESS was accounted for by ANGER and HOPE. The adjusted R square reflects a correction based on the number of subjects per variable. The standard error is 2.67682 and can be used for calculating confidence intervals around predicted scores for STRESS.

③ The ANOVA table reports 2 *df* associated with regression sum of squares, reflecting the two independent variables. The residual *df*s are calculated as $n - k - 1$, or $20 - 2 - 1 = 17$. The F value, reflecting the ratio of explained (regression) to unexplained (residual) variance, equals 27.56235 and is significant at 0.0000.

④ To evaluate the effect of each independent variable, we look at the table called "Variables in the Equation." The *b*-weight associated with HOPE is negative, indicating that as HOPE increases, STRESS decreases. The standard errors associated with the *b*-weights can be used to construct confidence intervals around each *b*-weight. The prediction equation based on this table is:

$$\text{Predicted score on STRESS } (Y') = 5.546645 - 0.582106(\text{HOPE}) + 0.967267(\text{ANGER})$$

The correlation between HOPE and STRESS with ANGER held constant is

TABLE 12-1
Data for Computer Example

Subjects	Anger	Hope	Perceived Stress
1	0	9	2
2	7	8	9
3	8	5	11
4	6	7	7
5	8	4	7
6	9	0	20
7	7	5	10
8	2	10	2
9	15	1	18
10	9	2	12
11	13	5	16
12	3	8	5
13	8	4	11
14	6	9	5
15	10	3	18
16	7	6	10
17	6	3	6
18	7	6	9
19	11	7	10
20	5	3	4

-0.311246, the beta weight. The correlation between ANGER and STRESS with HOPE held constant is 0.646052. Using the 0.05 level of significance, HOPE does not contribute significantly to the regression ($p = 0.0540$), but ANGER does ($p = 0.0005$).

To understand these relationships, it is helpful to examine the correlations among the variables (Fig. 12-6). Note that both HOPE and ANGER are significantly related to STRESS. For HOPE the correlation is -0.7129 ($p = 0.000$), and for ANGER the correlation is 0.8396 ($p = 0.000$). Why didn't HOPE make a significant contribution in the regression? It is because there is a high correlation between HOPE and ANGER (-0.6217); that is, these two variables overlap in their relationship to STRESS. The partial correlations clarify the overall relationship and indicate that the variance accounted for by ANGER with HOPE held constant is 41.7% (0.646052^2), and the variance accounted for by HOPE with ANGER held constant is only 9.7% (-0.311246^2).

CODING

Nominal level variables can be included in a regression analysis, but they must be coded to allow for proper interpretation. You might collect information on the marital status of your subjects, and when entering the information into the computer, you decide on

SPSS/PC+

① REGRESSION/VARIABLES ANGER STRESS HOPE/DEPENDENT STRESS/METHOD
ENTER.

* * * *   M U L T I P L E   R E G R E S S I O N   * * * *

Listwise Deletion of Missing Data

Equation Number 1   Dependent Variable..   STRESS

Block Number 1. Method: Enter

* * * *   M U L T I P L E   R E G R E S S I O N   * * * *

Equation Number 1   Dependent Variable..   STRESS

② Variable(s) Entered on Step Number
      1..   HOPE
      2..   ANGER

Multiple R   .87424
R Square   .76430
Adjusted R Square   .73657
Standard Error   2.67682

③ Analysis of Variance
                    DF   Sum of Squares   Mean Square
      Regression   2   394.98876   197.49438
      Residual   17   121.81124   7.16537

F =   27.56235   Signif F = .0000

* * * *   M U L T I P L E   R E G R E S S I O N   * * * *

Equation Number 1   Dependent Variable..   STRESS

---------------- Variables in the Equation ------------------

④ Variable   B   SE B   Beta   T   Sig T

   HOPE   -.582106   .281169   -.311246   -2.070 .0540
   ANGER   .967267   .225086   .646052   4.297 .0005
   (Constant)   5.546645   2.882870   1.924 .0713

End Block Number   1   All requested variables entered.

FIGURE 12-5
Multiple regression produced by SPSS/PC+.

some arbitrary code numbers, such as single = 1, married = 2, and divorced = 3. If you entered that variable into a regression equation, it would be treated as though the numbers really meant something, that 2 was twice as big as 1, and so on. Such coding is *not recommended*. Instead, coding methods have been developed to allow us to enter such variables; three of these techniques, *dummy, effect,* and *orthogonal* coding, are presented here.

SPSS/PC+

Correlations:	ANGER	HOPE
STRESS	.8396	-.7129
	(20)	(20)
	P= .000	P= .000
ANGER		-.6217
		(20)
		P= .002

FIGURE 12-6
Correlations among variables.

In all the coding methods variables are coded into *vectors*, and the rule is that $n - 1$ vectors are used to describe the categories. If the variable has two categories, such as sex, one vector $(2 - 1 = 1)$ is enough. With dummy coding, which is described below, all the members of one sex would be given a 1, and all the members of the other group would be given a 0 on the vector. If there were four categories, three vectors would be required, and so on.

Dummy Coding

This system uses 1s and 0s. If sex is a variable, you could code all males as 1 and all females as 0 (or vice versa). Correlational techniques applied to such a variable would tell you whether or not the sex of the individual was related to some measure. The 1 and 0 simply indicate that you belong to the chosen group or you do not. There is no distinction among members of a group; that is, all the 1s are considered equally male and all the 0s equally female. Suppose you had three groups, experimental group 1, experimental group 2, and a control group. You would need $n - 1 (3 - 1)$ vectors to describe those categories (Table 12-2). To code those groups start with the first vector, which we label $X1$. All the subjects in the first experimental group get a 1 on that vector, and all others get a 0. On the second vector, $X2$, all subjects in the second experimental group get a 1, and all the other subjects get a 0. The control group has received 0s on

TABLE 12-2
Dummy Coding

	Vectors	
Groups	*X1*	*X2*
Experimental 1	1	0
Experimental 2	0	1
Control	0	0

both vectors. On these two vectors each group has a different pattern; that is, the first experimental group has 1,0; the second experimental group has 0,1; and the control group has 0,0.

This form could be extended for any number of categories. When the regression is run, the vectors $X1$ and $X2$ are entered to represent group membership. When such dummy coding is used, the intercept constant, a, in the prediction equation equals the mean of the dependent variable for the group that is assigned 0s throughout. In our example that would be the control group. Therefore, in this form of analysis we are testing the means of the other groups against the mean of a control group. In addition to a, the prediction equation would contain a b-weight for each of the vectors; that is, the prediction equation would look like:

$$Y' = a + b_1X_1 + b_2X_2$$

The regression weight, b_1, represents the difference between the group assigned 1s on $X1$ and the group assigned 0s throughout. In our example testing b_1 for significance would be testing to see whether there is a significant difference between the first experimental group and the control group on some dependent variable, Y. Testing b_2 for significance tells us if there is a significant difference between the second experimental group and the control group. Although it is most clear when used with a control group, dummy coding may be used to code categorical variables, whether or not a control group exists. You can use dummy coding for race, marital status, and so on, but it is important that you understand what testing the b-weights means. In addition to comparing a group with the control group, you may want to compare it with some other group. In our example you may want to compare experimental group 1 with experimental group 2. To do that you would need to use a method that allows you to make multiple comparisons between means. Such comparisons are explained in Chapter 7.

Effect Coding

Effect coding looks like dummy coding except that the last group gets -1s throughout, instead of 0s (Table 12-3). Five categories of marital status are coded into four vectors. We proceed in the same way as with dummy coding, but we give the last group -1 on

TABLE 12-3
Effect Coding

	Vectors			
Marital Status	*X1*	*X2*	*X3*	*X4*
Single	1	0	0	0
Married	0	1	0	0
Divorced	0	0	1	0
Widowed	0	0	0	1
Separated	-1	-1	-1	-1

each vector. Vectors $X1$ through $X4$ would then be entered into the regression equation to represent marital status.

When using effect coding, the a in the prediction equation represents the mean of the dependent variable. It is not the mean of one particular group on the dependent variable, but the overall mean for all the subjects in the analysis. This is referred to as the *grand mean*. What you are testing with this type of coding is how each group's mean differs from the grand mean.

In our example the regression equation would be:

$$Y' = a + b_1X_1 + b_2X_2 + b_3X_3 + b_4X_4$$

If you tested b_1 for significance, you would be testing to see whether the mean score on the dependent variable for single people differed from the overall or grand mean. We could compare the means for single, married, divorced, and widowed against the grand mean, but what about the separated group? There is no b-weight to represent the fifth group. That b-weight can be calculated easily when you know that all the b-weights add up to zero; in the example this is $b_1 + b_2 + b_3 + b_4 + b_5 = 0$. Given the b-weights for the first four categories from the regression, the fifth b-weight can be obtained by subtracting the sum of the first four from zero. For example if the following b-weights were obtained: $b_1 = 1, b_2 = 3, b_3 = -2, b_4 = 2$, then $1 + 3 + (-2) + 2 = 4$, and $0 - 4 = -4$. So the b-weight for the "separated" category would be -4. To compare specific pairs of means, a test for multiple comparisons between means must be applied.

Orthogonal Coding

As previously mentioned when you hypothesize ahead of time, you are able to use more powerful statistical tests. Orthogonal coding allows you to code your hypotheses so they can be tested. To use this technique you must have hypothesized a priori (i.e., before the data were collected). Here, orthogonal means that the comparisons that you want to test are independent of each other; that is, knowing the answer to one does not give you the answer to the other.

To have comparisons that are independent, only $n - 1$ comparisons can be made; that is, if there were three groups (experimental 1, experimental 2, and control), there could only be two orthogonal contrasts. Suppose that you were trying to decrease the number of postoperative complications, and you had three groups. Subjects in experimental group 1 (EG1) were given special preoperative instruction by a nurse and a booklet that they could refer to later. EG2 received instruction only, and the control group just received the usual care. You would want to know whether the special instructions reduced postoperative complications and whether providing a booklet and instruction was better than instruction alone. We could compare the mean for groups EG1 and EG2 with the mean of the control group to see whether there was a difference between experimental and control groups. We also could compare the means of EG1 and EG2 to see whether the booklet made a difference. Table 12-4 contains the vectors necessary to code such a contrast. On vector $X1$ subjects in both experimental groups receive a -1, and the control group subjects receive a 2. That contrast tests the difference between the mean number of postoperative complications for all the experimental subjects and the mean for the control group subjects. Testing b_1 for significance

TABLE 12-4
Orthogonal Coding

Groups	Vectors	
	X1	X2
Experimental 1	−1	1
Experimental 2	−1	−1
Control	2	0

would tell you whether that difference was statistically significant. The second contrast is given in vector $X2$. The first experimental group is compared with the second. Testing b_2 for significance would tell you whether there was a significant difference in the mean number of postoperative complications between those within the experimental group who received the booklet and those who did not. To ensure that hypothesized contrasts are orthogonal, three tests must be applied (*see also* Chapter 7):

First, there must be only $n - 1$ contrasts.
Second, the sum of each vector must equal zero. In the example the sum of $X1$ is (-1) $+ (-1) + 2 = 0$, and the sum of $X2$ is $1 + (-1) + 0 = 0$.
Third, the sum of the cross-products must equal zero. In the example $(-1 \times 1) + (-1 \times -1) + (2 \times 0) = 0$.

Table 12-5 shows some other examples of possible contrasts, given three groups. Are they all orthogonal? The vectors $X1$ and $X2$ reflect an orthogonal contrast, as do the vectors $Y1$ and $Y2$. Vectors $Z1$ and $Z2$ do not reflect an orthogonal contrast; group 1 is compared to group 2 and to group 3. The sum of the cross-products does not equal zero $([-1 \times 1] + [0 \times -1] + [1 \times 0] = -1)$.

In the regression equation with orthogonal coding, a is the grand mean of the dependent variable, and each b represents a hypothesized contrast.

Summary of Coding

Regardless of the method of coding used, the overall R^2 will remain the same, and so will its significance. Predictions based on the resulting prediction equations will be identical. The differences lie in the meaning attached to testing the b-weights for significance. With *dummy coding* the b-weight represents the difference between the mean of the group represented by that b and the group assigned 0s throughout.

In *effect coding* the bs represent the difference between the mean of the group associated with that b-weight and the grand mean. With *orthogonal coding* the b-weight measures the difference between two means specified in an hypothesized contrast.

As pointed out in Chapter 8 one can study the interaction among variables. Interactions among variables may be coded and entered into the regression equation. Suppose you had two categorical variables to code, group membership and sex.

TABLE 12-5
Contrasts

	Pairs of Vectors					
Group	*X1*	*X2*	*Y1*	*Y2*	*Z1*	*Z2*
1	2	0	−1	1	−1	1
2	−1	1	2	0	0	−1
3	−1	−1	−1	−1	1	0

Dummy coding will be used in this example, but any of the coding methods could be used. Figure 12-7 shows the basic design of the study. There are six mutually exclusive groups. We can now look at the effects of group membership, the effects of sex, and whether there is any interaction between group and sex. For example does the booklet reduce postoperative complications for women but not for men? Coding of an interaction is demonstrated in Table 12-6. (M and F are used for male and female.) The six groups formed by the design are listed. First, we code group membership. To do that ignore the sex variable. We need two group vectors and will call them $G1$ and $G2$. All EG1 subjects will be assigned 1 on $G1$; all other subjects will be assigned 0. All EG2 subjects will receive a 1 on $G2$; all other subjects will receive a 0. Only one vector ($S1$) is needed to code sex. Males are assigned 1s; females are assigned 0s.

In this example there are two vectors for group and one for sex, so there must be two (2 × 1) vectors to code the interaction between these two variables. These vectors are labeled $I1$ and $I2$. For $I1$ multiply $G1$ by $S1$, and for $I2$ multiply $G2$ by $S1$.

As shown in these examples coding is the way categorical variables and interactions are entered into the regression equation.

Groups

FIGURE 12-7
Design of study.

TABLE 12-6
Coding Interactions

	Vectors				
Groups	*G1*	*G2*	*S1*	*I1*	*I2*
EG1, M	1	0	1	1	0
EG1, F	1	0	0	0	0
EG2, M	0	1	1	0	1
EG2, F	0	1	0	0	0
Control, M	0	0	1	0	0
Control, F	0	0	0	0	0

MULTIPLE COMPARISONS AMONG MEANS

None of the coding methods allows us to make all the comparisons among mean scores that we might like. If we have three groups *A, B,* and *C,* and use dummy coding, we can compare the means of *A* and *B* with the mean of the control group *C* to see whether they are statistically different; however, we cannot compare the means of *A* and *B* by testing the *b*-weights. With effect coding we could compare the means of each of the three groups with the grand mean, but we could not compare *A* with *B, A* with *C,* and so on. With orthogonal coding, we are restricted to $n - 1$ orthogonal hypothesized contrasts.

As is discussed in Chapter 7, some contrasts can be measured "after the fact," that is, after the overall *F* is found to be significant. Using these *post hoc* tests, we can then compare each group with every other group or compare two groups with one group and so on. Given our two experimental groups (preoperative teaching plus booklet and preoperative teaching alone) and a control group, we could compare each experimental group with the control group, the two experimental groups, the two experimental groups together with the control group, and so forth. Measures for multiple comparisons among means allow us to explore all interesting differences in our data once we have an overall *F* that is significant.

SELECTING VARIABLES FOR REGRESSION

Because there is so much intercorrelation among variables used in behavioral research, we may want to select a subset of variables that does the best job of predicting a particular outcome. Usually, we want to find the smallest group of variables that will account for the greatest proportion of variance in the dependent variable. Using such information we can make practical decisions. If two predictors are equally good, we will probably decide to use the one that is easiest to administer, most economical, and so forth. Outlined here are some of the commonly used methods for selecting variables, including *standard, hierarchical,* and *stepwise.*

Standard

All the independent variables are entered at once. This is the method used in the computer analyses presented in this chapter. All variables are evaluated in relation to the dependent variable and the other independent variables through the use of partial correlation coefficients.

Hierarchical

The researcher may want to force the order of entry of variables into the equation. Suppose you want to know whether a particular intervention would improve pregnancy outcomes. You already have some givens, such as age, socioeconomic status, and nutritional status, and you would like to know whether your intervention makes a difference over and above factors that you cannot change. You might then enter the givens first and add your intervention last. As is shown in Chapter 15, this technique is used in developing *path* models. The variables may be entered one at a time or in subsets, but there should always be a theoretical rationale for the order of entry.

For example Norbeck and Anderson (1989), in testing the multivariate effects of life stress and social support on anxiety during pregnancy, controlled for ethnicity and marital status by entering them into the equation on the first step, before the life stress and social support variables.

Stepwise

Forward Solution

The independent variable that has the highest correlation with the dependent variable is entered first. The second variable entered is the one that will increase the R^2 the most over and above what the first variable contributed. We have four independent variables, and we calculated the correlations between each independent variable and the dependent variable and found the highest correlation to be 0.50. That independent variable enters the equation and accounts for 0.50^2, or 25%, of the variance. Now we want to know which of the three remaining variables will add the most to the 25% that is already explained. We cannot simply select the one with the next highest correlation with the dependent variable, because there is intercorrelation among the independent variables. Therefore, we, or more likely the computer, calculate partial correlations between each of the three remaining independent variables and the dependent variable. Thus, the effect of the first variable is removed from the correlation. The variable that has the highest partial correlation with the dependent variable enters next. Then the partials between the two remaining independent variables and the dependent variable, taking out the effects of the first two variables in the equation, would be calculated. The one with the highest partial correlation would be entered next. Various criteria may be set for entry into the regression equation. The 0.05 level of significance is often used. In that case a variable would have to contribute a significant ($p = 0.05$) amount of variance to be included in the analysis. Once none of the remaining independent variables can contribute significantly to the R^2, the analysis is ended.

Backward Solution

In this method we start with the overall R^2 generated by putting all of our independent variables in the equation. Then each variable is deleted, one at a time, to see whether the R^2 drops significantly. Each variable is tested to see what would happen if it were the last one entered into the equation. With four independent variables the following differences would be tested:

$$R^2y.1234 - R^2y.234 \qquad \text{tests for variable 1}$$
$$R^2y.1234 - R^2y.134 \qquad \text{tests for variable 2}$$
$$R^2y.1234 - R^2y.124 \qquad \text{tests for variable 3}$$
$$R^2y.1234 - R^2y.123 \qquad \text{tests for variable 4}$$

If for any of these variables there is a significant drop in R^2, that variable is contributing significantly and will not be removed. If all the variables contribute significantly, the analysis would end with all four variables remaining in the equation. If one is not significant, there would be three variables left in the equation. Then, each of those three variables would be tested to see whether it would contribute significantly if entered last. The analysis continues until all variables in the equation contribute significantly if entered last.

Stepwise Solution

The stepwise solution combines the forward solution with the backward solution and therefore overcomes difficulties associated with the other two solutions. With the forward solution once a variable is in the equation, it is not removed. No attempt is made to reassess the contribution of a variable once other variables have been added. The backward solution remedies that problem, but the order of entry is not clear (i.e., Which variable enters first and contributes most to the explained variance?).

With the stepwise solution, variables are entered in the method outlined under the heading Forward Solution and are assessed at each step using the backward method to determine whether their contribution is still significant, given the effect of other variables in the equation.

Maximum R^2 Improvement Technique

This technique is available in the SAS package program but not in the SPSS program. It is considered superior to the stepwise method because in addition to what occurs with the stepwise method, at each step every variable in the equation is compared with each variable that has not yet been entered into the equation. If an exchange of a variable in the equation for one of the remaining variables would increase the R^2, that exchange is made. "With this method, *all* exchanges are evaluated before any change is made. In the stepwise method, the 'worst' variable may be removed without considering what adding the 'best' variable might accomplish" (Helwig and Council, 1979, p. 392).

Summary of Methods of Entry

Selecting a method for entering variables into the equation is an important decision, because the results will differ depending on the method selected. Stepwise methods were in vogue in the 1970s, but they are less popular today. Because the order of entry is based on statistical, rather than theoretical, rationale, the technique is criticized for capitalizing on chance (Tabachnick & Fidell, 1983, pp. 101–107). This is because the entry is based on the correlations among the variables, and these correlations are not stable with time because error is involved in their measurement. This becomes more of a problem when dealing with variables with low reliability. Stepwise may be useful in exploratory work where model building is the goal rather than model testing (Tabachnick & Fidell, 1983, pp. 105–106).

ISSUES RELATED TO REGRESSION

Relationship Between Number of Independent Variables and Sample Size

Multiple regression is a useful technique, but there are numerous examples of its misuse. A major problem is including too many variables for the number of subjects. On the computer printouts we saw an adjusted R^2. It was smaller than the first R^2, a more conservative estimate given the number of subjects and variables. It also has been called a *shrinkage formula*, because it predicts how much the R^2 is likely to shrink. There are several formulas for this adjustment; one is given here:

$$R^2 = 1 - (1 - R^2)\frac{n - 1}{n - k - 1}$$

As you can see the formula is based on the number in the sample (n) and the number of independent variables (k). The more variables compared to subjects, the greater the shrinkage will be. If you put in the same number of subjects as independent variables, you will get a perfect R (1) no matter which variables you use. (However, the *adjusted R* will be zero!) Thus, you must always consider the number of subjects and independent variables. Very high and seemingly impressive R^2s may be an artifact of too few subjects. Nunnally (1978) suggests 30 subjects per independent variable. With only 10 subjects per variable, chance can greatly distort the results.

Cohen (1987) provides a formula for determining sample size, given an effect size index, which he calls L. He defines a small effect as an R^2 of 0.02, a moderate effect as an R^2 of 0.13, and a large effect as an R^2 of 0.30. The formula is

$$N = \frac{L(1 - R^2)}{R^2} + u + 1,$$

where N = total sample size

L = effect size index

u = number of independent variables

R^2 = desired effect

L can be obtained from a table and is defined by Cohen as a Function of Power and number of independent variables at a given level of alpha. For our example we select a power of 0.80, alpha of 0.05, a moderate effect size, and two different numbers of independent variables to determine appropriate sample sizes.

For three independent variables the value of L is 10.90, and the formula is

$$N = \frac{10.90(1 - 0.13)}{0.13} + 3 + 1$$

$$N = 77.$$

For six independent variables the value of L is 13.62, and the formula is

$$N = \frac{13.62(1 - 0.13)}{0.13} + 6 + 1$$

$$N = 98.$$

Software programs also can calculate sample size. Sample size must be determined prior to data collection to ensure an adequate sample to conduct the proposed analyses.

It is possible to increase the accuracy of the prediction by adding predictor variables to the equation. The best additional variables to add are those that are highly correlated with the dependent variable but not highly correlated with the other independent variables. Usually four or five predictors are enough. Adding more than that adds little to the R^2 because of intercorrelations among the predictors.

Because the analysis uses error variance and true variance, the multiple correlation is usually inflated by such error variance. In addition to the shrinkage formula, another way to evaluate the R^2 is to calculate it with a second sample. This is called *cross-validation*. A weakness of multiple regression is a tendency to throw variables into the equation. There should be some rationale for each variable included.

Multicollinearity

A problem for behavioral researchers is the interrelatedness of the independent variables. These variables provide very similar information, and evaluation of results is problematic. Schroeder (1990) provides detail on diagnosing and dealing with multicollinearity. Indications of the problem include high correlations between variables (>0.85); substantial R^2 but statistically insignificant coefficients; unstable regression coefficients (i.e., weights that change dramatically when variables are added or dropped from equation); unexpected size of coefficients (much larger or smaller than expected); and signs ($+/-$) that are unexpected (Lewis-Beck, 1980).

The *tolerance* of a variable is used as a measure of collinearity. It is the proportion of the variance in a variable that is not accounted for by the other independent variables (Norusis, 1990d). To obtain measures of tolerance, each independent variable is treated as a dependent variable and regressed on the other independent variables. A high multiple correlation indicates that the variable is closely related to the other independent variables. If the R^2 were 1, then the independent variable would be completely related to the others. Tolerance is simply $1 - R^2$; therefore, a tolerance of 0 ($1 - 1 = 0$)

would indicate perfect collinearity. The variable is a perfect linear combination of the other variables. Tolerances may be requested as part of the STATISTICS subcommand in SPSS. By default, tolerances are set as criteria for entry into regression equations. These values may be changed by the investigator.

Testing Assumptions by Analyzing Residuals

You should check the data before they are submitted to a regression procedure. Frequency distributions are assessed for outliers and for violation of normality of distributions. Scattergrams between variables are helpful to assess the shape of the relationship. Additionally, an important tool for checking the assumptions is residual analysis. Verran and Ferketich (1987) present an overview of the use of residual analysis to test linear model assumptions.

The residual is the difference between the actual and the predicted score. If the analysis were perfect, there would be no residuals; they would be zero.

Normal Distribution

If the relationships are linear, and the dependent variable is normally distributed for each value of the independent variable, then the distribution of the residuals should be approximately normal (Norusis, 1990a). This can be assessed by using a histogram of the standardized residuals. See Figure 12-8 for an example. (The data came from measures of patient satisfaction submitted for review by Munro, Jacobsen, and Brooten.)

① N indicates the observed number of residuals.

② Exp N is the number of residuals expected in a normal distribution.

③ The third column contains measures of the normal curve from $+3$ to -3 standard deviations from the mean (0.00).

④ In this example we see that 2 residuals fell more than $+3$ standard deviations above the mean.

⑤ No residuals were more than -3 standard deviations below the mean. Residuals that are more than 3 standard deviations from the mean should be examined.

The observed numbers are indicated by asterisks. Superimposed on the histogram are the expected frequencies, which are indicated by a period. A colon indicates an overlap between observed and expected frequencies. Although fairly normally distributed, this example indicates more scores at the mean and 0.33 standard deviations above the mean than would be expected. It is possible to transform the data mathematically, if residual analysis indicates violation of the assumption of normality.

Homoscedasticity

To check this assumption the residuals can be plotted against the predicted values and against the actual values. If the assumption is met, the residuals should form a rectangular band (i.e., the spread should be equivalent across the values of the variable). In Figure 12-9 **A** is a plot of the residuals against the predicted scores, and **B** is a plot of the residuals against the actual scores on a measure of good impression (GOODIMPR)

SPSS/PC+

```
Histogram - Standardized Residual

 (1)(2)
     N Exp N    (3)  (* = 2 Cases,     . : = Normal Curve)
(4)  2   .22    Out  *
     1   .45   3.00  *
     1  1.14   2.67  :
     1  2.60   2.33  :
     3  5.31   2.00  **.
     5  9.73   1.67  *** .
     7 15.97   1.33  ****    .
    16 23.47   1.00  ********    .
    31 30.91    .67  **************:*
    51 36.46    .33  ******************:*******
    67 38.52    .00  ******************:***************
    38 36.46   -.33  ****************:*
    28 30.91   -.67  **************.
     7 23.47  -1.00  ****        .
     8 15.97  -1.33  ****     .
    10  9.73  -1.67  ****:
     5  5.31  -2.00  **:
     4  2.60  -2.33  :*
     3  1.14  -2.67  :*
     3   .45  -3.00  **
(5)  0   .22    Out
```

FIGURE 12-8
Histogram of standardized residuals produced by SPSS/PC+.

(Munro, Jacobsen, & Brooten, manuscript submitted for review). We see that the spread is fairly equivalent, except for the middle, around the mean, where the spread is wider.

Linear Relationship

In addition to plotting the dependent variable against the independent variable in a scatter diagram, you can plot the residuals against the predicted values and against the actual values, as was done to test for homoscedasticity. If there is a pattern and they deviate from a horizontal band, there may be a nonlinear relationship. Look again at Figure 12-9. Note that there is no obvious pattern in the scatterplots.

CALCULATIONS

Simple Linear Regression Equation

The example used here to demonstrate the calculation of the regression equation is the same example we used for the Pearson Product Moment Correlation (see Table 11-7). See Table 12-7 for the calculations. Table 12-8 contains the calculations of the confidence intervals.

(text continues on page 221)

SPSS/PC+

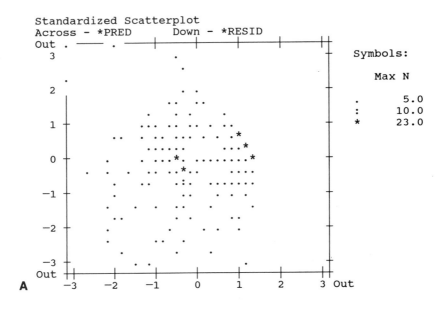

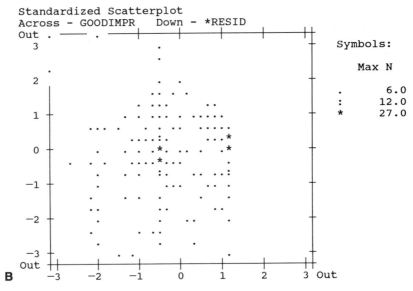

FIGURE 12-9
(**A**) Plot of residuals against predicted scores; (**B**) Plot of residuals against actual scores.

TABLE 12-7
Calculation of the Simple Linear Regression Equation

Subjects	Anger X	Perceived Stress Y	X^2	Y^2	XY
1	0	2	0	4	0
2	7	9	49	81	63
3	8	11	64	121	88
4	6	7	36	49	42
5	8	7	64	49	56
6	9	20	81	400	180
7	7	10	49	100	70
8	2	2	4	4	4
9	15	18	225	324	270
10	9	12	81	144	108
11	13	16	169	256	208
12	3	5	9	25	15
13	8	11	64	121	88
14	6	5	36	25	30
15	10	18	100	324	180
16	7	10	49	100	70
17	6	6	36	36	36
18	7	9	49	81	63
19	11	10	121	100	110
20	5	4	25	16	20
	147	192	1311	2360	1701

$$\overline{X} = 7.35 \qquad \overline{Y} = 9.6$$

CALCULATION OF SUM OF SQUARES

Sum of squares of X

$$\Sigma_x^2 = \Sigma X^2 - \frac{(\Sigma X)^2}{n}$$

$$= 1311 - \frac{(147)^2}{20}$$

$$= 230.55$$

Sum of squares of Y (total sum of squares)

$$\Sigma_y^2 = \Sigma Y^2 - \frac{(\Sigma Y)^2}{n}$$

$$= 2360 - \frac{(192)^2}{20}$$

$$= 516.80$$

Sum of squares of cross-products

$$\Sigma_{xy} = \Sigma XY - \frac{(\Sigma X)(\Sigma Y)}{n}$$

$$= 1701 - \frac{(147)(192)}{20}$$

$$= 289.8$$

(*continued*)

TABLE 12-7 (CONTINUED)
Calculation of the Simple Linear Regression Equation

CALCULATION OF REGRESSION WEIGHT AND CONSTANT

Regression weight	$b = \dfrac{\text{sum of squares of cross-products}}{\text{sum of squares of } X}$
	$b = \dfrac{\Sigma_{xy}}{\Sigma_{x}^{2}}$
	$b = \dfrac{289.8}{230.55}$
	$b = 1.26$
Constant	$a = \bar{Y} - b\bar{X}$
	$a = 9.6 - (1.26)(7.35)$
	$a = 0.339$

REGRESSION EQUATION

$$Y' = a + bX$$
$$Y' = 0.34 + 1.26X$$

CALCULATION OF R^2 AND F VALUE

Sum of squares for regression	$SS_{\text{regression}} = \dfrac{(\text{sum of squares of cross-products})^2}{\text{sum of squares for } X}$
	$SS_{\text{regression}} = \dfrac{(\Sigma xy)^2}{\Sigma_{x}^{2}}$
	$= \dfrac{(289.8)^2}{230.55}$
	$= 364.28$
Sum of squares for residual	$SS_{\text{residual}} = \text{total sum of squares} - \text{regression sum of squares}$
	$SS_{\text{residual}} = \Sigma_{y}^{2} - SS_{\text{regression}}$
	$= 516.8 - 364.28$
	$= 152.52$
Squared multiple correlation	$R^2 = \dfrac{SS_{\text{regression}}}{SS_{\text{total}}}$
	$= \dfrac{364.28}{516.80}$
	$= 0.70$
F value	$F = \dfrac{R^2/k}{(1 - R^2)/(n - k - 1)}$
	$= \dfrac{0.70/1}{(1 - 0.70)/(20 - 1 - 1)}$
	$= 41.92$

(*continued*)

TABLE 12-7 (CONTINUED)
Calculation of the Simple Linear Regression Equation

TABLED VALUES—APPENDIX D

With 1, 18 *df*
0.05 = 4.41
0.01 = 8.28

CALCULATION OF STANDARD ERROR OF ESTIMATE

$$S_{y \cdot x} = \sqrt{\frac{SS_{residual}}{n - k - 1}}$$

$$= \sqrt{\frac{152.52}{20 - 1 - 1}}$$

$$= 2.91$$

Summary

Multiple regression may be used for explanation and prediction. It is a flexible technique that allows the use of categorical, as well as continuous, variables. Overall, this is one of the most powerful techniques in our field, and if used wisely, it can be of great assistance in studying many problems related to human behavior and the health professions.

TABLE 12-8
Calculation of Confidence Intervals Around a Predicted Score

95% Y' ± 1.96 (standard error)
99% Y' ± 2.58 (standard error)

Example:

Susan scored 8 on the measure of anger. Her predicted score on perceived stress would be:

$$Y' = 0.34 + 1.26 (8)$$

$$= 10.42$$

95% Confidence interval

$$10.42 \pm (1.96) (2.91)$$

4.72 to 16.12

CANONICAL CORRELATION

When calculating a multiple correlation, you have more than one independent variable but only one dependent variable. Suppose, however, that you have more than one dependent variable. For example in a study of postmyocardial infarction (MI) patients, suppose we want to predict outcomes based on the patient's age, score on the Jenkins' Activity Survey, and type of MI. The outcomes (dependent variables) that we want to investigate are time to return to work and psychological adaptation. We could run two separate multiple regressions, with time to return to work as the dependent variable in one and psychological adaptation as the dependent variable in the other. That would not allow us to explore all the variation in the data, however. A method that takes all the information into account, thus giving a better understanding of all the relationships, is *canonical correlation*. This technique measures the relationship between a *set* of independent variables and a *set* of dependent variables. The method of least squares is used to give two composites, one for the independent variables, sometimes called the variables "on the left," and one for the dependent variables, or variables "on the right." (Many authors reserve the term *multivariate analysis* for situations in which there is more than one dependent variable.) Due to the complexity of the analysis, this technique was rarely used until sophisticated computer software became available. Use of the technique is increasing, and overviews of the method have been presented in the literature. For example Wikoff and Miller (1991) discussed the use of canonical analysis in a "Methodology Corner" in *Nursing Research*. Although the variables are weighted through the procedure of canonical correlation, the main emphasis of this technique is on assessing relationships, rather than on prediction. More than one canonical correlation coefficient can be generated from a single analysis, because each coefficient represents the relationship between one factor in one of the groups of variables and a related factor in the other group. In this way canonical correlation is like factor analysis. As is demonstrated in Chapter 14, there may be several factors in a group of variables. If there are three factors in one set of variables and three related factors in the second group of variables, three canonical correlation coefficients might emerge, one for each pair of factors. There cannot be more canonical correlation coefficients (Rcs) than there are variables in the smaller set. For example if you had four independent variables ($X1, X2, X3, X4$) and three dependent variables ($Y1, Y2, Y3$), the most Rcs that could be calculated is three. The variance accounted for by each Rc is unique. The first canonical correlation accounts for the largest amount of variance, the second accounts for the second largest amount, and so on. The procedure ends when no significant Rcs are left.

A *canonical variate* is a weighted composite of the variables in a set. It is a "new" variable or construct derived from the original variables. *Canonical weights*, which are in standard score form, are generated for each variable. Like standardized regression coefficients (betas), they are used more for explanation than for prediction. Because they are in standard score form, they indicate the relative importance of the variable with which they are associated. They must be interpreted with caution, however. Canonical weights, like the betas in regression equations, may be unstable because they may vary a great deal from one analysis to another. Because of this, many researchers prefer to interpret loadings called *structure coefficients*. These loadings represent the correlation between the canonical variates and the real (or original) variables. If there is a high correlation between the new variable (canonical variate) and the original variables, the canonical variate represents what the original variables were measuring. Loadings or structure coefficients of 0.30 or higher are treated as meaningful (Pedhazur, 1982, p. 732). They are interpreted like the loadings in factor analysis. The higher loadings give meaning to the canonical correlation and are used to name it. The square of a loading is the proportion of variance accounted for, so you can say how much of the variance is accounted for by an Rc.

To test the significance of a canonical correlation, Wilks' lambda (λ) is used. Lambda varies from 0 to 1 and stands for the error variance, the variance *not* accounted for by the independent variables. Thus, it is interpreted in an opposite way to the squared multiple correlation, R^2. A 1 means that the independent variables are *not* accounting for any of the variance in the dependent variable, and a 0 means that the independent variables are accounting for *all* of the variance. The *smaller* the lambda, the *greater* the variance accounted for. A $1 - \lambda$ would be equivalent to R^2. A chi-square statistic (called *Bartlett's test*) is used to test the significance of lambda.

The redundancy of the variables is often mentioned when canonical correlation results are presented. The higher the redundancy, or correlation, among a group of variables, the better the ability to predict from one group to another. Pender, Walker, Sechrist, and Frank-Stromberg (1990) used canonical correlation to determine the extent to which a set of six dimensions of health-promoting lifestyle could be explained by a set of seven cognitive–perceptual and modifying variables in the Health Promotion Model. Given six variables in the dependent set and seven in the independent set, the most canonical variates that could be extracted was six. In the analysis the criterion of meaningfulness was set at a squared canonical correlation (Rc^2) of greater than 0.10 (i.e., an explained variance of at least 10%). Using that criterion, three canonical correlates emerged (Table 12-9).

The first Rc accounted for 31.9% of the variance and indicated that higher levels of perceived personal competence, wellness, and overall health status and lower levels of control of health related to chance were related to the six dimensions of health-promoting lifestyle. The second Rc accounted for 18.4% of the variance and indicated that lower age, decreased belief that powerful others control health, and increased personal competence were related to higher self-actualization and interpersonal support and lower health responsibility. The third Rc accounted for 11.7% of the variance and consisted of a relationship between being female and interpersonal support.

Computer Analysis

The MANOVA program in SPSS/PC + was used to produce the canonical correlation. The data are from Munro, Jacobsen, and Brooten (manuscript submitted for review) (Fig. 12-10).

① The command line is for the procedure MANOVA. The variables before WITH (DISSATIS and GOODIMPR) are the dependent variables, and the other three variables (TALKING, RX, and GROUP) are the independent variables.

TABLE 12-9
Canonical Correlation Summary Table for Concurrent Measures of Health-Promoting Lifestyle Dimensions and Cognitive–Perceptual and Modifying Variables

Variable Sets	Canonical Variates		
	1	2	3
Health-Promoting Lifestyle Dimensions			
Self-actualization	.891*	.408	
Health responsibility	.720	−.601	
Exercise	.418		
Nutrition	.642		
Interpersonal support	.619	.367	.658
Stress management	.669		
Cognitive/Perceptual and Modifying Factors			
Control of health—chance	−.440		
Personal competence	.752	.492	
Definition of health—wellness	.508		
Health status overall	.529		
Control of health—powerful others		−.635	
Age		−.751	
Gender†			.956
Canonical correlation	.564	.429	.342
Explained variance	31.9%	18.4%	11.7%
Total variance explained 62.0%			
Canonical redundancy coefficient	.145	.024	.011
Total redundancy coefficient .180			

Note: N = 589.
* Structure coefficient.
† Coded as 0 = male, 1 = female.
(From Pender, Walker, Sechrist, & Frank-Stromberg [1990]. Predicting health-promoting lifestyles in the workplace. Nursing Research, 39[6], 330.)

② The subcommand DISCRIM requests the following coefficients:

RAW—raw coefficients
STAN—standardized coefficients
COR—correlations between the dependent and canonical variables

③ The PRINT command requests significance values for the multivariate analysis and for the univariate analyses. In the univariate analyses each dependent variable is regressed on the independent variables. EIGEN requests the canonical correlations and their associated eigenvalues.

④ No options are listed on the DESIGN command; therefore, this will be a

```
                                                 SPSS/PC+
(1) MANOVA DISSATIS GOODIMPR WITH TALKING RX GROUP

(2) /DISCRIM=RAW STAN COR

(3) /PRINT SIGNIF (MULTIV UNIV EIGEN)

(4) /DESIGN.
           291 cases accepted.
             0 cases rejected because of out-of-range factor values.
            16 cases rejected because of missing data.
             1 non-empty cells.

             1 design will be processed.

     * * ANALYSIS  OF  VARIANCE -- DESIGN   1 * *

     EFFECT .. WITHIN CELLS Regression
     Multivariate Tests of Significance (S = 2, M = 0, N = 142 )

(5)  Test Name            Value  Approx. F Hypoth. DF    Error DF  Sig. of F

     Pillais             .64052  45.07303      6.00      574.00      .000
     Hotellings        1.68104   79.84927      6.00      570.00      .000
     Wilks               .36932  61.53774      6.00      572.00      .000
     Roys                .62477

     Eigenvalues and Canonical Correlations

(6)  Root No.    Eigenvalue        Pct.    Cum. Pct.  Canon Cor.    Sq. Cor

            1         1.665      99.048      99.048        .790        .625
            2          .016        .952     100.000        .125        .016

     * * ANALYSIS  OF  VARIANCE -- DESIGN   1 * *

     EFFECT .. WITHIN CELLS Regression (CONT.)
     Univariate F-tests with (3,287) D. F.

(7)  Variable    Sq. Mul. R     Mul. R  Adj. R-sq.  Hypoth. MS    Error MS

     DISSATIS        .49270     .70192      .48739  5555.33786    59.79149
     GOODIMPR        .61727     .78566      .61326  8906.85288    57.72838

     Variable            F  Sig. of F

     DISSATIS     92.91185       .000
     GOODIMPR    154.28897       .000

(8) * * ANALYSIS  OF  VARIANCE -- DESIGN   1 * *
    Raw canonical coefficients for DEPENDENT variables
            Function No.

     Variable            1         2
     DISSATIS         .018      .164
     GOODIMPR        -.068      .129
```

FIGURE 12-10

Canonical correlation produced by SPSS/PC +. (*continued*)

⑨ Standardized canonical coefficients for DEPENDENT variables
               Function No.

Variable	1	2
DISSATIS	.198	1.771
GOODIMPR	-.830	1.577

⑩ Correlations between DEPENDENT and canonical variables
               Function No.

Variable	1	2
DISSATIS	.885	.466
GOODIMPR	-.994	.111

⑪ Raw canonical coefficients for COVARIATES
               Function No.

COVARIATE	1	2
TALKING	-.599	.706
RX	-.348	-.013
GROUP	-.335	-1.926

⑫ Standardized canonical coefficients for COVARIATES
               CAN. VAR.

COVARIATE	1	2
TALKING	-.466	.548
RX	-.630	-.024
GROUP	-.168	-.965

⑬ Correlations between COVARIATES and canonical variables
               CAN. VAR.

Covariate	1	2
TALKING	-.793	.327
RX	-.887	-.015
GROUP	-.429	-.851

FIGURE 12-10 (CONTINUED)

canonical correlation between the variables listed on the first line. With the smaller set containing two variables, the maximum number of canonical correlations that will emerge is two.

Dependent Variables

DISSATIS is a measure of patient dissatisfaction with care; a higher score indicates a higher level of dissatisfaction.

GOODIMPR is a measure of patient satisfaction with the overall impression of the nurse; a higher score indicates a better impression.

Independent Variables

TALKING is a measure of how talking with the nurse makes the patient feel better. A higher score indicates better results from talking with the nurse.

RX is a measure of how satisfied the patient is with the nurse's understanding of the treatment. A higher score indicates more satisfaction.

GROUP is a measure of group membership; 1 is the experimental group, and 0 is the control group.

⑤ All four of the multivariate tests of significance indicate that the analysis was significant. If there were only one dependent variable, all four of these measures would be equivalent to the overall F statistic in ANOVA or multiple regression. With more than one dependent variable, however, they are not always equivalent. Which one should you use? Norusis (1990b) states that two factors should be taken into account, power and robustness. In terms of power, from most to least powerful, the tests are Pillai's, Wilks', Hotelling's, and Roy's. (See the section on Multivariate Analysis of Variance in Chapter 8 for more detail on these measures.) In addition to being the most powerful, Pillai's trace also is the most robust; that is, it best withstands violations of the assumptions.

⑥ Two canonical correlations were produced. Eigenvalues are measures of the explained variance. In general an eigenvalue must equal at least 1 to represent a significant portion of the variance. See Chapter 14 for more information on this measure. The first canonical correlation squared (Rc^2) equals 0.625, which indicates that it explains 62.5% of the variance. The second canonical correlation explains less than 2% (0.016) of the variance.

⑦ The univariate F-tests are the regressions of each dependent variable taken separately on the independent variables. Both of those regressions were significant.

Next the coefficients associated with the dependent variables are presented.

⑧ The raw canonical coefficients are equivalent to the b-weights in regression and can be used to calculate predicted scores based on subjects' actual scores.

⑨ The standardized canonical coefficients are like the beta weights in regression. They are based on the standard scores of the variables and indicate the relative importance of each variable.

⑩ The correlations between the dependent and canonical variables are sometimes called structure coefficients and are what are usually interpreted when assessing the relationships between the two sets of variables. Values greater than 0.30 are treated as meaningful.

⑪, ⑫, and ⑬ These contain the coefficients for the independent variables (called COVARIATES on the printout).

The complete results of the regression of each of the dependent variables on the independent variables also is contained on the printout but has been eliminated here for ease of presentation. What would be examined to interpret these results in relation to the variables are the correlations between the variables and the canonical variables, sections 10 and 13. They are reproduced in Figure 12-11.

Using the rule that coefficients greater than 0.30 are meaningful, we can say that the first canonical variate indicates that being less satisfied with talking with the nurse and with the nurse's knowledge of the treatment and being in the control group are associated with being dissatisfied and having a lower overall impression of nursing. Being more satisfied with talking and the nurse's knowledge and being in the experimental group are associated with being more satisfied and having a higher overall impression of nursing.

```
Correlations between COVARIATES and canonical variables
        CAN. VAR.

Covariate              1               2

TALKING             -.793            .327
RX                  -.887           -.015
GROUP               -.429           -.851

Correlations between DEPENDENT and canonical variables
        Function No.

Variable               1               2
DISSATIS             .885            .466
GOODIMPR            -.994            .111
```

FIGURE 12-11

Coefficients for interpretation of canonical correlation.

Because the second variate has an eigenvalue of less than 1 and accounts for less than 2% of the variance, it would not be interpreted.

SUMMARY

Canonical correlation is an extension of multiple regression that enables the researcher to include more than one dependent variable in the analysis. It is a powerful technique that helps us study the complex relationships that exist in health-care research.

13 | Logistic Regression

*Barbara
Hazard Munro*

OBJECTIVES FOR CHAPTER 13

After reading this chapter you should be able to do the following:

1. **Determine when it is appropriate to use logistic regression.**
2. **Interpret a computer printout of a logistic regression analysis.**
3. **Evaluate research reports using this technique.**

As is described in the previous chapter, multiple regression has been used extensively by nurse researchers. It allows us to find the best fitting and most parsimonious model to describe the relationship between the dependent variable and a set of independent or predictor variables. While the independent variables can be of differing levels of measurement (nominal to ratio), the dependent variable is supposed to be measured at the interval or ratio level. Suppose, however, the outcome measure is categorical. For example in medical and epidemiologic studies, outcomes may be occurrence or nonoccurrence, mortality (dead or alive), and so forth. It is possible to code a dichotomous outcome variable as 1 or 0 and run a regression. In that case the statistics generated will be the same as if you ran what is called a discriminant function analysis. With more than two outcome categories, multiple regression cannot be used, and discriminant function or some other technique must be used. Until recently discriminant function analysis often was used to develop a model when the outcome measure was categorical. Today, more people are reporting logistic regression, especially when the outcome measure is dichotomous. People who have studied the methods report that logistic regression is better suited to the data, and the results include odds ratios that lend interpretability to the data. The odds of an outcome being present as a measure of association has found wide use, especially in epidemiology, because it approximates how much more likely (or unlikely) it is for the

Barbara Hazard Munro and Ellis Batten Page: STATISTICAL METHODS FOR HEALTH CARE RESEARCH, SECOND EDITION. © 1993, 1986 by J. B. Lippincott Company.

outcome to be present given certain conditions. For example when looking at lung cancer in smokers and nonsmokers, an odds ratio of 2 indicates that smokers had twice the incidence of lung cancer in the study population. The odds ratio approximates another indicator called relative risk. Before describing logistic regression, we present an overview of discriminant function analysis as the technique is reported in the literature.

DISCRIMINANT FUNCTION ANALYSIS

Discriminant function analysis allows us to distinguish among groups, based on some predictor variables. The mathematical function that combines information from predictor variables to obtain the maximum discrimination among groups is called the *discriminant function*. With two groups the results are the same as using multiple regression with a dummy-coded dependent variable.

What we are trying to find out using this technique is which set of predictors will most clearly distinguish among these groups. For example in a study of adaptation to chronic illness, Pollock, Christian, and Sands (1990) used discriminant function analysis to determine what factors differentiated among the following groups: rheumatoid arthritis, hypertension, and multiple sclerosis. They found that health promotion activities, psychological distress, physiological adaptation, and dependence on medications correctly classified 73% of the sample.

People who use this technique are interested in explanation and prediction. They want to know which factors are most related to these groups and how well they can predict group membership. The aim of the procedure is to find a way to maximize the discrimination among groups. As with canonical correlation, more than one statistic may be derived. The most discriminant functions that can be derived are one less than the number of categories in the dependent variable or the number of independent variables, whichever is smaller. The first discriminant function derived from the data is the one that explains most of the between-group variance. The second discriminant function explains the next largest piece of variance, and so on. These functions are not correlated with each other. All the variables may be entered at once, or a stepwise procedure may be used to select the most discriminating variables. Eigenvalues and their associated canonical correlations are used to judge the most discriminating variables. Eigenvalues represent the amount of variance explained by a discriminant function.

As with multiple regression each variable is weighted, and those weights may be used to calculate a discriminant score for each subject. The mean of the discriminant scores for a given group, for example the rheumatoid arthritis group (Pollock, Christian, & Sands, 1990), is called the *centroid*.

The discriminant functions are calculated by a method similar to factor analysis. Principal components analysis is used on a matrix of indices of discrimination between and within groups. This type of analysis discriminates among subjects, rather than among variables. Rotation may be used to increase the interpretability of the functions.

Wilks' lambda (Λ) is used to measure the association between the independent and dependent variables. Using the discriminant function scores the members of the known groups are classified to see how well the system works. We want to know what percent is classified correctly and what percent is classified incorrectly.

The analysis produces *raw coefficients* (like *b*s in multiple regression), *standardized coefficients* (like betas), and *structure coefficients* (like those in canonical correlation). The raw coefficients are commonly used for calculating scores for each individual. The standardized coefficients represent the relative importance of the independent variables with which they are associated. Like betas they should be interpreted with caution, however, because they tend to be unstable.

The correlations between the discriminant score for each individual and the scores on the original variables are called *structure coefficients*, or *loadings*. The square of that coefficient is the proportion of variance in a particular variable explained by the discriminant functions. Structure coefficients of 0.30 or greater are considered meaningful (Pedhazur, 1982, p. 704). These coefficients are used to interpret the discriminant functions.

Figure 13-1 contains results from the Pollock, Christian, and Sands (1990) study. Two discriminant functions were produced. The Figure (**A**) indicates that the first function discriminates between the rheumatoid arthritis group (RA) and the hyperten-

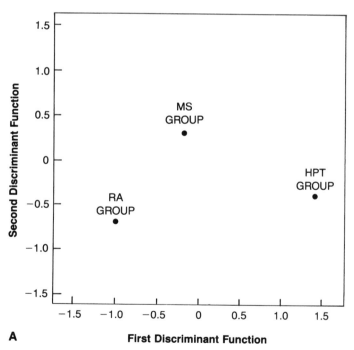

FIGURE 13-1
From Pollock, Christian, and Sands (1990, pp 302–303.) (*continued*)

Results of Discriminant Function Analysis of Predictor Variables for Three Diagnostic Groups (N = 208)

Predictor Variables	Correlations of Predictor Variables with Discriminant Functions	
	1	2
HLPRACT–Health Promotion	.24	.24
PSYDIS–Psych. Distress	.02	.41
PAXTOT–Physiological Adapt.	.17	.72
MEDS–Dependence on Meds.	.98	−.11

B

Discriminant Function Classification Results (N = 208)

Actual Group	No. of Cases	Predicted Group Membership		
		2	3	4
Group 2	43	34	3	6
Hypertension		79.1%	7.0%	14.0%
Group 3	42	3	32	7
Rheumatoid arthritis		7.1%	76.2%	16.7%
Group 4	123	6	31	86
Multiple sclerosis		4.9%	25.2%	69.9%
Percent of "grouped" cases correctly classified: 73.08				

C   Note: Three cases had at least one missing discriminating variable.

FIGURE 13-1 (CONTINUED)

sion group (HPT). (Their centroids are the farthest apart on that dimension.) Using the criterion of 0.30 or greater for the correlation of the predictor variables with the discriminant functions, we see that dependence on medications (0.98) is the variable contributing to the discriminating power of the first function (**B**). The arthritis group was much more dependent on medications than the hypertension group. Maximal separation on the second function occurs between the RA group and the multiple sclerosis group (MS). Psychological distress (0.41) and physiological adaptation (0.72) are contributing to this discrimination. The arthritis group had lower scores on physiological adaptation, and the multiple sclerosis group had higher psychological distress. The classification results are shown in (**C**). Overall, 73% of the cases were correctly classified.

When studying this method of analysis, the general conclusion is that discriminant function estimators are sensitive to the assumption of normality. In particular the estimators of the coefficients for non-normally distributed variables are biased away from zero. The practical implication for dichotomous independent variables is that the discriminant function estimators will overestimate the magnitude of the association (Hosmer & Lemeshow, 1989, p. 20).

According to Norusis (1990b), when the dependent variable has only two values—

either the event occurs or it does not—the assumptions underlying regression analysis are violated because the distribution of errors is not normal but binomial (because the outcome is either 1 or 0). Discriminant analysis does allow direct prediction of group membership, but the assumption of multivariate normality of the independent variables, as well as equal variance–covariance matrices in the two groups, is required for the prediction rule to be optimal. "Logistic regression requires far fewer assumptions than discriminant analysis; and even when the assumptions required for discriminant analysis are satisfied, logistic regression still performs well." (Norusis, 1990b, p. B-39). In logistic regression estimates of the probability of an event are given. As we will see, this provides information not obtainable from regression weights. The method of least squares is used in regression. The coefficients minimize the squared distances between the observed and predicted scores. (See Chapter 12, Regression, for more information.) In logistic regression the *maximum-likelihood method* is used. This means that the coefficients make our observed results most likely. The logistic model is nonlinear, when graphed the data assume an S-shaped curve. Because of this an iterative algorithm is necessary for parameter estimation. The reason this technique is used more often is that the computer software is now available.

LOGISTIC REGRESSION

Before giving an example of logistic regression, we need to explain some of the terms used with this analysis. An *odds ratio* is defined as the probability of occurrence over the probability of nonoccurrence. Table 13-1 contains fictional data to enable us to demonstrate calculations of an odds ratio. We see that of 450 women, 95 had a low birth weight infant (LBW), and 355 did not. Also, 200 of the women had prenatal care, and 250 did not. Table 13-2 contains probabilities based on the data in Table 13-1. The probability of having an LBW infant if no prenatal care was received is calculated as the number of LBW infants over the total number who received no prenatal care (75/250). The resulting probability is 0.3. In the same way the probability of a normal weight baby with no prenatal care is the number of normal weight babies over the total number in the no prenatal care group. Therefore, for women who have not received prenatal care the probability of having a normal weight baby is 0.7, and of having an LBW infant is 0.3. For those having prenatal care, the probabilities are 0.1 for LBW and 0.9 for normal weight. (Remember these numbers were simply contrived for this example.)

TABLE 13-1
Low Birth Weight

	Yes	No	Row totals
Prenatal Care			
No	75	175	250
Yes	20	180	200
	95	355	450

TABLE 13-2
Probabilities

PROBABILITY OF LOW BIRTH WEIGHT (LBW) WITH NO PRENATAL CARE

LBW
No prenatal care $\dfrac{75}{250} = 0.3$

PROBABILITY OF NORMAL WEIGHT WITH NO PRENATAL CARE

Normal weight
No prenatal care $\dfrac{175}{250} = 0.7$

PROBABILITY OF LBW WITH PRENATAL CARE

LBW
Prenatal care $\dfrac{20}{200} = 0.1$

PROBABILITY OF NORMAL WEIGHT WITH PRENATAL CARE

Normal weight
Prenatal care $\dfrac{180}{200} = 0.9$

The odds of an event are the probability of occurrence over the probability of nonoccurrence. The odds of these events are presented in Table 13-3. The odds of having an LBW infant with no prenatal care is 0.43 and with prenatal care is 0.11. The odds ratio, which is the ratio of one probability to the other, is calculated as 3.91 in Table 13-4. We can say then that the odds of having an LBW infant are almost four times greater when the woman has no prenatal care.

Odds ratios are used to estimate what epidemiologists call relative risk. A risk is the number of occurrences out of the total. Relative risk is the risk given one condition

TABLE 13-3
Odds

of (low birth weight) infant, when no prenatal care:

$$\frac{\text{Probability of occurrence}}{\text{Probability of nonoccurrence}} = \frac{0.3}{0.7} = 0.43$$

of LBW infant, with prenatal care:

$$\frac{\text{Probability of occurrence}}{\text{Probability of nonoccurrence}} = \frac{0.1}{0.9} = 0.11$$

TABLE 13-4
Odds Ratio

Ratio of one probability to the other

$$\frac{0.43}{0.11} = 3.91$$

versus the risk given another condition. Table 13-5 contains the calculation of the risks of LBW, with and without prenatal care. Table 13-6 contains a calculation of the relative risk. We see that the relative risk is three times higher for women with no prenatal care. The odds ratio is at least equal to relative risk but often overestimates it, especially if the occurrence of the event is not rare. Here the odds ratio was 3.91, and the relative risk was 3. Because odds ratios are generated by the logistic regression procedure, it is important to understand what they are and not confuse them with actual measures of relative risk.

Computer Analysis

In preparation for presentation at a conference held in Utah, the following example with fictitious data was contrived. The data are supposedly based on a survey of individuals attending this conference who have never skied before. See Figure 13-2 for the printout.

① The command line requests a logistic regression in which SKI is the dependent

TABLE 13-5
Risks of Low Birth Weight

Without prenatal care:

$$\frac{75}{250} = 0.3$$

With prenatal care:

$$\frac{20}{200} = 0.1$$

TABLE 13-6
Relative Risk

$$\frac{0.3}{0.1} = 3.0$$

① LOGISTIC REGRESSION SKI WITH ATHLETIC FEARHT MISTAKES.

> Total number of cases: 100 (Unweighted)
> Number of selected cases: 100
> Number of unselected cases: 0
>
> Number of selected cases: 100
> Number rejected because of missing data: 0
> Number of cases included in the analysis: 100

② Dependent Variable Encoding:

Original   Internal
Value   Value
0   0
1   1

Dependent Variable..   SKI   DECISION TO SKI

Beginning Block Number   0.   Initial Log Likelihood Function

③ -2 Log Likelihood   138.62944

* Constant is included in the model.

Beginning Block Number   1.   Method: Enter

④ Variable(s) Entered on Step Number
1..   ATHLETIC   ATHLETIC ABILITY
           FEARHT   FEAR OF HEIGHTS
           MISTAKES   WILLINGNESS FOR MISTAKES TO BE OBSERVED

Estimation terminated at iteration number 8 because
Log Likelihood decreased by less than .01 percent.

	Chi-Square	df	Significance
⑤ -2 Log Likelihood	15.986	96	1.000
Model Chi-Square	122.643	3	.0000
Improvement	122.643	3	.0000
Goodness of Fit	89.605	96	.6641

⑥ Classification Table for SKI
                    Predicted
                 NO   YES   Percent Correct
                 N   Y
Observed
   NO   N | 49 | 1 | 98.00%
                 |-------|-------|
   YES   Y | 1 | 49 | 98.00%
                 |-------|-------|
                      Overall   98.00%

⑦ --------------------- Variables in the Equation ---------------------

Variable	B	S.E.	Wald	df	Sig	R	Exp(B)
ATHLETIC	2.3238	.7539	9.5001	1	.0021	.2326	10.2148
FEARHT	-.3981	.2127	3.5023	1	.0613	-.1041	.6716
MISTAKES	3.7781	1.7323	4.7568	1	.0292	.1410	43.7346
Constant	-11.3533	3.8716	8.5992	1	.0034		

FIGURE 13-2

Logistic regression produced by SPSS/PC+.

or outcome measure, and ATHLETIC, FEARHT, and MISTAKES are the predictors or independent variables.

ATHLETIC (athletic ability) scored from 0 to 10, with 0 indicating no athletic ability and 10, highest ability.

FEARHT (fear of heights) also scored from 0 to 10, with 0 indicating no fear and 10, the greatest fear.

MISTAKES (willingness for mistakes to be obvious) scored as a dichotomous variable, yes or no.

There were 100 subjects.

② In dependent variable encoding, you can see that the original values and internal values are the same. The dependent variable was decision to SKI (yes or no). It was entered as 0 = no, and 1 = yes. This is appropriate coding for the logistic regression procedure, so the original (value given by the investigator) and internal (value assigned by the computer) are the same. If the data had been entered as yes = 1, and no = 2, for example, the variable would have been recoded.

Coding

Just as in multiple regression, categorical independent variables are coded. You can use dummy (indicator), effect (deviation), or orthogonal coding. In the new software for SPSS-PC, the computer will produce the dummy or effect coefficients for you. You name the variable and tell it what type of coding you want. You also can specify orthogonal contrasts.

Interaction terms also may be entered into the equation. This is especially important when considering risk factors. Does smoking and drinking coffee increase the odds of a myocardial infarction more than adding up odds of each taken separately?

−2 Log Likelihood

③ "The probability of the observed results given the parameter estimates is known as the *likelihood*. Since the likelihood measure is a small number, less than 1, it is customary to use −2 times the log of the likelihood as a measure of how well the estimated model fits the data" (Norusis, 1990, p. B-45). In regression we evaluate models with and without particular variables to determine if they are making a significant contribution to the explanatory power. In logistic regression comparison of observed to predicted values is based on the log likelihood (LL) function. A good model is one that results in a high likelihood of the observed results. This means a small value for −2 LL. The value for −2 LL is 138.62944.

④ The method is enter, which means that all the variables were entered in one step, not in a stepwise fashion. All three variables were entered on step 1. In the SPSS-PC program it is possible to use forward stepwise or backward stepwise or to enter variables in some particular order or by subsets.

Assessing the Overall Fit of the Model

⑤ This is the equivalent of the F test in the regression model. To test the null hypothesis that the observed likelihood does not differ from 1, the value of $-2LL$ is tested with a chi-square distribution with $N - p$ df, where N = number of cases, and p = number of parameters estimated.

We had 100 cases and four parameters estimated (three independent variables and one constant). So ours is $100 - 4 = 96$.

When the significance is large, you do not reject the null hypothesis that the model fits. In other words a nonsignificant result indicates that the model fits. A significant result indicates that it does not fit. Our probability is 1, indicating a perfect fit; obviously, contriving the data helps!

Model Chi-Square

The model chi-square is the difference between -2 LL for the model with only a constant and -2 LL for the complete model. In other words, Does adding our predictors do anything for the model? It tests the null hypothesis that the coefficients for all the independent variables equal 0. This is comparable to the overall F in regression. In our example we have 3 dfs for the difference in estimators between one model and the other. (We had 1 df in the first model and 4 in the second.) The result is significant ($p = 0.0000$). The null hypothesis is rejected, indicating that the three variables add to the model. The -2 LL was 138.62944 at the beginning step; after adding the variables it became 15.986. The difference between these two numbers, 122.643, is the model chi-square, or the explanatory power of the three independent variables.

Improvement

Improvement is the change in -2 LL between successive steps of building a model. It tests the null hypothesis that the coefficients for the variables added at the last step are 0. Because we had only one step, these numbers are the same. If we had requested a stepwise solution, these numbers would be different.

Goodness of Fit Statistic

This statistic compares the observed probabilities to those predicted by the model (like regression in which you compare the scores that would be predicted for each subject given the prediction equation with the scores they actually received). In other words it examines the residuals. This statistic also has a chi-square distribution, and the same df as -2 LL. In our example it also indicates a good fit of the model.

Classification Table

⑥ In our example we see that only two subjects were misclassified. One person the model predicted would ski did not, and one person who was not predicted to ski did. The model predicted equally well those who would and those who would not ski, 98% each. Many times models predict better in one category than the other.

The predicted classification is based on the probabilities, that is, greater than or less than 0.5. You cannot tell from the table whether the misclassified individuals had calculated probabilities that were close to the 0.5 level. You can change the rules if there are problems with misclassification in one direction or the other (i.e., you can change from 0.5 to some other value).

Variables in the Equation

⑦ The b-weights associated with each independent variable and the constant term are given in the first column. The b-weights in multiple regression are used to create a prediction equation; that is, knowing a person's score on each variable, we can use the weights and the constant term to predict the individual's score on some outcome measure. In logistic regression these weights are used to determine the probability of a subject doing one thing or the other. In our example this is the probability of skiing or not skiing. So instead of a score, as with the continuous variables used as dependent variables in regression, we will get a probability from 1 to 0. If the probability is greater than 0.5, the individual would be predicted to ski, if less than 0.5, not to ski. We demonstrate the formula for these calculations after explaining the other columns in this section.

The signs associated with the b-weights indicate the direction of the relationship. Because ski is coded 1 and do not ski is coded 0, we would predict that those who are more athletic and willing to let their mistakes be seen are more likely to ski, and those who are afraid of heights are less likely to ski.

The next column contains the standard errors for the predictors and the constant. In general a statistic is divided by its standard error to give the value that is tested for significance. For large sample sizes the test that a b coefficient is equal to 0 can be based on the Wald statistic, which has a chi-square distribution. When a variable has 1 *df*, the Wald statistic is simply the square of the result of dividing the b value by its standard error. For example the coefficient for ATHLETIC is 2.3238. Dividing that by the standard error of 0.7539 and then squaring the result equals the Wald value of 9.5001. (For categorical variables the Wald statistic has *df*s equal to one less than the number of categories.) The value is significant at the 0.0021 level.

Using the 0.05 level, two of the coefficients are significant, ATHLETIC ($p = 0.0021$) and MISTAKES ($p = 0.0292$), and one is not, FEARHT ($p = 0.0613$).

Unfortunately, the Wald statistic has a very undesirable property. When the absolute value of the regression coefficient becomes large, the estimated standard error is too large. This produces a Wald statistic that is too small, leading to nonsignificant results, even when the null hypothesis should be rejected. When you have a large coefficient, you should not rely on the Wald statistic for hypothesis testing. Instead, you should build a model with and without that variable and base your hypothesis test on the difference between the two likelihood-ratio chi-squares (Norusis, 1990b).

As is the case with multiple regression, the contribution of individual variables in logistic regression is difficult to determine. The contribution of each variable depends on the other variables in the model. This is a problem particularly when independent variables are highly correlated.

A statistic that is used to look at the partial correlation between the dependent variable and each of the independent variables is the R statistic. R can range in value from -1 to $+1$. A positive value indicates that as the variable increases in value, so does the likelihood of the event occurring. If R is negative, the opposite is true. Small values indicate small partial correlation.

In our example ATHLETIC has a partial correlation of .2326 with decision to ski, which means that with fear of heights and willingness to let mistakes be seen controlled, there is a correlation between SKI and ATHLETIC of .2326. Squaring that number indicates that 5.5% of the variance in SKI is contributed by perception of athletic ability.

Exp (B) is the odds ratio. Mathematically, this is e (the base of the natural logarithm, 2.718) raised to the power of b. In this example 2.718 raised to the power of 2.3238 (b for ATHLETIC) is 10.2148. Remember that the odds ratio is the ratio of one probability to the other. In this example it is the probability of deciding to ski over the probability of deciding not to ski. In linear regression b indicates the amount of change in the dependent variable for a one-unit change in the independent variable. To understand logistic coefficients, we need to think in terms of the odds of an event occurring. The logistic coefficient (b) is the change in the log odds associated with a one-unit change in the independent variable with the other variables held constant. Thus, if ATHLETIC went up one point, the log odds would go up 10.2148.

Example

We will use an example to help clarify the relationships expressed in this table of variables in the equation. The probability of an event is determined by the following formula:

$$\frac{1}{1 + e^{-z}}$$

e = base of the natural logarithm, 2.718

z = constant + $b1X1$ + $b2X2$ + $b3X3$ + ...

In our example:

$z = -11.3533 + 2.3238 \text{ (ATHLETIC)} - 0.3981 \text{ (FEARHT)} + 3.7781 \text{ (MISTAKES)}$

Ratings of two individuals:

	Jane	*Susan*
Athletic	6	4
Fearht	5	6
Mistakes	1	0

Looking at the ratings we see that Jane rates herself as slightly better than average (6) in athletic ability, with a moderate fear of heights (5) and an ability to let others see her mistakes (1). Susan rates herself lower in terms of athletic ability (4), has a greater fear of heights (6), and does not like people to see her mistakes (0). Let's see what the probability of each of these deciding to ski is, given the data collected.

First, the z-scores for each individual are calculated as:

Jane	$z = -11.3533 + 2.3238(6) - 0.3981(5) + 3.7781(1)$
Susan	$z = -11.3533 + 2.3238(4) - 0.3981(6) + 3.7781(0)$
Jane	$z = 4.3771$
Susan	$z = -4.4467$

The formulas for determining the estimated probabilities of these individuals deciding to ski are:

Jane	$\dfrac{1}{1 + 2.718^{-4.3771}}$
Susan	$\dfrac{1}{1 + 2.718^{-(-4.4467)}}$
Jane	$1/1.0126 = 0.9876$
Susan	$1/86.3055 = 0.0116$

Because Jane's probability is greater than 0.5, we would predict that she would decide to ski. Susan's probability is less than 0.5, so she would be predicted to stay off the slopes.

As we pointed out the odds of an event are the probability of occurrence over the probability of nonoccurrence. Thus, for our subjects the odds of deciding to ski are:

| Jane | $\dfrac{0.9876}{1 - 0.9876} = 79.65$ |
| Susan | $\dfrac{0.0116}{1 - 0.116} = 0.0117$ |

and the odds ratio is:

$$\frac{79.65}{0.117}$$

The odds ratio is 6807.69; Jane is more than 6000 times as likely to ski as Susan!

If the score on a given variable goes up 1 point, the log odds go up by the amount listed under exp (B), which is the odds ratio. For example suppose a third individual, Harry, had the same scores as Susan, except on MISTAKES he scored 1 instead of 0. His z-score would be calculated as:

$z = -11.3533 + 2.3238(4) - 0.3981(6) + 3.7781(1)$
$z = -0.6686$

Estimated probability:	$\dfrac{1}{1 + 2.718^{-(-0.6686)}} = 0.3388$
Odds for Harry:	$\dfrac{0.3388}{1 - 0.3388} = 0.5124$
Odds ratio for Harry and Susan:	$\dfrac{0.5124}{0.0117} = 43.7$

The odds for Harry skiing are 43.7 times higher than the odds for Susan skiing (odds ratio), even though the only change in their scores was a 1-point change on the variable, MISTAKES. If we had changed his score 1 point on ATHLETIC only, then his odds would have been 10 times higher than Susan's.

Comparing Susan and Harry

	Susan	Harry
Probability	0.0116	0.3388
Odds	0.0117	0.5124 (up by 43.7346)
Log odds	− 4.448	− .6686 (up by 3.7781)

If you take the natural log of the odds and compare them by subtracting − 0.6686 from − 4.448, Harry's log odds went up by 3.7781, which is the value for the *b*-weight associated with MISTAKES.

The clearest use of the odds ratio is when the independent variable is categorical. Then the odds ratio tells us what happens when you change one variable from 0 to 1. It is not as interesting when the change is just 1 point on a scale (say from 1 to 20). You can calculate the odds for some more meaningful change, perhaps 5 points by multiplying the *b* value by the change you want and then performing an exponentiation on that number.

For ATHLETIC if 3 points was of interest, $2.3232 \times 3 = 6.9696$. Raising 2.718 to the power of $6.9696 = 1063.8$, so for every 3-point increase in ATHLETIC, the odds go up 1064 times.

Because the odds ratio is usually the parameter of interest in a logistic regression, due to its ease of interpretation, it is important to be aware that as a point estimate, the distribution is skewed, because it is bounded away from zero. If the sample size is large enough, this is not a problem. Confidence intervals often are used to demonstrate more clearly the odds ratio. These interval estimates are provided in some software packages. (You perform an exponentiation on the usual formula; that is, you raise 2.718 to a power derived from the *b*-weight $\pm 1.96 \times$ the standard error.)

Example from the Literature

Logistic regression was used to determine the probability of having a premature or LBW infant based on predictors, including maternal education, race, weight gain, and mother's age at birth (Ketterlinus, Henderson, & Lamb, 1990). Using the results of this analysis the investigators constructed a table listing the estimated probabilities. This is a good example of the use of the odds ratios (Table 13-7). A practitioner, making note of a client's demographics, could determine the probabilities from this table. For example a 16-year-old African-American woman with 12 years of education and light weight gain would have a 0.27 probability of having a premature birth and a 0.23 probability of having an LBW infant.

TABLE 13-7

Estimated Probabilities of Giving Birth to a Premature or Low Birth Weight (LBW) Infant by Maternal Race, Education, Age, and Pregravid Weight and Pregnancy Weight Gain

| Race | Maternal Education (Year) | Age at Birth (Year) | Premature Birth* | | LBW | |
			Light Weight Gain	Normal Weight Gain	Light Weight Gain	Normal Weight Gain
Black	0–11	13–15	.47	.41	.29	.13
		16–18	.30	.26	.28	.13
		19–21	.29	.24	.23	.10
		22–30	.29	.24	.33	.16
	12	13–15	.43	.37	.25	.11
		16–18	.27	.22	.23	.10
		19–21	.26	.21	.19	.08
		22–30	.25	.21	.28	.13
	13+	13–15	.39	.33	.20	.09
		16–18	.24	.20	.19	.08
		19–21	.23	.18	.16	.06
		22–30	.22	.18	.23	.10
White	0–11	13–15	.42	.36	.18	.08
		16–18	.26	.22	.17	.07
		19–21	.25	.20	.14	.06
		22–30	.25	.20	.21	.09
	12	13–15	.38	.32	.15	.06
		16–18	.23	.19	.14	.06
		19–21	.22	.18	.11	.05
		22–30	.22	.18	.17	.07
	13+	13–15	.34	.29	.12	.05
		16–18	.20	.17	.11	.05
		19–21	.19	.16	.09	.04
		22–30	.19	.15	.14	.06

Coefficients are adjusted for memory bias.

SUMMARY

Logistic regression is now more commonly reported when the outcome measure is categorical. As with all methods of regression it is of utmost importance to select variables for inclusion in the model based on clear scientific rationale. One can use a stepwise method (forward or backward) in which variables are selected strictly on statistic criteria. An alternative selection method is *best subsets*. Stepwise, best subsets, and other mechanical selection procedures have been criticized because they are based solely on correlations derived from variables measured with some error. Following the fit of the model, the importance of each variable included in the model should be verified (Norusis, 1990b). This should include the examination of the Wald statistic for each variable and a comparison of each estimated coefficient with the coefficient from the univariate model containing only that variable. Variables that do not contribute to the model based on these criteria should be eliminated and a new model fit. The new model should be compared to the old model through the likelihood ratio test. Once you have obtained a model that you believe contains the essential variables, you should consider whether to add interaction terms.

As with regression, residuals may be examined to evaluate the model. The residuals in logistic regression are the differences between the observed and predicted probabilities of an event. They should be normally distributed with a mean of 0 and a standard deviation of 1.

Deviance compares the predicted probability of being in the correct group based on the model to the perfect prediction of 1. It can be viewed as a component of -2 LL, which compares a model to the perfect model. Large values for deviance indicate that the model does not fit the case well.

Logistic regression programs are available with most of the software packages for the personal computer; they manage model building with a dichotomous outcome variable very well and provide the additional benefit of odds ratios, which lend interpretability to the data. Programs for managing outcomes with more than two categories are not as widely available.

14

Grouping Techniques

Jane Karpe Dixon

OBJECTIVES FOR CHAPTER 14

After reading this chapter you should be able to do the following:

1. **Identify research situations in which factor analysis would be appropriate.**

2. **Describe the steps involved in carrying out a factor analysis procedure.**

3. **Interpret factor analysis results from a computer printout or published study.**

4. **Appreciate the potential value of confirmatory factor analysis or cluster analysis in supplementation of the results of exploratory factor analysis.**

FACTOR ANALYSIS

Researchers in the health-care fields often focus their attention on multiple variables. This is a direct result of the nature of the problems under study, which are complex in the real world of patient care. For example with regard to major causes of illness and death in the developed world (e.g., cancer, heart disease, stroke, diabetes, accidents), we have learned to speak of risk factors rather than one single cause. In some cases a particular disease may exist only in the presence of a particular agent (e.g., clinical mononucleosis with the Epstein-Barr virus). Even then, however, variables describing personal and environmental characteristics are crucial in influencing the course of the illness or even whether symptoms occur. Also, multiple issues affect such nursing concerns as recuperation following surgery and compliance with health-care recommendations. In other chapters of this book we discuss how multivariate strategies can be used to

Barbara Hazard Munro and Ellis Batten Page: STATISTICAL METHODS FOR HEALTH CARE RESEARCH, SECOND EDITION. © 1993, 1986 by J. B. Lippincott Company.

understand the way multiple causes may lead to a single event. Factor analysis is often an early step in the process of achieving a multivariate perspective on a clinical research problem.

This chapter addresses the understanding of *concepts*. Often, when labeling variables, a single word or phrase is used to represent a phenomenon with multiple parts. Our language may be overly general, blending together the multiple aspects of the phenomenon of interest. Consider, for example, the term *satisfaction* with care. Superficially, it seems logical to measure this with a single rating. ("Rate your satisfaction with the care you received.") However, with thought we realize that such a rating might involve opinions on a variety of matters, such as perceived competence of caregivers, convenience, and pleasantness of the environment. (As an exercise, think of at least two other aspects of satisfaction with care.) It is hard to know which of these influences are reflected in a subject's satisfaction rating and what such a rating really means. Instead of a global rating, should several aspects be measured separately? There are so many potentially important variables, we may feel at a loss to decide which should be measured and which should not. Factor analysis can help us make such decisions.

The amount of information on which our minds can focus simultaneously is limited. As a convenience we may concentrate on factors thought to be primary. This will reduce the data burden. In some research endeavors, however, simplicity of questionnaire may not be necessary, because we have techniques for organizing such data. Factor analysis is one of these techniques. Factor analysis and related techniques serve the purpose of *data reduction*. In factor analysis a large number of variables are "reduced" (grouped) into a smaller number of factors. This is analogous to univariate approaches in which a mean, variance, or correlation coefficient is calculated to reduce individual scores on one or two values. In this chapter the purposes of factor analysis are explained, and the steps used to carry out a factor analysis are introduced. Because factor analysis is a very complex technique, almost exclusively carried out by computer, this chapter emphasizes interpretation rather than calculation. Confirmatory factor analysis, an advanced form of factor analysis, is introduced. The chapter concludes with a brief section on the related technique of cluster analysis.

For further information regarding factor analysis, the reader may consult Child (1990).

HYPOTHETICAL EXAMPLE OF A FACTOR ANALYSIS

A hypothetical example of a factor analysis situation may be helpful. Suppose a researcher measures six variables within a sample of adult male participants in a health maintenance organization (HMO). Three of these variables are aspects of body size: height, arm length, and leg length. Three are derived from a health history in which the subject is asked to report the number of specific episodes occurring in the last year. These variables are number of sore throats, number of headaches, and number of earaches. In the matrix of correlations for these six variables, we will probably see that the three size variables have high intercorrelations and that the three history variables also have high intercorrelations; that is, a man with longer than average legs, also may

TABLE 14-1
Six by Six Correlation Matrix: Size and History Variables

	Height	Arm Length	Leg Length	Number of Sore Throats	Number of Headaches	Number of Earaches
Height	—	high	high	low	low	low
Arm length		—	high	low	low	low
Leg length			—	low	low	low
Number of sore throats				—	high	high
Number of headaches					—	high
Number of earaches						—

High means correlation of high magnitude, regardless of direction (approaching + 1.00 or approaching − 1.00). Low means correlation of low magnitude (near zero).

have longer than average arms. He is also likely to be taller than average. A person reporting frequent sore throats also may report other discomforts. On the other hand it would be surprising if the size variables and the history variables were highly related.

A simplified representation of a correlation matrix is shown in Table 14-1. If such a matrix is factor analyzed, a factor matrix defining the two groups of variables would be derived, as shown in Table 14-2. Each column in this table reflects one of the variable groupings or factors. The size variables have high values in one column, and the history variables have high values in the other column. This table, indicating the presence of two distinct groups of variables—two factors—summarizes the information contained in the larger correlation matrix. It reduces the data. Much of the information from a 6 × 6 correlation matrix is conveyed in a 6 × 2 factor matrix.

TABLE 14-2
Abbreviated Factor Matrix: Size and History Variables

	Factors	
Variables	*I*	*II*
Height	high	low
Arm length	high	low
Leg length	high	low
Number of sore throats	low	high
Number of headaches	low	high
Number of earaches	low	high

High means above 0.40 or blow − 0.40—especially approaching 1.00 or − 1.00.
Low means between − 0.40 and + 0.40—especially near zero.

You may object that the groupings derived were already easily apparent from the correlation table and that one does not need an advanced statistical technique to show what is already obvious. This is true, but in the usual case, factor analysis does help us know what we would not otherwise know. Suppose that we had a 20 × 20 correlation matrix with widely ranging correlation coefficients, and the groupings among the variables were subtle. The variables would appear in random order, rather than neatly arranged according to grouping. Then patterns will not be obvious. Factor analysis is a tool through which we may study groupings of variables that are *not* obvious. A more realistic example follows.

EXAMPLE FROM PUBLISHED RESEARCH

A study by Walker, Sechrist, and Pender (1987) was designed to support development of an instrument to measure health-promoting lifestyle. Factor analysis was used as one aspect of the instrument development process.

For this instrument items were originally created to fit into 10 categories—all components of a health-promoting lifestyle. These 10 original categories are as follows: general health practices, nutrition, physical or recreational activity, sleep, stress management, self-actualization, sense of purpose, relationships with others, environmental control, and use of the health-care system. A 4-point response format was used so that for each item the subject would indicate frequency of the described behavior through choice of the responses *never, sometimes, often,* or *routinely.* The researchers approached individuals and groups in a variety of community settings; 952 subjects were obtained.

When creating an instrument it is common practice to write many more items than will eventually be kept as a part of the instrument; those that do not perform well are eliminated. In this study the researchers began with 107 items, but only 48 items were included as variables in the final factor analysis. (A correlation matrix of 48 × 48 may seem small but would still boggle the mind.) This factor analysis yielded six groupings or factors, rather than the 10 that were expected. The researchers point out that each of these six was conceptually similar to one of the original categories or to a combination of two of the original categories; however, one of the 10 original categories was not represented in the six final factors.

Table 14-3 represents the factor analysis results from the article. Note that this table presents 48 items (rows) and six factors (columns). However, the actual number associating the item with the factor is listed only if it is above a certain cutoff point—in this case 0.35 or higher. Based on the way the items grouped together, the researchers labeled each factor with a name, as shown in the footnote at the bottom of the table. However, the meaning of each factor is best conveyed by the items within it. That is why the authors present this information in such detail in their article. The name of the factor is simply the researchers' attempt to summarize this meaning.

As an exercise, take a few minutes to think about each grouping of items. If this were your study, what names would you have chosen?

Because of this analysis, Walker, Sechrist, and Pender (1987) changed their ideas

TABLE 14-3
Example of Published Factor Analysis Results

FACTOR LOADINGS AND FACTOR STRUCTURE FOR THE HEALTH-PROMOTING
LIFESTYLE PROFILE (*N* = 952)

Items	Factors*					
	1	2	3	4	5	6
Enthusiastic/optimistic	.70				.38	
Like myself	.70					
Growing/changing	.68				.37	
Long-term goals	.59					
Feel happy/content	.72					
Aware of strength/ weakness	.55					
Look forward to future	.61					
Set realistic goals	.55					
Know what is important	.62				.41	.38
Respect accomplishments	.68					
Find days challenging	.71					
Life has purpose	.71				.37	
Satisfying environment	.58					
Check cholesterol level		.45				
Report symptoms to M.D.		.54				
Read books about health		.45	−.40			
Question M.D./second opinion		.42				
Discuss health concerns		.69			.42	
Check blood pressure		.60				
Seek information		.75			.40	
Attend environmental programs		.49				
Observe body for changes		.48			.44	
Attend health care programs		.49	−.43			
Do stretching exercise			−.78			
Vigorous exercise 3 times/ week			−.82			
Supervised program		.37	−.63			
Recreational activities			−.55			
Check pulse rate		.40	−.57			
Eat breakfast				.75		
Eat 3 meals daily				.85		
No preservatives				.38		
Read labels		.39		.39		
Eat roughage/fiber				.47		
Basic 4 food groups				.50		.39
Discuss concerns/problems					.53	

(continued)

TABLE 14-3   (CONTINUED)
Example of Published Factor Analysis Results

FACTOR LOADINGS AND FACTOR STRUCTURE FOR THE HEALTH-PROMOTING
LIFESTYLE PROFILE (*N* = 952)

	*Factors**					
Items	1	2	3	4	5	6
Praise others easily	.36				.53	
Enjoy touching	.37				.70	
Maintain meaningful interpersonal relationships	.60				.59	
Time with close friends	.44				.56	
Express concern/love					.49	
Touch/am touched	.36				.69	
Daily relaxation time						.44
Aware of stress sources						.35
Meditation/relaxation						.51
Relax muscles before sleep						.54
Pleasant bedtime thoughts	.38					.48
Express feelings	.55				.43	.51
Use stress control methods	.55					.53

Factors are: 1, Self-Actualization; 2, Health Responsibility; 3, Exercise; 4, Nutrition; 5, Interpersonal Support; 6, Stress Management.

(From Walker, S. N., Sechrist, K. R., & Pender, N. J. [1987]. The health promoting lifestyle profile: Development and psychometric characteristics. Nursing Research, 36, 76–81.)

about the structure of their instrument, concluding that it consists of six subscales, as shown in Table 14-4 (also from the published article). As shown in the right-hand column labeled "alpha" (for alpha coefficient), internal consistency reliabilities of the subscales were acceptable. That is, within each subscale, the items correlated with each other; they seem to be measuring approximately the same thing. Based on these analyses the researchers concluded that the health-promoting lifestyle profile could be used effectively with other populations and that it measures six dimensions of healthy lifestyle.

TYPES OF FACTOR ANALYSIS

Factor analysis is a statistical tool for analyzing scores on large numbers of variables to determine whether there are any identifiable dimensions that can be used to describe many of the variables under study. One assumes that observed covariation between variables is due to some underlying common factors. This collection of intercorrelations are treated mathematically in such a way that underlying traits are identified.

TABLE 14-4
**Subscales Derived through Factor Analysis
and Their Alpha Reliabilities**

INTERNAL CONSISTENCY OF THE HEALTH-PROMOTING LIFESTYLE PROFILE
AND ITS SUBSCALES ($N = 952$)

Subscales	Number of Items	Alpha
Self-actualization	13	.904
Health responsibility	10	.814
Exercise	5	.809
Nutrition	6	.757
Interpersonal support	7	.800
Stress management	7	.702
Health-Promoting Lifestyle Profile	48	.922

(From Walker, S. N., Sechrist, K. R., & Pender, N. J. [1987]. The health promoting
lifestyle profile: Development and psychometric characteristics. Nursing Research,
36, 76–81.)

As implied in the chapter objectives, factor analysis may be exploratory or confirmatory. In exploratory factor analysis one summarizes data by grouping together variables that are intercorrelated. This occurs in the early stages of research. Confirmatory factor analysis tests hypotheses about structure of variables. This may follow an exploratory analysis, or it may come directly from theory.

Another way of thinking about the type of factor analysis focuses on what is being correlated by using the correlation matrix. Most commonly, the correlations are between variables and across subjects. This is referred to as R-type. This type of factor analysis dominates the research literature of nursing and other health-care professions.

However, it is also possible to construct a correlation matrix based on correlation between subjects and across variables. (That is, a data matrix is transposed so that each row represents a variable, and each column represents a subject prior to calculation of correlations; this can be done easily in some software programs.) A factor analysis performed on such a correlation matrix is Q-type. In such an analysis subjects, rather than variables, are grouped together. However, a superior alternative to such a factor analysis of subjects is cluster analysis, which is described later in this chapter.

In P-type factor analysis correlations represent relationships across time (repeated measures from a single person). P-type factor analysis reveals groupings of variables across time.

Except in the brief section on cluster analysis, this chapter focuses on R-type factor analysis, which is the most common type used in research within the health-care professions.

USE OF FACTOR ANALYSIS

The direct purpose of factor analysis is to reduce a set of data so that it may be described and used easily. Other purposes include instrument development (as indicated in the previous example), and theory construction (described in more detail in Chapter 16).

Instrument Development

In the research literature of nursing and other health-care professions, factor analysis is most often used as a part of the instrument-development process. Factor analysis may be a vital part of creating a new measurement tool. It is a method for organizing the items into *factors*. A factor is a group of items that may be said to belong together. A person who scores high on one item is likely to score above average on others, and vice versa. Such an item has high correlations with other items of the same factor and not so high correlations with items of different factors. This principle provides the mathematical basis for assignment of items to factors through the statistical technique of factor analysis.

Factor analysis is often used to test the validity of ideas about items to decide which items should be included. Such factors justify our use of *summated scales* (sets of items summed into a single scale score). In the study by Walker, Sechrist, and Pender (1987) described previously, some items were dropped out based on preliminary factor analysis results. Factor analysis is the most important statistical tool for validating the structure of our instruments. In most cases, as in the Walker, Sechrist, and Pender (1987) study, the establishment of validity through factor analysis is followed by computation of Cronbach's alpha coefficient, which is a measure of internal consistency reliability. Such reliability is an alternative way of looking at the extent to which items go together, similar to the factor analysis itself; however, in computation of reliability only one set of items is dealt with at a time. Also, reliability computations are useful for further identifying weak items that may be omitted in subsequent analysis. In any case items found to form a strong factor in factor analysis generally may be expected to yield acceptable alpha coefficients, thus providing evidence of internal consistency reliability, as well as evidence of construct validity for a developing scale.

Theory Development

The building of theory is a principal purpose of research, and factor analysis may support such efforts in a variety of ways—to describe clinical phenomena, to explore relationships, to identify (name) constructs that unite a set of elements, to create units of classification for systems construction, and even to test hypotheses. All of these are theory building functions.

Most basically, approaches to factor analysis may be distinguished as exploratory or confirmatory or in some intermediate position between these poles. Although the emphasis in this chapter is on exploratory approaches (because this is the most reasonable starting point for the beginning user of factor analysis), confirmatory approaches also are addressed, and Chapter 16 shows that structural modeling with latent variables incorporates factor analysis into a series of procedures with confirmatory purposes. In a truly exploratory approach a researcher uses factor analysis to discover a structure that can be meaningfully interpreted. The researcher begins without preconceived expectations about the nature of the structure that will emerge; rather, the structure is allowed to unfold from the data. In a truly confirmatory approach a hypothesis is developed, and variables relevant to that hypothesis are then identified and (once data are collected) submitted to factor analysis. The researcher asks whether the data fit the hypothesized model better than they fit alternative models. Confirmatory factor analysis has received increasing attention in nursing and other health-care research areas in the last decade. More details on this approach appear later in this chapter.

Data Reduction for Subsequent Analysis

Sometimes factor analysis is used solely for data reduction, because such reduction may be needed for subsequent analysis. One goal of scientific inquiry is *parsimony*, simplicity of explanation; that is, it is preferable to use one variable, rather than many, to explain a phenomenon. Factor analysis provides a means for creating a single composite variable out of many variables. Often, it is used to identify several composite variables, which taken together summarize the sources of variance contained in all (or most) variables included in a study (or at least of those variables of a particular type). These composite variables are mathematically constructed through a combination of the measured variables. The several composite variables, rather than the larger number of measured variables, are then used in subsequent data analysis. Data reduction of this sort may serve a highly pragmatic function. The researcher may collect a large amount of data, reduce the data through factor analysis, and conduct other analyses (such as regression or analysis of variance) on the reduced data. In these subsequent analyses the number of variables relative to the number of subjects is kept within reasonable bounds, reliability is augmented, and, provided that the meanings of factors are clearly defined and communicated, interpretation of the analysis may be simplified. Often, such purpose is combined with instrument development or theory development. Brown and Tanner (1990) used four subscales, derived through factor analysis, as independent variables in a regression analysis. These concerned various aspects of Type A behavior in preschool children. The dependent variable in the regression was a measure of change in systolic blood pressure occurring with challenge.

Type of Data Required and Assumptions

You are already familiar with the correlation matrix, the beginnings of many of our statistical treatments. In such a matrix (as in Fig. 12-6) the two halves are identical; that is, the correlation of X with Y is the same as the correlation of Y with X. We call such a matrix *symmetrical*. Factor analysis may be performed with any symmetrical matrix of correlations. There are no special assumptions or requirements beyond those applicable to the calculation or interpretation of correlation, or both. Remember, however, that a curvilinear relationship between two variables cannot be detected using the Pearson Product Moment Correlation. Also, if the correlation matrix is smaller than 10 × 10, some special considerations may be appropriate.

In addition, although factor analysis is especially appropriate when working with a large amount of data, the number of variables that may be included in a factor analysis procedure is limited. It is tied to sample size. Certainly, the number of cases should always exceed the number of variables. A ratio of at least 10 subjects for each variable is desirable to generalize from the sample to a wider population. With smaller ratios the influence of relationships based on random patterns within the data becomes more pronounced. Another perspective on sample size is that because it is based on correlation, 100 to 200 subjects are enough for most purposes. In any case it is well understood that sample size may be problematic, and the need for replication of factor studies is increasingly emphasized. In a recent article Teel and Verran (1991) present a variety of approaches through which factor solutions obtained in various studies may be compared.

Six Matrices

The mathematics of factor analysis is complex. It is based on *matrix algebra*—the branch of mathematics that deals with the manipulation of matrices. However, matrix algebra is beyond the scope of this book, and you do not need an understanding of matrix algebra to conduct a factor analysis. All mathematics can be done by computer.

The process of conducting a factor analysis, as experienced by the clinical researcher working within the structure of a packaged statistical program for the computer such as SPSSX, is now presented. This process may involve as many as six matrices. Each matrix is derived from a previous one through the computer program. But the researcher should still *understand* each matrix.

Raw Data Matrix

These are the data that the researcher collects about the study subjects. They are entered into the computer by the researcher in the form of data lines, each containing information about one subject. In such a matrix each row represents a single subject, and each column represents a variable. The reader is already familiar with this sort of matrix; it is the beginning of any data analysis. Table 11-2 provides an example of the structure of a raw data matrix. A raw data matrix to be factor analyzed would, by definition, contain many variables. (*Note*: For a Q-type analysis the data matrix would be transposed so that each row is a variable, and each column is a subject.)

Correlation Matrix

The reader also is familiar with the correlation matrix. When fully depicted the correlation matrix is a square, symmetrical matrix in which the number of rows and the number of columns each equal the number of variables. Because the correlation matrix is symmetrical (therefore containing much duplication), it is often depicted in one of several abbreviated forms. Figure 12-6 is one example of a correlation matrix. The correlation matrix summarizes information in the raw data matrix. It is smaller, with fewer rows and elements than the raw data matrix. This is the beginning of the data reduction process.

Factor Matrix, Unrotated

Based on the correlation matrix, the first of two (or more) factor matrices is calculated. In a factor matrix (Table 14-5) each row represents one variable included in the factor analysis. There are fewer columns, each column representing one factor. In the unrotated factor matrix, the elements within the matrix are the unrotated *factor loadings*—numbers ranging between -1 and $+1$, which may be thought of as "correlations" of the variable with the factor. The square of a factor loading represents the proportion of variance that the item and the factor have in common; in other words this is the proportion of item variance explained by the factor. For example in Table 14-5, illustrating an unrotated factor matrix, the first variable (1) has a loading of .85 on Factor I; approximately 72% of variance is accounted for by this loading ($[.85]^2 = .7225$). Adding the squared loadings across a row, you arrive at the item communality (b^2). This is the portion of item variance accounted for by the various factors. For variable 1 of Table 14-5, the squared factor loadings are totaled as follows: $.85^2 + .22^2 + .03^2 = .72 + .05 + .00 = .77$. The item communality is .77; that is, 77% of item variance is "explained" by the three factors.

Likewise, if you add the squared loadings contained in a single column, you will obtain the *eigenvalue* for the factor. The eigenvalue represents the total amount of variance explained by a factor. The average of the squared loadings in a column is obtained by dividing the eigenvalue by the number of items in the column (eigenvalue/n). This average represents the percent of inter-item variance accounted for by the factor. For the first factor in Table 14-5, the eigenvalue is calculated as follows: $.85^2 + .15^2 + .51^2 + .83^2 + .26^2 = .72 + .02 + .26 + .69 + .07 = 1.76$. This eigenvalue of 1.76

TABLE 14-5
Factor Loading Matrix

| | | Factors | | | |
		I	II	III	b^2
Variables	1	.85	.22	.03	.77
	2	.15	•	•	•
	3	.51	•	•	•
	4	.83	•	•	•
	5	.26	•	•	•
Eigenvalues		1.76			
% of variance		.35			

is divided by 5 (because there are five variables), yielding .352. Thus, approximately 35% of total item variance is accounted for by the first factor. Adding up the percent of variance accounted for by each factor tells us how much variance was explained by all the factors.

Factor eigenvalues and variance accounted for are the most important figures contained in the unrotated factor matrix. One may be especially interested in how much variance is accounted for altogether by the important factors; this is simply the sum of variance accounted for by individual factors. Either factor eigenvalues or the variance accounted for by factors may be used to determine the number of potentially interpretable factors contained in the data. Typically, researchers want to interpret the number of factors that each account for at least 5% of variance or similarly the number of factors for which the eigenvalue is 1 or greater. Determination of the appropriate number of factors paves the way for the next matrix of the factor analysis process. However, before moving on to this next matrix, a diversion is needed.

A Note on Extraction Models

For the ambitious reader further explanation is provided here concerning the choices facing the researcher who is conducting a factor analysis. (If you are a less ambitious reader, you may want to skip this section.) The unrotated factor matrix is obtained through use of an extraction method, and the statistical software packages that are generally used offer a choice of extraction methods. Most basically, two general approaches are based on two very different assumptions about the data (Ferketich & Muller, 1990).

The distinction has to do with the nature of the variance in the data. One possible assumption is that all measurement error is random. In this case the means of deviations (representing the error) is zero. Based on this assumption a researcher chooses to use the extraction method known as principal components. Using this method of extraction, new variables are exact mathematical transformations of the original data. When this method of extraction is used, *all* variance in the observed variables contributes to the solution. Because each variable correlates perfectly with itself, the ones (unities) in the diagonal of the correlation matrix are a part of the variance that is analyzed. The goal is to convert a given set of variables into a new set of variables that is an exact mathematical transformation of the original data.

The other possible assumption to be made is that measurement error consists of a systematic component as well as a unique component. The systematic component is of particular interest because it may be explored to determine unmeasured factors in the data. These may be described as *latent* factors. Based on this assumption, a researcher chooses to use any of a class of extraction methods categorized as "common factor analysis." This includes methods named principal axis, image, alpha, generalized least square, and unweighted least square. Because the researcher making this assumption wants to focus on the common variance, it is not appropriate to use the full correlation matrix. Instead, the diagonals are altered so that instead of consisting of unities (ones), an estimate of the communalities (h^2) is used. Such modification of a matrix may seem surprising to someone new to factor analysis. However, as has been pointed out by Gable (1986), "We should appreciate that the choice of these diagonal values consumed many years of research by psychometricians." In any case in common factor analyses the matrix analyzed does not reflect the full variance in the data; rather, the covariance is analyzed.

While some research methodologists place strong emphasis on the distinction between principal components and common factor analysis (Ferketich & Muller, 1991), others point out that there is little practical difference in results obtained (Child, 1990; Nunnally, 1978). Undoubtedly, this will remain a point of contention for some time to come.

Later in this chapter we return to the problem of choosing a specific extraction model. Now, we return to discussion of the fourth of six matrices.

Factor Matrix, Rotated

The unrotated factors are created (based on the correlations between variables) so that the amount of variance accounted for by each successive factor is maximized. This means that factors may (in geometric terms) run between independent groups of related variables, rather than accurately reflecting the meaning of a group of variables. The consequence of this fact is that unrotated factors rarely can be meaningfully interpreted. However, just as one may alter an algebraic equation by performing the same operation on both sides, one may transform or "rotate" a factor matrix into any one of an infinite number of mathematically equivalent matrices. If factor rotation is conducted according to the criterion of *simple structure* as described by Thurstone in 1947, the result is a set of factors that are distinct from one another and that, in most situations, can be meaningfully and creatively interpreted by the researcher. In simple structure factors are set to maximize the number of loadings of great magnitude (near + 1 and − 1) and loadings of small magnitude (near 0.00) for each factor; that is, a distinct pattern emerges in the factor matrix so that each factor has certain variables that go with it, while other variables do not. Likewise, as simple structure is approached, each variable is identified with *only one* factor. According to Thurstone (1947), the following occur in a factor matrix:

1. Each row should have at least one loading close to zero.
2. Each column should have at least as many variables with near-zero loadings as there are factors.
3. For pairs of columns (factors), there should be several variables that load on one and not on the other.

The essence of interpreting factor analytic results is the process of identifying, from the rotated factor matrix, which variables go with a factor and then naming the factor based on whatever meanings these variables with high loadings have in common. The criterion for considering a loading high varies from study to study, with some researchers using cutoff points as low as 0.35; others use cutoff points as high as 0.55. In their figure, Walker and associates (1987) used 0.35 as their cutoff point.

When naming and describing factors, the researcher uses not only knowledge of the statistical technique and how it works, but also an understanding of the subject matter under study, especially an ability to construct new understandings of that subject matter. By facilitating the organization of individual variables into variable groupings, factor analysis opens the door to new conceptualizations and new ways of thinking, provided that the researcher is ready to discover these in the data. More than any other statistical technique, factor analysis requires the full exercise of one's creative potential.

Factor Score Matrix

Based on the rotated factor matrix, a score for each subject on each factor may be computed. To calculate such *factor scores*, an individual's score on each variable included in a factor is multiplied by the factor loading for the particular variable. The sum of these products is the individual's factor score. The general formula is:

$$\text{Factor score} = \text{sum of} \begin{pmatrix} \text{individual's} \\ \text{score on} \\ \text{variable} \end{pmatrix} \times \begin{pmatrix} \text{factor loading} \\ \text{of variable} \\ \text{on factor} \end{pmatrix}$$

Factor scores can be calculated automatically within factor analysis procedures in statistical packages for the computer, such as SPSSX. Consider an individual included in the data of Table 14-5 who received scores as follows:

Variable	Scores
1	2
2	4
3	1
4	5
5	2

This person's factor score on factor 1 would be calculated as follows:
$(.85)(.2) + (.15)(4) + (.51)(1) + (.83)(5) + (.26)(2) = 1.7 + .6 + .6 + .51 + 4.15 + .52 = 7.48$.

This factor score, based on the strength of the correlation of each variable with the factor, could be used instead of the individual's unweighted (i.e., summative) score on the factor. The factor score is based on the relative "importance" of each variable as indicated by that correlation. This individual's unweighted score would be the sum of the scores on the five variables ($2 + 4 + 1 + 5 + 2 = 14$).

The factor score matrix has as many rows as subjects, with each column representing one factor. The structure of such a matrix is illustrated in Table 14-6. The factor score matrix is smaller than the raw data matrix because there are fewer factors than variables. The data have been reduced.

TABLE 14-6
Factor Score Matrix

		Factors			
		I	*II*	•	•
Subjects	1	7.48	•	•	•
	2	•			
	•	•			
	•	•			
	•	•			
	n	•			

Factor Correlation Matrix

Factor Rotation

Factor rotation is often *orthogonal*, with resulting factors uncorrelated with each other. This is usually desirable for instrument development, in which the researcher seeks to determine subscales that are independent of one another. Alternatively, factor rotation also may be *oblique*, with factors that are not totally unrelated to each other. Advocates of oblique rotation assert that in the real world important factors are likely to be correlated; thus, searching for unrelated factors is unrealistic. Novice factor analysts should probably plan to use an orthogonal, rather than oblique, rotation because it is easier to interpret. The *Varimax* (variance maximized) method, available on all widely used computer packages, may be recommended for orthogonal rotation. Other alternatives are *Quartimax*, which is likely to yield a first, very general factor with many high loadings, and *Equimax*, which combines characteristics of *Quartimax* and *Varimax*, balancing the advantages and disadvantages of each.

With orthogonal rotation, one factor loading matrix is produced. It represents regression weights (called a *pattern matrix*) and correlation coefficients (called a *structure matrix*). Because the solution is orthogonal, the regression weights are equal to the correlation coefficients. The loadings are interpreted as were those in the unrotated factor matrix. A squared loading represents the variance accounted for in a variable by a particular factor. The squared loadings may be added across a row to determine total variance accounted for in a variable by all the factors, and so on.

Because with oblique rotation there is correlation among the factors, the *factor pattern matrix* (the regression weights) and the *factor structure matrix* (containing correlation coefficients) are not the same. The two matrices are produced and interpreted differently. The pattern matrix is generally considered preferable as a basis for interpreting the meanings of factors. The square of a loading in a factor pattern matrix represents the variance accounted for by a particular variable, but because other factors may share some of this variance (due to intercorrelation among factors in an oblique

TABLE 14-7
Factor Correlation Matrix

	Factor 1	Factor 2	Factor 3
Factor 1	1.00	0.65	0.30
Factor 2		1.00	0.45
Factor 3			1.00

solution), the total variance in an item accounted for by all the factors *cannot* be determined by adding the squared loadings in a row (h^2).

Factor Correlations

In oblique rotation a matrix displaying the correlation of each factor with every other factor is displayed in a factor correlation matrix. The structure of such a matrix is displayed in Table 14-7.

STEPS OF A FACTOR ANALYTIC STUDY

The steps of a factor analytic study are as follows:

1. Formulate a research question or hypothesis. If factor analysis is the appropriate statistical technique for answering research questions or testing the hypothesis, proceed with the following steps.
2. Collect data of interest.
3. Calculate and examine univariate data on a variable-by-variable basis, identifying variables that should not be included in the factor analysis because of failure to meet initial assumptions or criteria.
4. Calculate and examine bivariate relationship data—again with an eye toward identifying variables and relationships that should not be included in the factor analysis.
5. "Run" the factor analysis. Unless you have a good reason to do otherwise, use an orthogonal rotation. If you have predicted certain factors, specify in the computer program how many factors you expect; otherwise, let the computer determine the number of factors in the course of the factor analysis, based on eigenvalues in the unrotated factor matrix. Note the total proportion of interitem variance accounted for by the factor solution and the number of factors involved.
6. Name and interpret factors from the rotated factor loading matrix. (Sometimes researchers experiment with several factor solutions to choose the one that can be most meaningfully interpreted.)
7. If subsequent analyses are planned, use factor analysis results to decide how to combine variables; calculate these new or combined variables for each subject.

(Usually, factor scores can be easily calculated on the computer.) Remember to consider the reliabilities of the derived scores. Then conduct the subsequent analyses.

8. Relate findings to the existing literature and disseminate results through presentation and publication. If appropriate, repeat the analysis with other available populations.

COMBINING FACTOR ANALYSIS WITH OTHER APPROACHES

When used for its data-reduction purpose, factor analysis is often an early stage of a multistage analysis, as indicated by steps 7 and 8 above. Subsequent analyses also may be conducted in studies involving an instrument development process. For example Brown and Tanner (1990) factor analyzed data from the Matthews Youth Test for Health, a 17-item teacher report instrument to assess type A behavior in young children. They obtained four factors that were named competitiveness, hostility, impatience, and leadership. These four factors were used for the creation of four subscales. After determining that internal consistency and test–retest reliabilities were adequate, subscales were related to measures of cardiac reactivity. In univariate analysis competitiveness, hostility, and impatience each related to systolic blood pressure response to challenge. However, when the various subscales were used as independent variables in a stepwise multiple regression, only competitiveness entered the regression equation; it accounted for 12% of variance in systolic blood pressure response. This finding suggests a physiological link relating childhood behavior to possibility of future cardiovascular disorder.

Such findings have important substantive and instrument development implications. Generally, factor analysis tends to be most useful when combined with other analyses within a single study.

EXAMPLE OF A COMPUTER PRINTOUT

As an example an edited computer printout of a principal components analysis is shown in Figure 14-1. The data analyzed are from a 10-item scale designed to measure self-assessed health. Responses were obtained from 311 subjects. The 10 × 10 correlation matrix was submitted to principal components analysis with Equamax rotation using the SPSSX computer package. (Equamax rotation was used to balance the need for interpretable factors with the need for simplified, interpretable variables.)

① The first four lines reprint the procedure commands needed to implement the computer run. So few command statements are needed because of heavy use of default options. For example principal components is the default extraction method in SPSSX. (Alternatively, any one of six methods of common factor analysis could have been used.)

② The table that follows the label "initial statistics" presents two types of information: (1) Because the extraction method was a principal components analysis, the

(*text continues on page 264*)

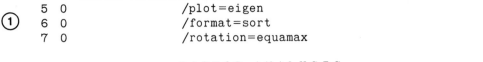

```
  4  0   factor variables=all
  5  0              /plot=eigen
① 6  0              /format=sort
  7  0              /rotation=equamax
```

———————————————————— F A C T O R   A N A L Y S I S ————————————————————

ANALYSIS NUMBER 1 LISTWISE DELETION OF CASES WITH MISSING VALUES

EXTRACTION 1 FOR ANALYSIS 1, PRINCIPAL–COMPONENTS ANALYSIS (PC)

INITIAL STATISTICS:

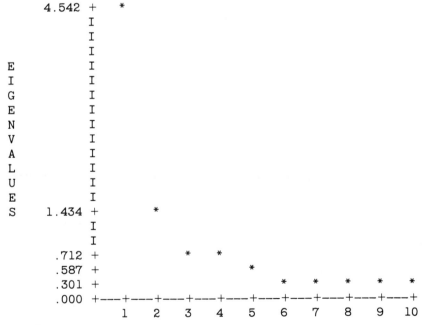

② VARIABLE	COMMUNALITY	*	FACTOR	EIGENVALUE	PCT OF VAR	CUM PCT
PURPOSE	1.00000	*	1	4.54230	45.4	45.4
ENERGY	1.00000	*	2	1.43410	14.3	59.8
SYMPTOM	1.00000	*	3	.88429	8.8	68.6
CHRONIC	1.00000	*	4	.71156	7.1	75.7
EMOTION	1.00000	*	5	.58654	5.9	81.6
SPORATIC	1.00000	*	6	.45276	4.5	86.1
DISABIL	1.00000	*	7	.38327	3.8	89.9
MAJILL	1.00000	*	8	.36480	3.6	93.6
SOCTIES	1.00000	*	9	.33923	3.4	97.0
ACCEPT	1.00000	*	10	.30113	3.0	100.0

```
        4.542 +   *
              I
              I
              I
   E          I
   I          I
   G          I
   E          I
   N          I
   V          I
   A          I
   L          I
   U          I
   E          I
   S    1.434 +       *
              I
              I
         .712 +           *   *
         .587 +               *
         .301 +                   *   *   *   *   *
         .000 +---+---+---+---+---+---+---+---+---+
                1   2   3   4   5   6   7   8   9   10
```

FIGURE 14-1
Edited computer printout of a principal component analysis.

PC EXTRACTED 2 FACTORS

(3) FACTOR MATRIX:

	FACTOR 1	FACTOR 2
ENERGY	.78644	.00606
EMOTION	.76618	−.27295
PURPOSE	.75584	−.30671
ACCEPT	.74274	−.42868
SOCTIES	.67430	−.55553
CHRONIC	.66493	.47268
SYMPTOM	.66435	.43335
MAJILL	.60852	.21185
DISABIL	.54621	.46797
SPORATIC	.45500	.31310

FINAL STATISTICS:

(4)

VARIABLE	COMMUNALITY	*	FACTOR	EIGENVALUE	PCT OF VAR	CUM PCT
		*				
PURPOSE	.66537	*	1	4.54230	45.4	45.4
ENERGY	.61852	*	2	1.43410	14.3	59.8
SYMPTOM	.62915	*				
CHRONIC	.66556	*				
EMOTION	.66153	*				
SPORATIC	.30506	*				
DISABIL	.51734	*				
MAJILL	.41517	*				
SOCTIES	.76329	*				
ACCEPT	.73542	*				

EQAMAX   ROTATION 1 FOR EXTRACTION   1 IN ANALYSIS   1−KAISER NORMALIZATION.

EQUAMAX CONVERGED IN 3 ITERATIONS.

(5) ROTATED FACTOR MATRIX:

	FACTOR 1	FACTOR 2
SOCTIES	.87278	.03934
ACCEPT	.83860	.17936
PURPOSE	.76662	.27869
EMOTION	.75167	.31068
ENERGY	.57979	.53138
CHRONIC	.17696	.79639
SYMPTOM	.20288	.76680
DISABIL	.09198	.71336
MAJILL	.30983	.56496
SPORATIC	.12802	.53728

FIGURE 14-1 (CONTINUED)

263

diagonals in the correlation matrix to be analyzed were kept as unities; this is indicated by the repetition of 1.000 in each row for the second column. Had any type of common factor analysis (e.g., principal axis, maximum likelihood) been used, rather than principal components analysis, communality estimates would have replaced ones in the diagonal. The multiple R^2 of the regression equation that predicts the variable from other variables would be used as the default communality estimate for each variable. Alternatively, the researcher could use communality estimates obtained in some other way (e.g., item reliabilities) and simply specify these into the program.

Moving toward the right, the next four columns under "initial statistics" contain the information needed relative to general characteristics of the unrotated factors. Note that 10 factors are listed. This is because the number of unrotated factors obtainable equals the number of variables included in a principal components analysis. The purpose of this part of the analysis is, however, to determine how many of the 10 factors should be rotated for conceptual interpretation. Eigenvalues and percent of variance accounted for are given. The first two factors each have an eigenvalue greater than 1 (default on SPSSX), and each of these accounts for 10% of variance or more. The right-hand column gives cumulative percent of variance accounted for; the first two factors together account for 59.8% of the interitem variance.

In this printout a plot of eigenvalues was requested in line 5 of the procedure commands (/plot = eigen). This provides a graphic representation of the relative values of eigenvalues. Because eigenvalues often are the key criteria for determining number of factors to be rotated, this can be useful.

③ In this analysis two factors were extracted. These are displayed in the next table labeled, "factor matrix," which contains the unrotated factor matrix. As usual, the first factor is a generalized factor on which all variables load. The second factor, containing positive and negative loadings, has a bipolar quality. Typically, no attempt is made to derive conceptual interpretations of these unrotated factors. Next, the two factors with eigenvalues greater than 1 are rotated, and the final solution is derived.

④ Under the heading "final statistics" the second column shows final communalities achieved for each variable in the rotated factor matrix. The next column repeats information already given concerning the rotated factors only.

⑤ The last table, "rotated factor matrix," represents the culmination of this effort. These rotated factors are to be conceptually interpreted. Note that the items are now listed by strength of loading, rather than by the order in which they were listed previously. This reordering was requested in line 6 of the procedure commands (/format = sort); use of this option on SPSSX is highly recommended. Otherwise, the researcher must reorder items by loading manually.

After inspecting the items that load on a factor and their respective loadings, the investigator gives each factor an appropriate name as a way of capturing its meaning. In the naming process one gives most emphasis to the three or four variables with the highest loadings. In this analysis factor 1 was named psychological health, and factor 2 was named physiological health. Subjects could receive a score on each of these factors. Often, a factor analysis includes more variables and more factors than that shown here. The researcher who wants to include a tabular presentation of a factor analysis in a research thesis or article should take care to present it in an easily readable format, such as that shown in Table 14-3.

Other Options

A factor analysis may be more complicated than the one shown here—not simply because of the inclusion of more variables and more factors.

Rather than principal components analysis (on SPSSX, the default), any of six types of extraction method representing common factor analysis may be used. Principal axis factoring differs from principle components mainly in that the correlation matrix diagonals are squared multiple correlations, rather than ones, in the first step. Following this initial step, communalities are estimated from the factor matrix, and factoring is repeated with these communalities in the diagonal. Each such step is one iteration. This is repeated until the estimated communalities and calculated communalities are approximately the same.

Another important method of extraction within the class of common factor analysis is alpha factoring, which is designed to maximize the alpha reliability of the factors. It is assumed that the particular variables measured are a sample of the universe of variables represented by the factor. One wishes to generalize, not to the population of cases from which research subjects were drawn, but to the universe of variables from which the measured variables were sampled. Ferketich and Muller (1990) point out that this method is highly appropriate for instrument development efforts—particularly the early stages.

Other extraction methods available on SPSSX are image factoring, unweighted least squares, and generalized least squares. These may be less important to the sort of applications discussed here; however, the interested reader can find an excellent discussion of the characteristics and underlying assumptions of these methods in Norusis (1990d) and in Ferketich and Muller (1990). Finally, the maximum likelihood method of extraction is an available option. This method lays the groundwork for a confirmatory factor analysis process, and it is discussed in the following section.

INTRODUCTION TO CONFIRMATORY FACTOR ANALYSIS

The maximum likelihood method of extraction is distinct from those previously described in the inclusion of a test for goodness of fit. That is, the adequacy of the factor model is tested using a test of statistical significance. While researchers using other methods of extraction may rely on such statistical criteria as magnitude of eigenvalues or percent of variance accounted for in determining the appropriate number of factors, a researcher using the maximum likelihood technique may determine number of factors through the chi-square statistic. (The generalized least square method of extraction also allows the calculation of a goodness of fit statistic.)

In this process the adequacy of the factor model is tested. This is based on the assumption that the sample is from a multivariate normal population. Any factor model is an attempt to summarize or reduce a multivariate dataset. In the maximum likelihood method, the hypothesis tested is that the factor model derived is a good fit with the original data. Because statistical significance would indicate a difference between the factor model and the full data, the researcher hopes to obtain a chi-square that is nonsignificant, indicating that a good fit is obtained.

In any case initial results can be used to guide continued refinement of the factor model. What does one do if statistical significance is obtained on the chi-square value, indicating significant difference between the factor model and the full data, an inadequate fit? One reruns the analysis, making adjustments in the criteria governing number of factors to be derived. In SPSSX this is done with the CRITERIA command. (To obtain three, rather than two, factors, CRITERIA = FACTORS [3]). In any factor solution increasing the number of factors will increase the statistical adequacy of factor model; the goal is to obtain the number of factors that is the smallest number necessary to achieve an acceptable fit. One may repeatedly run analyses, adding a factor with each repetition until the chi-square statistic obtained is nonsignificant. Alternatively, if on the first run the chi-square statistic is nonsignificant, one repeats the analysis with one factor fewer to determine the smallest possible number of factors that will yield a nonsignificant chi-square.

The development of confirmatory factor analysis in recent decades is due largely to the work of K.G. Jöreskog and is based on maximum likelihood techniques. Made accessible to researchers through the LISREL family of computer programs (Jöreskog & Sörbom, 1989), complex forms of confirmatory factor analysis not only guide the researcher as to the appropriate number of factors, but also allow the researcher to specify what variables relate to which factors and to identify relationships between variables that are not captured by the factors. (However, they may conceivably indicate the existence of an additional factor). Modifications are suggested by how much a factor model may be improved, and changing goodness of fit statistics aid in interpretation of the value of the improvement. Remember that the goal of confirmatory factor analysis is to identify latent (unmeasured) variables that underlie the set of variables that are measured. These latent variables are considered to be the reason behind the specific measured values obtained. Thus, in figures depicting confirmatory factor models, either hypothesized or obtained, the direction of arrows leads from the latent variable to the measured variable. Confirmation of the nature of these latent variables is achieved through confirmatory factor analysis; these latent variables may then become the foundation of subsequent analysis, as in structural equation modeling.

Confirmatory factor analysis can be applied to the health-care professions research literature in three major ways: (1) Confirmatory factor analysis may directly follow exploratory factor analysis. In two studies by Gulick (1987, 1989) designed to evaluate instrumentation for use with people with multiple sclerosis, factor models obtained through exploratory factor analysis were improved by means of confirmatory factor analysis. (2) Confirmatory factor analysis has been recommended for studies using the multitrait–multimethod approach to construct validity. This is because of its ability to handle systematically hypotheses that posit that some sources of variation are due to content distinctions between variables; however, this is crossed with other sources of variation due to method distinctions in the same variables. (The reader should consult Figueredo, Ferketich, & Knapp [1991] for elaboration of this recommendation.) (3) Confirmatory factor analysis is used as the first step of structural equation modeling— establishing the measurement model so that the latent (i.e., unmeasured) variables are identified. An example of this usage may be seen in study of the impact of emotions on the interrelationship between creative intelligence and conventional skills (Dixon, Hickey, & Dixon, 1992). This is discussed further in Chapter 16.

One important distinction between exploratory factor analysis and confirmatory factor analysis is that in exploratory analysis it is assumed that all observed variables are related to (i.e., affected by) all of the common factors. In confirmatory approaches one may develop specific expectations, such that each variable is assumed to relate to some common factors but not to others (Long, 1983). Hypotheses about the relationships in the data may be specific. However, as pointed out by Goodwin and Goodwin (1991), "the exploratory–confirmatory distinction is often tenuous" (p. 239); exploratory techniques often are used by researchers with well-specified expectations, and confirmatory techniques may be applied in a highly exploratory manner.

The process of confirmatory factor analysis is illustrated with an example from the literature. Gulick (1989) examined the structure of the multiple sclerosis-related symptoms checklist, consisting of 26 signs and symptoms thought to be characteristic of multiple sclerosis. Subjects provided self-report data indicating the frequency with which they experienced each symptom on a 6-point scale ranging from never (0) to always (5). Data from 491 subjects who completed the third year of a longitudinal study were first submitted to a principal components analysis with Varimax rotation. This was an exploratory factor analysis. A five-factor solution incorporating 22 of the 26 items and accounting for 59.3% of interitem variation was derived. The factor loading matrix is represented in Table 14-8. (Note that the format of this published factor loading matrix is in some ways different from the format of the published factor loading matrix displayed in Table 14-3. As an exercise identify three differences, and for each think about which format communicates most easily to the reader.)

Based on these results a graphic model was constructed, which was evaluated in a confirmatory factor analysis. This is reprinted in Figure 14-2 with circles used to illustrate the latent variables (the factors) and rectangular boxes used to represent measured variables. Arrows from the latent variables to the measured variables represent the assumption that the latent characteristics form the foundation of the obtained measurement. The numbers accompanying these arrows are the factor loadings obtained, and correlations obtained between factors also are shown. The three numbers in the lower left corner of the figure provide an evaluation of the model. The coefficient of determination may be thought of as a reliability. This is not problematic. However, the chi-square value (984.87) is statistically significant, and the goodness of fit ratio of 0.801 is not high enough. Ideally, this should be 0.9 or higher. The relationships between measured variables have not been fully captured by this model.

Modification indices obtained in the computer printout suggested a number of modifications. In all, seven changes were made. One of these involved associating an observed variable (falling) with a second factor (elimination). The other six involved the pairing of measured variables due to relationships between their residual variances. That is, there was a relationship between arm weakness and leg weakness, over and above their common connection with the latent variable, skeletal. The modified model is displayed in Figure 14-3. The researcher points out that the chi-square value decreased by more than half (= 405.08), and the goodness of fit index also improved (0.910), suggesting a satisfactory model. Although the chi-square value remains statistically significant in the modified model, the author points out its sensitivity to sample size, and she suggests an alternative criterion—the ratio of chi-square to df. The ratio of 2.11 to 1 obtained is within acceptable range.

TABLE 14-8
Factor Loading Matrix of Exploratory Factor Analysis

MS-Related Symptom	Skeletal	Varimax Rotated Factor Analysis			
		Elimination	Emotions	Kinesthetic	Head
X_1 Arm weakness	.511	.040	.065	.218	.308
X_2 Leg Weakness	.693	.104	−.009	.186	.122
X_3 Spasms	.583	.079	.141	.358	.113
X_4 Tremors	.482	.022	.191	.231	.222
X_5 Knee locking	.721	.022	.085	.220	.023
X_6 Balance problems	.719	.132	.048	−.048	.020
X_7 Falling	.657	.293	.176	−.130	.079
X_8 Urine frequency: day	.046	.772	.001	.272	.101
X_9 Urine frequency: night	−.006	.786	−.022	.281	.105
X_{10} Trouble making bathroom: day	.247	.802	.125	−.025	.047
X_{11} Trouble making bathroom: night	.235	.811	.144	−.022	−.014
X_{12} Loneliness	.110	.041	.835	.056	.112
X_{13} Depression	.140	.110	.877	.096	.143
X_{14} Anxiety	.081	.040	.821	.196	.152
X_{15} Pain	.216	.074	.302	.542	.062
X_{16} Burning	.203	.173	.142	.642	.021
X_{17} Numbness	.122	.076	.024	.785	.147
X_{18} Pins and needles	.068	.096	.009	.754	.112
X_{19} Double vision	.133	−.040	.033	.112	.744
X_{20} Blurred vision	.140	.031	.045	.108	.793
X_{21} Difficulty swallowing	.174	.138	.192	.094	.590
X_{22} Forgetfulnees	−.010	.149	.391	−.002	.557
Percent of explained variance	26.600	1.220	8.600	7.500	6.300
Eigenvalue (principal component method)	3.184	2.702	2.372	2.233	2.064
Theta reliability coefficient	.800	.840	.867	.736	.687

Note: Item-factor loadings are underlined.
(From Gulick, E. E. [1989]. Model confirmation of the MS-related symptom checklist. Nursing Research, *38, 147–153.)*

The use of confirmatory factor analysis by nonstatisticians is a relatively new development in the research literature, but clearly this is a trend for the future. Structural equation modeling, described in Chapter 16, builds further on the application of maximum likelihood methods in the discovery of causal patterns between latent variables.

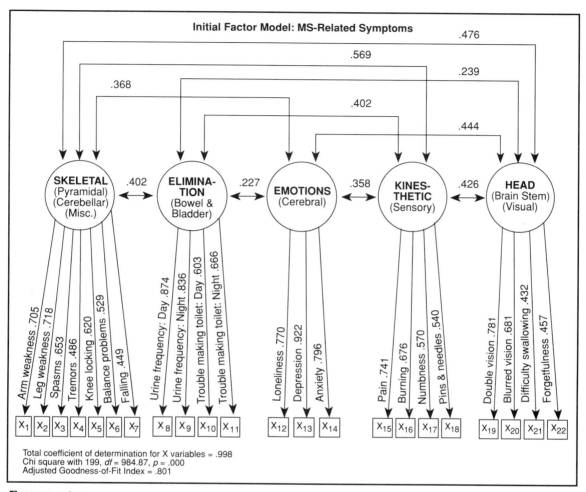

FIGURE 14-2

Graphic depiction of initial model by confirmatory factor analysis.

(From Gulick, E.E. [1989]. Model confirmation of the MS-related symptom checklist. *Nursing Research, 38*, 147–153.)

CLUSTER ANALYSIS

A brief note on clustering of subjects, as mentioned previously, concludes this chapter. Although factor analysis is the technique of choice for summarizing a correlation matrix to determine how the study variables tend to group together, cluster analysis is the technique of choice for obtaining empirical groupings of subjects based on the subjects' values on selected variables. Cluster analysis is used to identify homogeneous subsets of subjects or patients. Individuals within each of such subsets are more similar to each other than they are to individuals in other subsets.

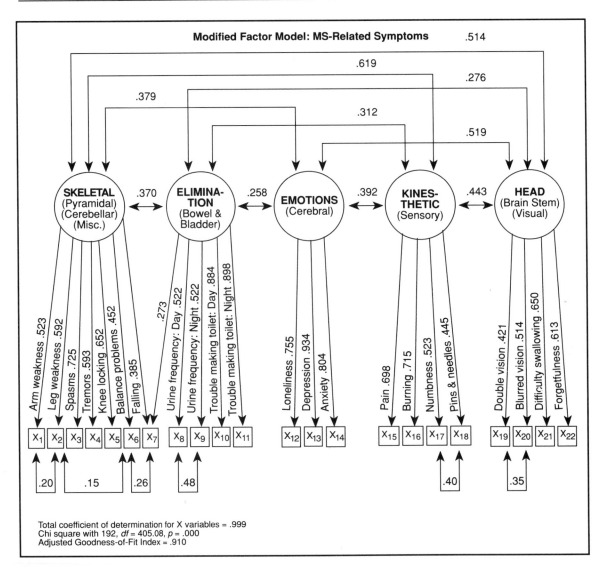

FIGURE 14-3

Graphic depiction of improved model by confirmatory factor analysis.

(Gulick, E.E. [1989]. Model confirmation of the MS-related symptom checklist. *Nursing Research, 38*, 147–153.)

In health-care professions this offers the possibility of developing clinical interventions specific to the needs of a particular group. Because individuals within a homogeneous subset or cluster may respond to a particular nursing intervention differently from individuals in other clusters, cluster analysis also may be a useful first step in any evaluative study; the way individuals cluster into groups may help to explain variance between individuals in response to treatment. The very process of diagnosis, whether within the realm of medicine or of nursing, is a clustering process. Based on observable indicators, an individual is classified as a member of a group made up of people who are similar, but probably not identical, on certain characteristics. To the extent that this grouping helps us understand the individual or to predict future events and responses of the individual, the grouping may be considered useful. Cluster analysis is simply an empirical method of arriving at such groupings or diagnoses.

Although it is much less commonly used than factor analysis, cluster analysis is applicable to many problems studied by health-care researchers. In the recent nursing research literature, it has been used to cluster women relative to life-span illness history (Dixon, Dixon, Spinner, Sexton & Perry, 1991) and relative to women's decision making concerning hormone replacement therapy (Rothert, Rovner, Holmes, Schmitt, Talarczyk, Kroll, & Gogate, 1990). Stuifbergen (1990) used cluster analysis to group families experiencing a chronic illness. She concludes the following:

> It seems clear that unidimensional analysis of families in clinical practice or research is not sufficiently complex to yield an accurate picture of what is occurring in families. The cluster analysis method of conceptualizing family environments is particularly useful because it allows one to consider not only how families with a chronically ill parent vary from others in one particular dimension of family functioning, but also how these specific dimensions of family functioning may covary with one another. The information gained from this empirically derived taxonomy of family environments may add to our understanding of the impact of chronic illness on family members and may help explain how different family environments are linked to different family outcomes. (p. 43)

Given such support among health-care researchers who use the technique of cluster analysis, one wonders why it is not used more often.

INDEX OF SIMILARITY

Cluster analysis is based on the premise that a valid measure of similarity between any two individuals can be obtained. Thus, one can construct a square, symmetrical matrix in which study subjects are represented by rows and by columns; the elements of the matrix are indices of similarity of each subject with each other subject. This similarity index may take any one of several forms.

It may take the form of a correlation; that is, you may compute the Pearson Product Moment Correlation between two individuals across a variety of variables by using the standard formula. Simply consider one person's values on all measures to represent the X variable, while the other person's values on all measures represent the Y variable. However, because it emphasizes the pattern that emerges, not actual magnitude of values, correlation is flawed as a measure of similarity between individuals. For example, in Figure 14-4 because Mary and Alice each did best on test 2 and worst on test 3, a high correlation between these individuals would be obtained, even though overall Mary scored much higher than Alice. In contrast although Mary's and Sue's scores on each test are close in magnitude, these individuals followed different patterns; Mary's best test is Sue's worst, and vice versa. A high correlation between these individuals would not be obtained.

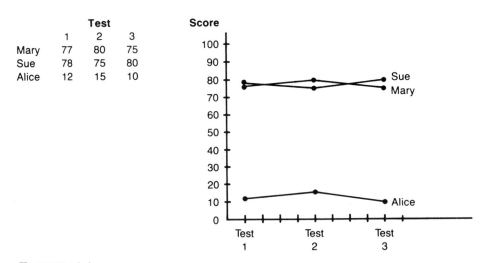

	Test		
	1	2	3
Mary	77	80	75
Sue	78	75	80
Alice	12	15	10

FIGURE 14-4
Three sets of test scores for determining distances between individuals.

These problems can be avoided by using Euclidian distance as the measure of similarity between individuals. With this measure, similarity is determined by how far apart two individuals are on each test. The distance between Mary and Sue would be small, and the distance between Mary and Alice would be large.

EXAMPLES OF CLUSTER ANALYSIS

As part of an evaluation study of a graduate nursing program, 106 employed graduates submitted information about their current roles. Data included the percentage of working time spent in a variety of activities, including clinical duties, teaching, administration, research, and consultation. Cluster analysis was based on these time variables. A three-cluster solution comprising all but one of the employed respondents emerged. Within each of these main clusters, at least one subcluster could be identified; two sets of second level subclusters also were discovered. A brief description of the primary clusters was constructed as follows:

Cluster I was characterized by a usually high administrative emphasis ($\overline{X} = 53\%$). The 18 individuals falling into this cluster spent more of their other working time on teaching ($\overline{X} = 22\%$) than on clinical activities ($\overline{X} = 8\%$) and more time on consultation ($\overline{X} = 11\%$) than on research ($\overline{X} = 6\%$).

Cluster II individuals were involved predominantly in activities of a clinical nature ($\overline{X} = 66\%$). Teaching occupied only 11% of these individuals' time, followed by administration (6%), consultation (4%), and research (3%). With 57 subjects this was the largest of the main clusters.

Cluster III was characterized primarily by teaching activity ($\overline{X} = 84\%$). Clinical activity occupied only 7% of the time of respondents classified into this cluster, followed by administration ($\overline{X} = 5\%$), research ($\overline{X} = 2\%$), and consultation ($\overline{X} < 1\%$).

The fact that alumni of a graduate program in nursing would fall into three categories based on a primary emphasis of clinical practice, teaching, or administration should not surprise any observer of the nursing profession. It is, however, always gratifying to find that data analysis results confirm our most common assumptions. They also provide a basis for further research using these clusters.

In another study cluster analysis was used to identify groups of women with varying histories of illness over their life spans (Dixon, Dixon, Spinner, Sexton, & Perry, 1991). Women in their 50s and 60s had submitted information concerning the three most serious illnesses experienced in each decade of life. "Illness" was broadly defined to include accidents or discomforts (such as headaches) if they were considered among the most serious. Responses given were quantified with a number representing decade impact of illness. Quantification used a scale ranging from 10 to 50, with higher numbers representing more serious illness effects. A five-cluster solution was obtained. Table 14-9 displays these results. There are distinctly different patterns of illness seriousness across time for the different clusters. For example cluster 1 is distinct from other clusters in showing improved health in the seventh decade (age 61 to 70). In contrast cluster 3 shows a pattern of worsening health beginning abruptly in the fifth decade (age 41 to 50), following good health in the teen and early adult years. The chronological patterns revealed in these data may shape response to health promotion efforts in middle and later adulthood; individuals with different illness histories may require different health promotion interventions. Cluster analysis is a useful tool for exploring such patterns.

TABLE 14-9
Example of Published Cluster Analysis Results

Cluster Analysis of Mean Decade Impact by Decade, including Cluster Frequencies, Cluster Means by Decade, and F values for Mean Differences between Clusters by Decade

Cluster	Frequency	Mean Decade Impact By Decade						
		1	2	3	4	5	6	7
1	54	23.2	18.9	15.7	16.4	22.6	21.1	16.9
2	48	21.8	18.8	25.5	24.9	18.0	16.1	22.4
3	23	25.0	19.1	17.8	14.3	32.7	36.1	38.5
4	36	23.1	10.9	15.0	21.9	18.8	32.6	32.6
5	49	27.6	25.5	28.6	30.4	29.7	31.6	32.6
F-value		7.6	23.1	33.0	32.5	24.8	61.4	64.0

Note: All values significant at p <0.001

(From Dixon, J. K., Dixon, J. P., Spinner, J., Sexton, D., & Perry, C. [1991]. Psychometric and descriptive perspectives of illness impact over the lifespan. Nursing Research, 40, 51–56.)

CONCLUSION

The variety of factor analysis techniques (including cluster analysis) presented in this chapter are distinct from many other statistical techniques in the potential for researcher creativity to shape understanding of the results obtained. Through application of statistical techniques, one arrives at numbers that indicate groupings in the data—grouping of variables in factor analysis and grouping of cases in cluster analysis. These groups must then be named or described by the researcher, a creative process in which clinical wisdom, knowledge of the literature, and research sophistication must be integrated. Most often, this creative process is the key element on which the value of all of the statistical analysis must rest. The factor analysis solution is designed to inform the creative process. Factor loadings and goodness of fit indices are only as valuable as the interpretation of the factors is insightful.

15

Path Models of Cause

*Ellis
Batten Page*

OBJECTIVES FOR CHAPTER 15

After reading this chapter you should be able to do the following:

1. **Draw a path model of a problem, of the recursive sort, with appropriate arrows or curved lines.**

2. **Set up a decomposition table for the path analysis, calculating the direct and indirect cause from one variable to another.**

3. **Reduce the path model according to some decision rule, eliminating the unimportant paths.**

We use statistics to understand our world. The last century has witnessed great strides in deepening our understanding. Our first step toward understanding has typically been *description*, and statistics began as a way of describing things and events. Following description, statistics have been used to show *relationships*, and once relationships are established, science has been concerned with *causes*. Which frequencies are dependent on which others? Which correlations are caused by unseen, hidden variables we have not considered?

Ultimately, scientists use the growing knowledge of cause to try to control events. We predict weather to ensure an adequate food supply. We seek to understand monetary supply to curb inflation. The history of science, then, has been from description to relations to causes to decisions. However, before such decisions are made, we must be concerned with causes.

The world of science has two principal methods of approaching the problem of cause. One method is the use of experiments; the other method is the use of observational models. In true experiments subjects are assigned randomly to treatments, and the effects of these treatments are then observed. These subjects may be bacteria, and the treatments

Barbara Hazard Munro and Ellis Batten Page: STATISTICAL METHODS FOR HEALTH CARE RESEARCH, SECOND EDITION. © 1993, 1986 by J. B. Lippincott Company.

might be different antibiotics. The subjects may be student nurses, and the treatments might be types of audiovisual instruction, with the goal of improving the training in some procedure. Experiments are a magnificent method for discovering important causes, and experimental design, the study of arranging experiments for the greatest information, is a major branch of applied statistics. The most common method for analyzing experiments has been analysis of variance (ANOVA), as described in Chapters 7 and 8.

Such advanced experimental methods are, like most of modern science, very new. The father of such complex experimental designs, which answer many questions at once, is the late R. A. Fisher, whose great work was *The Design of Experiments* (1935).

Unfortunately, countless important questions cannot be readily explored by experiments. Many events cannot be controlled (such as travel of the planets or the evolution of species) or would be too dangerous to apply (pollution in drinking water) or too expensive (large experiments in hospital administration). Thus, we seek more practical methods for studying causes. We want techniques that imitate experiments so that we may study the events we are curious about without actually controlling them.

PATH MODELS

Like experimental design, path analysis is very new; it began with the writings of geneticist Sewall Wright (1921). Paths have been heavily used in economics, sociology, and now other social sciences. They often are the favored method of explanation whenever we have large datasets available for analysis and we seek causal connections. For researchers paths provide a wonderful method for organizing data, for making sense out of variables that might otherwise confuse and overwhelm. This chapter first presents path analysis as a set of simple diagrams and as a way to think about research. Along with these diagrams, some special vocabulary required for path analysis is presented. Further, we show how we may use ordinary correlation or regression to "solve" these path models. Finally, we learn how to use path models to revise our hypotheses and improve our causal theories.

ELEMENTS OF PATH ANALYSIS

Correlated Variables

By now you should be familiar with the idea of one variable correlating with another, and you should know how to find such a correlation. Suppose, for the following examples, that we are interested in the achievement of student nurses and have certain background information on a group of such students. In the dataset there is a positive relation ($r = 0.40$) between student achievement (grades) and the student's family income. In path analysis this relation is represented as in Figure 15-1. Each part of this simple diagram has a meaning. When a variable is in a square, it means that it has been measured and has scores or numbers in our dataset. (Later we note variables in circles, which means that they are unmeasured.) Note that the line is curved (not straight) and

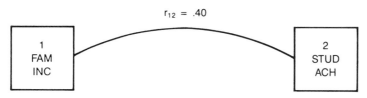

FIGURE 15-1
Correlated variables.

that there is no arrow point at either end. We have simply the correlation here, no causal path, and we are agnostic about which is the cause, family income or student achievement, and which is the effect.

The problem with such a diagram is that we cannot draw any important conclusions from it. In general, to draw benefits from statistical analysis, we must build in some assumptions.

Simplest Path Diagram

By adding some assumptions, such a diagram of correlation can be transformed into the simplest possible model of cause. In Figure 15-2 these very important changes in the model are explained.

First, we ask ourselves a question about the weak causal ordering of these two variables, the income of the parents, and the achievement of the student nurse. By saying "weak" we deny that we know one to be an influence on the other. Rather, we are answering the question, "If one is the cause of the other, which would it be?" When the question is so put, virtually everyone will agree that the arrow must be drawn from family income to student achievement, not the other way around. This is because one major consideration is temporal order, when these events took place, because causality must work forward in time, not backward. Clearly, family income was established before the student went into the nursing education program, ruling out a reversed arrow.

Notice that the decision about weak causal ordering is an important decision in the design and analysis of cause, but it is not a statistical decision. Rather, it depends on reason, logic, and some background knowledge of the variables. Making such decisions is largely a matter of consensus, close to using persuasion, rather than any inexorable technical conclusion. However, such agreements are easy to find in most of the situa-

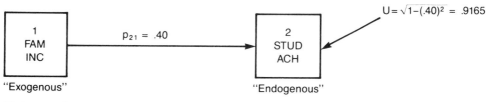

FIGURE 15-2
A path diagram.

tions that we study. When they are not logically obvious, it often will make little difference to the outcome of interest (because they are embedded in the diagram and because the outcome variables of greatest interest are not much affected by the arrow direction). Having drawn the arrow in this simplest path diagram, some new vocabulary is required, and some new possibilities for analysis emerge.

Exogenous Versus Endogenous Variables

Variable 1, family income, has now become the origin of the causal model (see Fig. 15-2). Because it has an arrow coming from it but no arrow leading to it, it is termed an *exogenous* variable. We are stating that any of the causes of family income must come from outside the model. On the other hand student achievement has an arrow pointing to it; thus, some of its variance is explained by a variable in the model. Such internal variables are called *endogenous* variables.

Path Coefficients

Note that in Figure 15-1 there was a curved line for the equation, $r_{12} = 0.40$. For Figure 15-2 the correlation between these variables has not changed, but instead of $r = 0.40$, we have $p_{21} = 0.40$. Because there are no other influences in the model, the correlation has simply been transformed into the path coefficient. Note that the order of the subscripts is changed, because path coefficients are traditionally expressed with the effect variable first and the cause variable second. Hence, p_{21} expresses the direct influence of family income (1) on student achievement (2).

What does a path of 0.40 mean? All the numbers are based on correlations, so they should be thought of in terms of standard scores. Thus, a path of 0.40 means that if family income is changed 1 standard deviation, student achievement will change 0.40 of a standard deviation.

There is one more addition in the transformation to a path model. We have added another arrow bearing on the endogenous variable—this arrow comes from U outside the model. The U may be thought of as *u*nexplained or *u*nknown influences that are pooled together and computed as the influences *not* explained by the paths leading to student achievement. (Some authors use R instead of U.) In this example with only two variables, U is solved as follows:

$$U = \sqrt{1 - r^2} \quad \text{or} \quad U = \sqrt{1 - (0.40)^2} = 0.9165$$

Almost 92% of the variance in student achievement is *not* explained by family income. Note that $(0.9165)^2$ plus $(0.40)^2$ is equal to 1, accounting for 100% of the variance in student achievement. Since the U expression does not add new information, why do we bother putting it in our model? Sometimes we do not, but here it serves the following purpose: Because there is no line connecting U with variable 1, we are indicating that this unexplained (or disturbance) variable is uncorrelated with any causes of student achievement in the model. Later these assumptions become clearer.

A Three-Variable Model

The power of path analysis becomes much more important when the problem is expanded to three variables. In Figure 15-3 parent education is added to the other two variables. The straight arrows indicate causal direction. The origin of the model is now parent education. This is because parent education is ordinarily prior to family income and may be thought of as contributing to it. Both of these background variables, parent education and family income, are possible causes of student achievement, and we are therefore granting the weak causal ordering. In this model parent education (1) is an exogenous variable, whereas family income (2) and student achievement (3) are endogenous.

A Recursive Model

The path model in Figure 15-3 is called *recursive*, because it may be analyzed in the same way as each new variable is added. Note that there are no loops in it. Flow is from left to right, with no doubling back. This particular model is called *complete recursive*, because no paths are omitted from the diagram. (We see later that often a goal of path analysis is to reduce the number of paths.) Some nonrecursive models are discussed later.

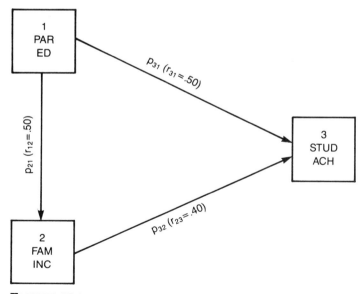

FIGURE 15-3
Three-variable model.

The Logic of Causal Models

In Figure 15-3 the coefficient for the path between variables 1 and 2 (p_{21}) equals the correlation between these two variables (r_{12}). This is true because no other causes in the model influence this correlation between the first and second variables. Therefore, because $r_{12} = 0.50$, $p_{21} = 0.50$.

The other two paths in Figure 15-3 leading to student achievement are not so simple, because there must be some adjustment made for the confusion of the two causes of student achievement and their own correlation with each other.

In the logic of path analysis the correlation of any two variables is explained by the tracing rule:

> A correlation between variables is the sum of the products of all path tracings from one variable to the other (except that there may be no entering the same variable twice on a tracing and no entering *and* leaving a variable through arrowheads).

In Figure 15-3 we see that for the path between 1 and 2, p_{21}, we count a tracing from 1 to 2 directly. We may not count the tracing 1 to 3 to 2, because that would require entering and leaving 3 through arrowheads. Thus, as already shown, $p_{21} = 0.50$ and represents r_{12}. The correlation between 1 and 3, however, consists of the direct path (1 to 3) and the indirect path (1 to 2 to 3). The direct path is p_{31}. Indirect paths are calculated as the product of the paths contained within them; therefore, here the indirect path from 1 to 3 is the product of $p_{21} \times p_{32}$, or $p_{21}p_{32}$.

The correlation between 2 and 3, r_{23}, consists of the direct path from 2 to 3, p_{32}, and the two-step tracing from 2 to 1 to 3, or $p_{21}p_{31}$. This indirect tracing is not immediately clear from looking at the model, because moving from 2 to 1 seems to be contrary to the arrow on that path. However, such a tracing is included under the tracing rule, because no variable is entered twice; although $p_{21}p_{31}$ enters and leaves 1, it does not enter *and* leave 2 through an arrowhead. This noncausal tracing helps us to understand the *correlation* between 2 and 3, because part of this correlation is caused by the fact that 1 has a common impact on both 2 and 3 (Asher, 1983). (For another method of determining which paths to include in the indirect path, see Pedhazur, 1982.) In path analysis we decompose, or break down, the correlations into direct causal, indirect causal, and noncausal components. *Note*: all *causal* paths must follow the arrows. From the example we can write:

	Direct Causal		Indirect Causal		Noncausal
$r_{12} =$	p_{21}	+	—	+	0
$r_{13} =$	p_{31}	+	$p_{21}p_{32}$	+	0
$r_{23} =$	p_{32}	+	0	+	$p_{21}p_{31}$

The path coefficients are calculated by using multiple regression analysis in which each endogenous variable is regressed on the variables that are prior to it in the model and assumed to have a causal effect on it, as indicated by the arrows in the model. The standardized or beta weight is the value most commonly used for the path coefficients

TABLE 15-1
Regressions Used to Compute Path Coefficients

Regression	Dependent Variable	Independent Variable(s)	Betas
1	Family income (2)	Parent education (1)	0.50 (p_{21})
2	Student achievement (3)	Parent education (1)	0.40 (p_{31})
		Family income (2)	0.20 (p_{32})

(although some researchers use the unstandardized or b-weights). In this example two regressions would be run. Family income (2) would be regressed on parent education (1), and student achievement (3) would be regressed on family income (2) and parent education (1). The results of these regressions are given in Table 15-1. Substituting these path values in our equation, we can determine the direct, indirect, and total causal effects, as presented in Table 15-2.

Direct and Indirect Paths

In Table 15-2 examine the decomposition of r_{13}, and note that variable 1 has two ways of influencing variable 3. It influences variable 3 directly with a path of 0.40. It also influences variable 3 indirectly with a path of 0.10, by influencing variable 2, which in turn influences variable 3. The total influence of variable 1 on variable 3 is $0.40 + 0.10$, or 0.50, which is the original correlation between variables 1 and 3. The tracing rule is thus demonstrated—that a correlation between two variables is the sum of the products of the tracings, subject to certain exceptions. In this simple example the other causal and noncausal covariation also is shown. The path analysis allows calculation of causal and noncausal components. If there is a difference between the total causal effect and the original correlation, that indicates that a portion of the original correlation was noncausal or spurious. For example the original correlation between variables 2 and 3 is 0.40, the total causal influences are 0.20, and the noncausal component of the correlation equals $0.40 - 0.20 = 0.20$. Path analysis, then, gives us the direct, indirect, and noncausal components of correlation coefficients.

TABLE 15-2
Calculation of Direct, Indirect, and Total Causal Effects

r	Direct Effect	Indirect Effect	Total Causal Effect (Direct + Indirect)	Noncausal Covariation
$r_{12} = 0.50$	$p_{21} = 0.50$	—	0.50	0.00
$r_{13} = 0.50$	$p_{31} = 0.40$	$p_{21}p_{32} = (0.50)(0.20) = 0.10$	0.50	0.00
$r_{23} = 0.40$	$p_{32} = 0.20$	0	0.20	0.20

Importance of Indirect Paths

Often in path models, the indirect paths may be more important than the direct paths. The total causal influence of a variable also is likely to be of great interest. Thus, the way we draw some of the arrows in a diagram can be central to the apparent findings. It is important that the model be based on reasonable deductions.

In Figure 15-4 a frequent event is diagrammed. The investigators do not declare the priority of the causal variables, preferring to show a curved, two-headed arrow pointing between them. This is essentially an *agnostic* diagram, as far as this relation is concerned. Causal influence is acknowledged, but there is no clear preference of one direction over the other and no willingness to exclude either influence.

In the published literature this may be the most usual position. Often, researchers are concentrating on the criterion or outcome variable and do not want to quibble about the causal variables and their relation to each other. Often, too, they may be principally interested in the direct causal influence on the outcome variable and, rightly or not, less interested in the indirect influence.

Such a position is understandable, but you should realize what is lost—any possibility of recovering the indirect influences, some of which may frequently be larger than the direct influences. Just as drawing paths allows far more interpretation than plain correlations, so one-directional arrows allow more interpretation than two-headed, ambiguous arrows.

For these reasons we strongly encourage students to try, whenever possible, to draw one-directional arrows. Our own research experience supports this. For example in studying the effects of origins of leadership, the importance of intelligence was operating mostly indirectly, through high school grades. Without a willingness to declare intelligence prior to grades, this influence would have been buried.

In general how may such arrows be validated? First, we recognize that we are

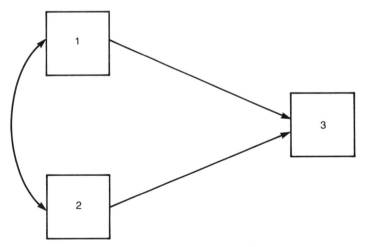

FIGURE 15-4
Lack of causal ordering between variables 1 and 2.

dealing with matters of logic, background knowledge, and persuasion through evidence. Thus, for one solution we may declare the directions that appear most wise to us and see whether there is any objection, or we may ask knowledgeable people their opinions and take majority opinion as support. Often, there is background literature or published opinion to support one direction. If these efforts still fail to satisfy us, we may calculate it both ways (one trial with the arrow pointing from A to B and the other with the arrow reversed). Sometimes, there will be no important differences in results, and the direction will therefore be unimportant. Other times, both results may be published, and the decision is left to the informed reader.

THEORY TESTING FROM A PATH MODEL

One of the overriding purposes of research is the development of theory. An example from the literature will help clarify the use of path analysis for testing theoretical relationships.

Identification

Muhlenkamp and Sayles (1986) sought to study the relationships among selected demographic variables (age, education, and gender), social support, self-esteem, and positive health practices among adults. Figure 15-5 contains the model they tested. As

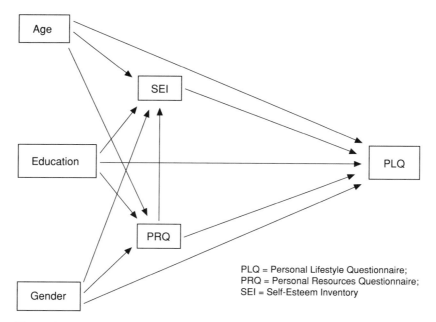

FIGURE 15-5
Adapted from Muhlenkamp and Sayles (1986), p. 336.

you can see, all possible paths have been drawn from the exogenous to the endogenous variables. This is called a *just-identified model*. Table 15-3 contains the results of the analyses on this model. Lifestyle (PLQ) is the final variable in the model. It is regressed on all of the preceding variables. Looking at the direct effects in Table 15-3, we see that the effect of social support (PRQ) is equal to zero. Because of this, the investigators dropped that path from their final model, which is seen in Figure 15-6. Self-esteem (SEI) was regressed on the four preceding variables. As we can see in Table 15-3, the path between education and self-esteem equaled zero, and that path also was dropped from the final model. Finally, social support (PRQ) was regressed on the three demographic variables. The path between age and social support was equal to zero and therefore was dropped from the final model.

Dropping paths from a just-identified model results in an *overidentified model*. The advantages of such a model include theory development, parsimony, and the ability to test the model for significance. A just-identified model cannot be tested for significance, because the correlation matrix will always be perfectly reproduced when all the parameters are included (Pedhazur, 1982, p. 616). An overidentified model may be

TABLE 15-3
Effects of Independent Variables on Lifestyle, Self-Esteem, and Social Support

	Effect			
	Causal			
Variables	Direct	Indirect	Total	Noncausal
On Lifestyle				
Self-esteem	.21	0	.21	0
Social support	0	.11	.11	.08
Age	−.17	−.03	−.20	.11
Education	.18	.02	.20	0
Gender	−.33	.02	−.31	.01
On Self-Esteem				
Social support	.54	0	.54	−.05
Age	−.15	0	−.15	−.03
Education	0	.11	.11	0
Gender	.21	−.11	−.10	.05
On Social Support				
Education	.20	0	.20	0
Age	0	0	0	.07
Gender	−.21	0	−.21	0

(From Muhlenkamp, A. F., & Sayles, J. A. [1986]. Self-esteem, social support, and positive health practices. Nursing Research, 35[6], 336.)

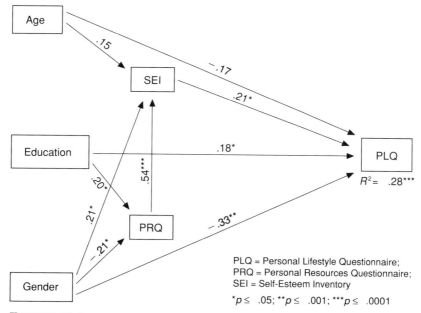

FIGURE 15-6
Overidentified causal model.

(From Muhlenkamp, A. F. & Sayles, J. A. [1986]. Self-esteem, social support, and positive health practices. *Nursing Research, 35*[6], 336.)

developed in two ways: by *hypothesizing* that certain paths are equal to zero or (as in this example) by dropping paths based on *analysis* of the just-identified model.

Trimming a Causal Model

In this example *trimming* of the model was quite clear, because the paths equaled zero. This is not usually the case. Because the path coefficients equal betas in the regression equation, testing the betas for significance provides a significance test of the paths. In Figure 15-6 asterisks are used to identify the significant paths. If Muhlenkamp and Sayles (1986) had used statistical significance at the 0.05 level as a criterion for deleting paths, they would have deleted two more. Can you see which two? Instead, they dropped all paths with significance levels greater than 0.10. In addition to statistical significance, meaningfulness also has been used in the deletion of paths. This is a judgmental criterion that depends on a variety of factors. As Pedhazur (1982) points out, "In the absence of guidelines many researchers select a criterion for the deletion of paths arbitrarily—say, all Betas less than .05 are deleted" (p. 617).

Once paths are dropped, the analyses must be rerun with only the retained variables. For example lifestyle (PLQ) is regressed on all the variables preceding it, except social support. Excluding a path or paths changes the betas for the other variables, so new regressions must be run.

Statistical Tests of the Model

The overidentified model can be tested using a chi-square goodness of fit test. A significant result (probability level less than 0.05) indicates that the model *does not fit*. It indicates that there are differences between the model as specified and the data. The larger the probability level, the better the data fit the model. Thus, a probability of 0.99 indicates a perfect fit, whereas a probability of less than 0.05 indicates lack of fit. A difficulty that arises with this method of assessing the fit is that with the large sample sizes required for such analyses, the null hypothesis may be rejected, even when the model fit is relatively good. Pedhazur (1982) suggests the Q statistic, because it is not affected by sample size. Again, the larger the probability level, the better the fit. In the example given the level of significance associated with the chi-square goodness of fit test was 0.983, and that associated with the Q statistic was 0.977. Both of these indicate a very good fit.

EXPERIMENTS IN PATH ANALYSIS

Such path models may help in identifying the nature of experiments and in understanding their results. In this section two expansions of the former example of achievement in nursing school are presented. First, our subjects attend different types of nursing schools (i.e., 2-year versus 4-year), and we add the variable (type of nursing school) to our model. Such a model may be drawn as in Figure 15-7.

Again, how we draw this model is important and depends on our reasoning about the way education works. In the sense of "weak causal ordering," we are entitled to place the family influences prior to the school selection.

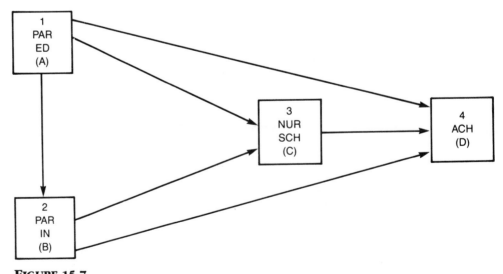

FIGURE 15-7
Four-variable path model.

False Experiments

Too often, investigators regard just one relationship by itself, such as that between nursing school type and achievement, and may draw conclusions filled with errors and exaggerations. For example suppose that the correlation between school type and achievement is 0.30. The implication might be that by simply changing school type, we would increase achievement nearly one third of a standard deviation, on the average. Suppose, however, that the more complete, four-variable model had correlations as in Table 15-4.

Note that school type is correlated 0.30 with achievement but that the prior variables are correlated with both school type and Achievement. So we may be properly inquisitive about the causal relations among these four variables.

A Computer Analysis of the Problem

Let us use SYSTAT, a large statistical system (of which Mystat is a smaller offshoot). SYSTAT is one of the most widely used packages for the personal computer. We may gain some feel for recursive path models from our example and how they may be solved by your own computer.

In the nursing school model we are mainly interested in the path coefficients, and these are produced by Systat in the form shown in Figure 15-8. In this example a correlation matrix, as if produced by previous analysis, was our input. More commonly, statistical systems work directly with individual data, but the use of the correlation matrix is easy, and the resulting analysis takes only a few seconds.

In Figure 15-8 we see the kinds of commands we might use for a four-variable path model. The second part of the figure shows the output produced by these commands, from the correlation matrix for the nursing school question.

The important path weights are found under the two headings of "COEFFICIENT" and "STD COEF." (Because we worked from correlations, rather than covariances, these two are the same.) For the first model regressing B on A (parent income on parent education), we find 0.500 to be the path. This is not changed from the correlation, but we have learned new information, that the T ratio is very high and is significant beyond the 0.001 level. Do you see this information for the first model?

TABLE 15-4
Correlations of Hypothetical Data for Effects of Nursing School Type

Variables	A	B	C	D
A. Parent education	1.00			
B. Parent income	0.50	1.00		
C. Nursing school type	0.30	0.40	1.00	
D. Achievement test	0.50	0.40	0.30	1.00

I. WHAT YOU MIGHT TYPE AT THE COMPUTER, USING SYSTAT:
>MGLH (This calls up the programs for ''multiple general linear hypothesis.''
    MGLH is very wide in its use and solves many kinds of problems, including
    path models.)
>USE NURSCOR (This is a filename you have given to the correlation matrix for the
    nursing problem)
>MODEL B = A / N = 100
    (This model asks about predicting B from A. Since these correlations were
    entered by hand, the ''N = 100'' tells Systat how many cases are involved.)
>ESTIMATE
    (This command tell Systat to estimate this first model. Systat would
    produce the result immediately.)
>MODEL C = A + B / N = 100
>ESTIMATE
>MODEL D = A + B + C / N = 100
>ESTIMATE

WHAT YOUR SYSTAT OUTPUT WOULD LOOK LIKE:
COMPUTER OUTPUT FROM THE THREE MODELS ABOVE
Output from the first model: MODEL B = A / N = 100

DEP VAR: B   N: 100 MULTIPLE R: 0.500   SQUARED MULTIPLE R: 0.250
ADJUSTED SQUARED MULTIPLE R: .242   STANDARD ERROR OF ESTIMATE: 0.870

VARIABLE	COEFFICIENT	STD ERROR	STD COEF	TOLERANCE	T	P(2 TAIL)
A	0.500	0.087	0.500	1.000	5.715	0.000

ANALYSIS OF VARIANCE

SOURCE	SUM-OF-SQUARES	DF	MEAN-SQUARE	F-RATIO	P
REGRESSION	24.750	1	24.750	32.667	0.000
RESIDUAL	74.250	98	0.758		

Output from the second model: MODEL C = A + B / N = 100

DEP VAR: C   N: 100 MULTIPLE R: 0.416   SQUARED MULTIPLE R: 0.173
ADJUSTED SQUARED MULTIPLE R: .156   STANDARD ERROR OF ESTIMATE: 0.914

VARIABLE	COEFFICIENT	STD ERROR	STD COEF	TOLERANCE	T	P(2 TAIL)
A	0.133	0.107	0.133	0.750	1.251	0.214
B	0.333	0.107	0.333	0.750	3.127	0.002

ANALYSIS OF VARIANCE

SOURCE	SUM-OF-SQUARES	DF	MEAN-SQUARE	F-RATIO	P
REGRESSION	16.987	2	8.493	10.169	0.000
RESIDUAL	81.013	97	0.835		

FIGURE 15-8
Input and output for SYSTAT analysis of the nursing school problem (Fig. 15-7).

Output from the third model: MODEL D = A + B + C / N = 100

```
DEP VAR:      D     N:      100  MULTIPLE R: 0.540      SQUARED MULTIPLE R: 0.292
ADJUSTED SQUARED MULTIPLE R: .270        STANDARD ERROR OF ESTIMATE:      0.846

VARIABLE   COEFFICIENT   STD ERROR   STD COEF   TOLERANCE    T      P(2 TAIL)
A             0.384        0.100       0.384      0.738    3.841     0.000
B             0.160        0.104       0.160      0.681    1.535     0.128
C             0.121        0.094       0.121      0.827    1.281     0.203

                ANALYSIS OF VARIANCE

SOURCE        SUM-OF-SQUARES    DF    MEAN-SQUARE    F-RATIO    P

REGRESSION         28.333        3       9.444       13.204    0.000
RESIDUAL           68.667       96       0.715
```

FIGURE 15-8 (CONTINUED)

In the second model, nursing school (*C*) is regressed on parent education (*A*) and parent income (*B*). The resulting paths are 0.133 for *A* and 0.333 for *B*. These, then, are our "causal" forces bearing on selection into nursing school type. In this model parent income appears much stronger than parent education.

For the third model the paths bearing on achievement (*D*) are 0.384 from parent education (*A*); 0.160 from parent income (*B*); and 0.121 from nursing school type (*C*). We may draw these paths into a new diagram, as shown in Figure 15-9. With all the causal variables having influences on each other, we expect to see the path coefficients considerably smaller than the correlations. Such is the case in Figure 15-9. Note that no paths are eliminated from the model, because no paths fell below the arbitrary test of 0.05. Observe that the effect of school type has shrunk to about one third of the power that we might previously have estimated. Even without eliminating such a path, we have greatly altered our theoretical understanding of it. Although these are fictitious data, this analysis illustrates a common finding in path models: We must control for preexisting causes and not be misled by variables that might have caught our attention or that come under our own control.

A True Experiment

The previous study of nursing school type may illustrate a common error in understanding: When seen in a path model, we observed that selection into nursing schools will not be random, but rather will be correlated with other variables of importance. Nursing school selection will seldom be a true experiment. Suppose, however, that we used a true experiment, such as a film aimed at improving the instruction of certain practices, and we wish to find out whether it improves the general achievement test scores for the field. By true experiment we mean that every subject has an equal chance of being

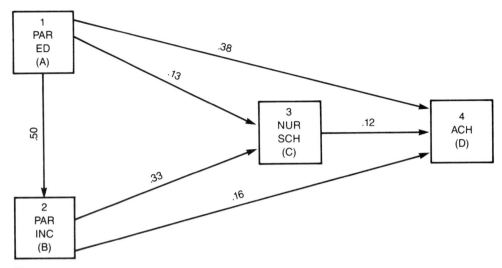

FIGURE 15-9
Model for nursing school study, with causal paths included.

placed in a particular experimental group. A true experiment would be drawn as in Figure 15-10.

In Figure 15-10 note that variable 4, our experimental variable, has no lines connecting it with parent education, parent income, or nursing school type. This is because, if the assignment is truly random, there will be no important correlations with any prior variables. One test of whether the treatments were assigned randomly is to inspect the correlations and the resulting paths. After the analysis is completed, the correlation of EXP and ACH should be close to the path coefficient for the same two variables.

If the effects of the experiment were overlapping the background variables, we might redraw the model, showing the apparent influences of the background variables on the experimental assignment. In the real world of experimentation with human subjects, frequently compromises with availability, self-selection, and other soft influences may distort true randomness. In such cases there is a great power in including all the available variables that might influence the apparent outcomes.

TIME-LAGGED MODELS

Usually, researchers find it more profitable and productive to work with recursive models, in which one variable points clearly to others and there is an assumed hierarchy leading from the first variable to the last. Needless to say, life is not always so simple, and some pairs of variables are difficult to sort into cause and effect. Does depression lead to illness, or does illness lead to depression? Does self-esteem lead to achieve-

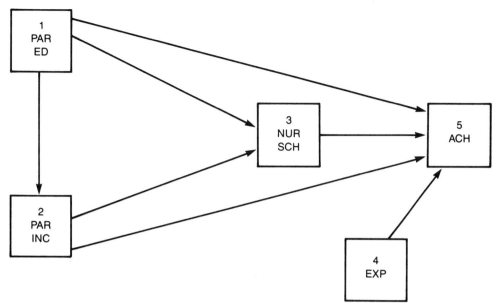

FIGURE 15-10
Inclusion of a "true" experiment in the nursing-school model.

ment, or is it the other way around? We could ask many such questions for which, given our present knowledge, we might be doubtful about the cause-effect relationship, or we might argue that the causes work both ways. How should such problems be handled? This brings us to a new approach called time-lagged models.

When the Problem Is Minor

First, depending on where our doubtful path occurs, it may not make any important difference in our outcome whether A causes B or B causes A. For example if our main concern is on other relationships and the questionable path occurs earlier in a large model, the direction of such an early arrow may be trivial in its later effects. The doubtful path may be weak and thus unimportant. We should be aware that any importance of earlier paths is typically in estimating indirect effects, and these will usually be small later in the causal chain. In any case we can often directly resolve the question of importance: The model can usually be run both ways, first with A influencing B, then with B influencing A. This will frequently show that the principal concerns are not importantly affected by the arrow. The results of such trials may be briefly reported, to satisfy the critical reader, so that questioning of some disagreement about cause will not be a barrier to the acceptance of the research as a whole.

Cross-Lagged Designs

On the other hand suppose that such a question of causal direction is close to the heart of our research. How may we find an answer? One type of solution has been used extensively and may, like a straight recursive model, be analyzed by simple methods. This type of model is often termed *cross-lagged panel correlation* (CLPC). It is so named because there is a lag of time between the two periods, and the interest is in the cross-correlations across time and variable. Such a case is shown in Figure 15-11.

In Figure 15-11 note that there are two variables, A and B, measured on two occasions, 1 and 2. From the four measures there are six correlations, and they may be separated into three different types:

1. $rA1B1$ and $rA2B2$ are synchronous correlations (with A and B measured at the same time).
2. $rA1A2$ and $rB1B2$ are autocorrelations (the same variables measured twice).
3. $rA1B2$ and $rB1A2$ are cross-lagged correlations (different variables at different times).

Figure 15-11 is drawn differently from the previous diagrams, showing the model with some straight lines but without any arrows. The straight lines are shown because, in the logic of causality, we believe that the earlier events might cause the later events, or at least the reverse would not be defended. On the other hand two curved lines are used for the synchronous correlations, because we are being agnostic about the direction of cause. But this notation is not standard. There are various ways of drawing such CLPC designs and various ways of analyzing them.

Method of Simple Difference

Such designs attracted much attention when explained in a classic early work on research design (Campbell & Stanley, 1963). In the earliest suggestion a researcher was mainly interested in the following question: Does A cause B more than B causes A?

This question was answered by a comparison of $rA1B2$ and $rB1A2$. If $rA1B2$ was greater than $rB1A2$ and this contrast was statistically significant, A (at time 1) was possibly causing B (at time 2) more than B1 was causing A2.

Doubts About the Simple Method

In the last decades there have been increasing doubts about the simple comparison of the cross-lagged correlations. If the reliability of B2 is greater than that for A2, all correlations with B2 might be expected to be relatively higher, including $rA1B2$, but this would say little about causality. For the cross-lagged correlations to be a good index of relative causality, it is expected that the whole construct of relations remains stable from time 1 to time 2 (the principle of stationarity), and this condition is not easy to verify. Many researchers would now urge that such data be set forth in more of an explicit and defensible path model and be solved by the use of multiple regression and other

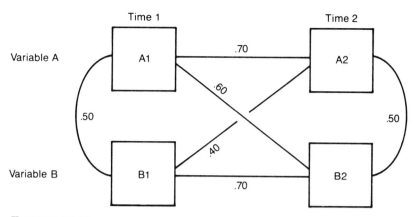

FIGURE 15-11
Cross-lagged panel design in its simplest form.

methods (Campbell, 1988; Cook & Campbell, 1979; Glymour, Scheines, Spirtes, & Kelly, 1987; Kenny, 1979, 1987; Kerlinger, 1986; Marascuilo & Levin, 1983).

For these reasons we do not describe such cross-lagged designs further in this book, but you should be aware that this is one method of exploring the possible direction of influence between two variables or their possible mutual influence. Even when you decide to use the straight recursive models, you should be aware of such time-lagged alternatives and sometimes consider using them.

PATH ANALYSIS AS A TOOL: A FINAL WORD

Path models can become complex and lead the researcher to almost endless questions of method and justification. The last thing we want to do is to intimidate a researcher who is seeking to understand and explain some of the interesting data in the health professions. Rather, we offer path models as a way of placing a great deal of material into some meaningful pattern. Data are clearly useless unless we have some general organizing principle. Often, simple diagrams can help us decide what we are looking for, what data we need to collect or examine, and how we may present our case.

For most of your uses you will probably be content with the completely recursive models, in which you are willing to draw causal arrows from some beginning variable to the intermediate variables, and on to the final variables. In such models you will frequently want to set forth correlation matrices, path coefficients for the diagrams, and tables of decomposition. Frequently, you may want to combine a number of variables into single measures using factor analysis or some other principle, so you can see the important relations more clearly. Another way of managing multiple measures is presented in the following chapter on structural equation modeling.

16 Structural Equation Models: *Latent Variables*

Mairead L. Hickey

OBJECTIVES FOR CHAPTER 16

After reading this chapter you should be able to do the following:

1. Describe the three conditions necessary for making causal statements.

2. Describe the role of theory in the structural equation modeling (SEM) process.

3. Compare latent variable measurement models and SEMs.

4. Describe the steps in the latent variable modeling process.

5. Interpret the findings of a latent variable SEM.

As mentioned in Chapter 15, causal modeling is a relatively new methodology to the social and health sciences. During the recent years of its development and refinement, causal modeling has been referred to by many names, including path analysis, structural modeling, structural equation modeling, and covariance structure analysis. Path analysis was first introduced by biometrician Sewall Wright in 1918 (Wright, 1918); however, it was not until the 1960s that sociologists (Blalock, 1961, 1963, 1964; Boudon, 1965; Duncan, 1966) realized the benefit of path analysis as a method of data analysis and the 1970s that Jöreskog (1973) and Wiley (1973) developed structural equation models (SEMs) with path analysis diagrams and features. SEMs first appeared in the nursing literature in the

Barbara Hazard Munro and Ellis Batten Page: STATISTICAL METHODS FOR HEALTH CARE RESEARCH, SECOND EDITION. © 1993, 1986 by J. B. Lippincott Company.

1980s with studies by such investigators as Aaronson (1984), Cox and Roghmann (1984), and Murdaugh and Verran (1986).

SEM techniques are attractive because they permit scientists to test hypotheses and make causal inferences about the effects of certain variables on other variables without adhering to experimental manipulation and random assignment, constraints often unrealistic in studies with human subjects. These techniques allow scientists to make causal inferences about SEMs with correlation data, rather than with experimentally manipulated data.

The focus of this chapter is on the process of SEM with latent, or unobserved, variables. The basic conditions of causation are presented along with the essential role of theory in the SEM process. The latent variable SEM process is described, and examples of latent variable analysis using LISREL VI (Jöreskog & Sörbom, 1986) are provided. As a note the fundamental elements of path analysis described in Chapter 15 also apply to latent variable SEMs and therefore are not be repeated in this chapter.

Before specific aspects of SEMs and the SEM process are described, it is necessary to present two major conditions that underly SEM—causation and adequacy of theory.

CONDITIONS OF CAUSATION

SEMs are composed of several causal statements that hypothesize causal relationships between several variables. Causal statements are composed of a cause (X) and an effect (Y). For example X causes Y, or $X \rightarrow Y$.

Three conditions are necessary to hypothesize causal statements (Kenny, 1979). The first condition is temporal ordering, which means that for X to cause Y, X must occur before Y. An example of temporal ordering is found in the causal relationship between hemorrhage (X) and hematocrit level (Y). In terms of temporal order, hemorrhage precedes a drop in hematocrit. The second condition necessary for making causal statements is the presence of an observed and measurable relationship between the variables X and Y. Clearly, in the example described, an inverse relationship exists between hemorrhage and hematocrit level.

Nonspuriousness between X and Y is the third condition required before making causal statements. A nonspurious relationship between variables implies that a relationship exists between X and Y when a third variable (Z) is controlled for. In the previous example, hemorrhage, in and of itself, affects hematocrit, even when spurious variables such as age, sex, and baseline blood volume are controlled for. Thus, a nonspurious relationship exists between hemorrhage and hematocrit.

THEORETICAL BASIS OF THE STRUCTURAL EQUATION MODEL

In addition to meeting the conditions of causation described previously, the causal statements in SEMs also must be supported by adequate theory. Theory provides the basis and context for the relationships between the variables in the SEM. Although the conditions of causation may warrant making causal statements, the SEM should be tested only when adequate theory or research findings exist to support and guide the causal statements in the SEM.

It is important to note that even when the conditions of causation and theory are adequately met and the causal statements within the SEM are subsequently tested, causal statements are never proven; they are only confirmed or unconfirmed. The validity of the confirmatory evidence gained through model testing is dependent on the adequacy of the SEM's theoretical foundation.

STRUCTURAL EQUATION MODELS

An SEM is a causal model that hypothesizes causal relationships between variables to explain a phenomenon. For example we may wonder what causes some cardiac patients to adjust well after cardiac surgery, while others do not. After a review of the available research and theory on surgical adjustment, we may identify variables that are expected to have a causal influence on surgical adjustment, place them in a theoretical SEM of surgical adjustment, and test the extent to which they explain the surgical adjustment phenomenon.

As mentioned in Chapter 15, the relationships between variables in an SEM may be graphically depicted in a path diagram. In addition each causal relationship also can be expressed as an algebraic equation, which provides the mathematical structure for the SEM. There are as many structural equations as there are endogenous (effect or dependent) variables in the model. Endogenous variables are presumed to be caused by or explained by other variables in the model. Exogenous (cause or independent) variables, on the other hand, are variables presumed to be caused by factors outside the model.

In each structural equation the endogenous variable is expressed as the sum of the products of each exogenous variable with its structural coefficient. Thus, in the structural equation

$$Y = a + b_1 X_1 + b_2 X_2 + \ldots b_n X_n + e,$$

the endogenous variable Y is the sum of the exogenous variables, denoted by X_1, $X_2, \ldots X_n$, weighted according to their respective structural coefficients. The structural coefficients, denoted by b_1, $b_2, \ldots b_n$, are regression coefficients and represent the expected amount of change in the endogenous variable with a 1-unit change in the respective exogenous variable. Disturbance, or error, denoted as e in the structural equation above, represents all unspecified causes on the endogenous variable.

Manifest and Latent Variables

SEMs can express causal relationships between two types of variables—observed (measured or manifest) and unobserved (latent). Traditionally, studies have examined manifest variables. Manifest variables are measured by one observed indicator variable. Latent variables, on the other hand, are hypothetical constructs that are not directly

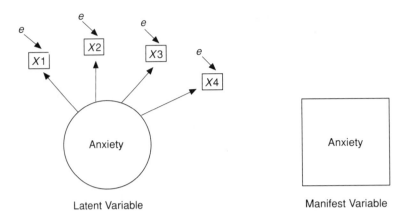

Note: X1 = Heart rate   X3 = Blood pressure
       X2 = Hand taps   X4 = Anxiety score
       e = measurement error

FIGURE 16-1
Anxiety as a latent and manifest variable.

measured or observed. Instead, a latent variable is measured by more than one observed indicator.

Figure 16-1 presents anxiety as a latent variable and a manifest variable. As a manifest variable anxiety is the score on an anxiety instrument. As a latent variable, however, anxiety is measured by four observed indicators (heart rate per minute, blood pressure, number of hand taps per minute, and score on an anxiety instrument). In graphic diagrams manifest variables are represented in boxes, while latent variables are depicted by circles, and their multiple observed indicators (i.e., manifest variables) are in boxes. Also, because the observed indicators of a latent variable are directly influenced by the latent variable, observed indicators are connected to their respective latent variable through causal paths with arrows coming from the latent variable and leading to the observed indicators.

STATISTICAL ANALYSIS PROCEDURES FOR STRUCTURAL EQUATION MODELS

The statistical analysis technique used to estimate SEMs is determined by the type of causal variables in the SEM. Models with manifest variables of cause are tested through multiple regression procedures within the rigid assumptions of ordinary least squares (OLS). Models with latent variables usually are tested through the more relaxed maximum likelihood estimation (MLE) procedures found in such analysis packages as LISREL 7 (Jöreskog & Sörbom/SPSS, 1989), EQS (Bentler, 1989), or CALIS (SAS, 1990). The value of MLE comes from its ability to account for measurement error in the SEM.

Unlike OLS, MLE does not assume that variables are perfectly measured; therefore, it is not subject to the distorting effect of measurement error on causal inference found in OLS procedures. Other valuable features of MLE, which are not found in OLS, follow:

1. MLE does not assume recursive (one-way) relationships between variables. It can test nonrecursive models that hypothesize feedback between variables.
2. MLE does not assume that all relevant variables are specified in the model. It can account for unspecified cause on the endogenous variable by estimating the error or disturbance associated with the endogenous variable.

MLE *does* include the following assumptions:

1. The coefficient matrix of dependent variables is nonsingular.
2. Endogenous and exogenous variable measurement errors are uncorrelated (Lomax, 1982).

LATENT VARIABLE MODELING PROCESS

Theoretical Model

As already mentioned SEMs are created to explain certain phenomena. Within the context of theory, the model's variables and causal relationships are hypothesized. The variables and relationships within theoretical models are operationalized and tested through a modeling process. This section presents the latent variable SEM process—the process through which the theoretical latent SEM is transformed into a model that can be tested and evaluated.

Operationalizing the Theoretical Latent Model: Measurement Models and Structural Equation Models

A major part of the latent variable modeling process involves operationalizing, or specifying, the theoretical latent SEM for testing. As mentioned previously the SEM hypothesizes causal relationships between latent variables. Before the causal hypotheses in the SEM can be operationalized, however, the SEM's underlying measurement model must be specified and tested. Due to the unobserved nature of the latent variables in an SEM, preliminary evidence about how well the latent variables and their observed indicators fit together is required before the SEM can be tested empirically. This preliminary evidence is provided through measurement model specification and testing. Unlike the SEM, which hypothesizes and tests causal relationships between latent variables, the measurement model hypothesizes and tests the following:

- Causal relationships from each latent variable to its observed indicators
- Correlations between latent variables
- Correlations among the errors associated with the observed indicators

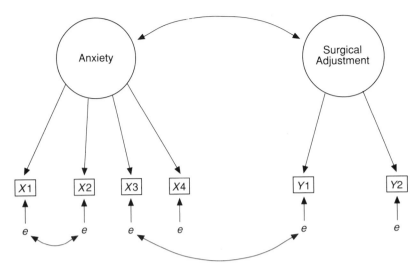

FIGURE 16-2
Hypothetical latent measurement model of surgical adjustment.

The measurement model may be considered a factor analytic model (Loehlin, 1987). Although measurement model estimation is an a priori, confirmatory process in which the indicators of latent variables are hypothesized, it is similar to exploratory factor analysis in that the indicators of latent variables are evaluated on how well they load on their latent variable factors. Also, the latent variables in a measurement model, like factors in a factor analytic model, are hypothesized to share a relationship as they explain the phenomenon.

Figure 16-2 presents a graphic representation of a hypothetical latent variable measurement model of surgical adjustment. The latent variables, anxiety and surgical adjustment, are depicted in circles. The curved line with an arrow at each end connecting the latent variables suggests a correlational, noncausal relationship between latent variables. The causal paths leading from the latent variables to their observed indicators demonstrate the causal influence of each latent variable on its observed indicators. Correlated measurement error is depicted as curved lines with arrows at each end between observed indicators.

As a comparison Figure 16-3 presents the SEM of surgical adjustment. This SEM can be tested only after the measurement model of surgical adjustment is evaluated and demonstrates a good fit with the data. Note that although the SEMs in Figure 16-3 include the observed indicators of the latent variables, SEMs can be graphically represented with or without observed indicators.

Modeling Process

The latent variable modeling process has two phases: measurement model specification, identification, estimation, and fit; and SEM specification, identification, estimation,

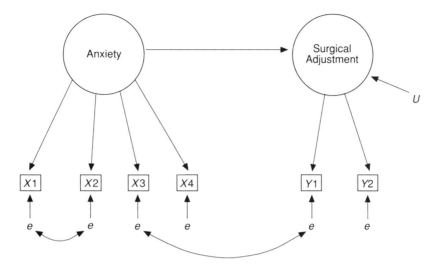

Note: *U* = disturbance or unexplained variance.

FIGURE 16-3
Hypothetical latent SEM of surgical adjustment.

and fit. The four sequential steps within each phase are described and later applied to a hypothetical latent variable SEM.

Measurement Model

Specification

Specification is the translation of ideas, theory, and hypotheses about the interrelationships between a set of theoretical latent variables and their indicators into a measurement model. The measurement model specifies noncausal relationships between the latent variables, causal relationships from latent variables to their observed indicators, and correlated error between observed indicators.

Identification

Identification is the existence of sufficient information to estimate the parameters in the model. Two types of identification (theoretical and statistical) must be considered. Theoretical identification is determined through a judgmental process that evaluates if the theoretical underpinnings of the model sufficiently support its specifications. Statistical identification means there is adequate information to uniquely solve the unknown parameters implied in the measurement model. The conditions of measurement model identification are quite complex and beyond the scope of this chapter. Readers interested in conducting latent variables modeling procedures are referred to the excellent discussion of measurement model identification by Kenny (1979).

Estimation

Estimation is the analysis of the specified model. Once the specified measurement model is considered identified, it is "run" with data from the study sample using a statistical analysis package (e.g., LISREL 7 [Jöreskog & Sörbom/SPSS, 1989], EQS [Bentler, 1989], CALIS [SAS, 1990]) that applies MLE approaches to test hypotheses about the unknown parameters in the measurement model.

Model Fit

Model Fit evaluates the theoretical and statistical fit of individual parameter estimates, as well as measuring the model as a whole. If the measurement model's individual parameters are significant and if the overall model fit is good, its hypotheses are supported, and the SEM can be tested. However, if the specified measurement model does not fit the data well, it needs to be respecified within the reason of theory. Respecification of the measurement model usually involves adding or deleting observed indicators and adding or deleting correlated measurement error parameters. Once respecified, the measurement model must undergo identification, estimation, and model fit until it fits the data.

Structural Equation Models

Specification

Specification is the translation of ideas, theory, and previous research within the theoretical model into an SEM with implied structural equations. The SEM specifies causal paths between latent variables.

Identification

Identification is the existence of sufficient information (theoretical and statistical) to estimate the unknown causal parameters between latent variables in the SEM. The basic premise of statistical identification of the SEM is that the known parameters (correlations or covariances) between latent variables in the model must equal or exceed the number of unknown parameters (paths between variables, correlations between exogenous variables, and correlated disturbance between variables) in the model (Kenny, 1979).

When a model contains more unknown parameters than known parameters, it is underidentified; conversely, when the number of known parameters exceeds the number of unknown parameters, the model is overidentified. When the number of known parameters equals the number of unknown parameters, the model is considered to be just-identified. Underidentified models, which have more unknown parameters than known parameters, cannot be estimated.

The number of known parameters is calculated by the following formula:

$$\frac{N(N-1)}{2},$$

N equals the total number of exogenous and endogenous variables in the model. The number of unknown parameters is the sum of all paths, correlations, and correlated disturbances between variables. To use this formula on the SEM of surgical adjustment in Figure 16-3, in which there are two latent variables ($N = 2$), the number of known parameters equals:

$$\frac{2(2-1)}{2} = 1.$$

The number of unknown parameters, determined by adding the number of paths, correlations, and disturbances between latent variables, equals 1. Thus, the SEM of surgical adjustment is just-identified and can be estimated.

Another example is found in Figure 16-4, which presents an overidentified SEM with four latent variables. Applying the model in Figure 16-4 to the formula described previously:

$$\frac{4(4-1)}{2} = 6,$$

The number of known parameters equals 6. The number of unknown parameters (i.e., the sum of the paths, correlations, and disturbances between latent variables) equals 4. Thus, the SEM in Figure 16-4 is overidentified and can be estimated.

Estimation

SEM estimation means "running" the SEM using a statistical package with data from the study sample to provide information about the unknown causal parameters.

Model Fit

SEM fit is the assessment of the theoretical and statistical fit of the individual causal parameters in the SEM and the overall fit of the SEM. If the SEM's fit is poor, it can be respecified, within the reason of theory, to undergo further estimation and evaluation of fit. Respecification of the SEM usually involves deleting or adding causal paths in the specified SEM.

The overall empirical fit of the measurement model and SEM is reported as a

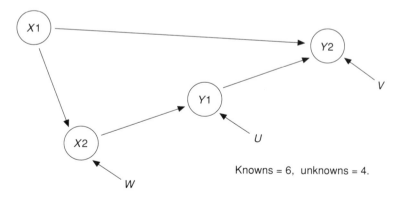

Knowns = 6, unknowns = 4.

Note: *U*, *V*, and *W* represent disturbance.

FIGURE 16-4
Overidentified SEM.

maximum likelihood chi-square (X^2) goodness of fit measure. Low, nonsignificant X^2 values are sought, suggesting that the specified model is consistent with the sample's observed data. Because the chi-square measure is dependent on sample size, other measures of model fit are sometimes used (Hayduk, 1987). In addition to the chi-square measure, LISREL also provides a goodness of fit index (GFI) that is independent of sample size (Jöreskog & Sörbom, 1986) and an adjusted goodness of fit measure (AGFI) that is adjusted for the *df*s in the model. With either measure, a value of 0.90 or greater indicates that the model fits the sample's data well. Another measure used to evaluate the overall fit of the model is the relative likelihood ratio (RLR), which is the ratio of the chi-square value to its *df*s (X/df). Models with RLRs of 2 : 1 or 3 : 1 are considered to have a good fit (Carmines & McIver, 1981).

Although the statistical validation of a model is essential, the importance of the SEM's theoretical basis cannot be underscored, because for every SEM that fits the data well, competing SEMs also may be statistically consistent with the data. Theory provides essential validity evidence for the model throughout all stages of the latent variable modeling process.

HYPOTHETICAL EXAMPLE OF THE LATENT VARIABLE MODELING PROCESS

A hypothetical latent variable SEM of college success was created for this chapter and is presented according to the latent variable modeling process just described. Based on a review of literature and theory, a latent variable SEM of college success was specified. Specifically, this model hypothesized that the exogenous latent variable high-school grades had a direct causal influence on the mixed latent variable academic self-confidence, which in turn had a direct causal influence on the latent variable college success (Fig. 16-5).

Measurement Model

Specification

Based on the review of literature and the theoretical underpinnings of this model, the following measurement model of college success was specified according to the three main objectives of measurement model specification:

1. The purely exogenous latent variable high-school grades was measured by three observed indicators (high-school math grade [X1], high-school verbal grade [X2], and high-school analytic ability [X3]). The mixed latent academic self-confidence was measured by two observed indicators (math self-confidence [Y1] and verbal self-confidence [Y2]). The endogenous latent variable college success was measured by four observed indicators (college students' perceptions of their math [Y3] and verbal success [Y5] and faculty's perception of each student's math [Y4] and verbal [Y6] success).
2. The latent variables high-school grades, academic self-confidence, and college success were correlated in the measurement model.

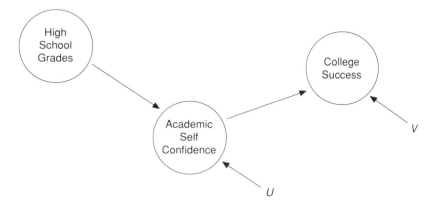

Note: *U, V* = disturbance or unexplained variance.

FIGURE 16-5
Hypothetical SEM of college success.

3. Measurement error, due to hypothesized method or measure variance, were correlated between seven observed indicators. As an example due to the potential method and measure variance associated with one individual completing two similar instruments, correlated error was hypothesized between the measure of math self-confidence ($Y1$) and students' perceptions of math success in college ($Y4$)(Fig. 16-6).

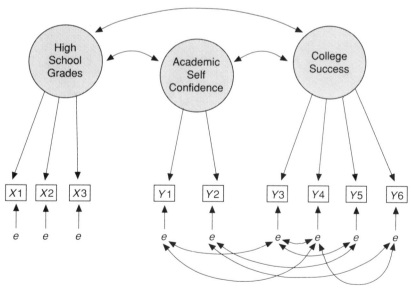

FIGURE 16-6
Hypothetical measurement model of college success.

Identification

The measurement model of college success was judged to be theoretically identified, and it met the conditions of statistical identification as described by Kenny (1979).

Estimation and Model Fit

The specified measurement model was analyzed using LISREL VI (Jöreskog & Sörbom, 1986). Figure 16-7 presents the LISREL computer printout for the measurement model of college success. This section provides a description of individual parameter estimates, followed by a description of the fit of the overall measurement model.

(*text continues on page 311*)

```
20-Mar-92
13:04:13    Yale University C&IS      IBM 3083     VM/CMS


DISSERTATION DATA/MEAS MODEL/REMOVAL
OF INDICATORS/ADD TE


STANDARDIZED SOLUTION


        LAMBDA Y

                HSGRADES        SLFCON          SUCCESS
    HSMATH        0.531          0.000            0.000
    HSVERBAL      0.487          0.000            0.000
    HSANALYT      0.731          0.000            0.000
    SCMATH        0.000          0.729            0.000
    CSVERB        0.000          0.736            0.000     (1a)
    SCCOLMTH      0.000          0.000            0.939
    TCHCOLMT      0.000          0.000            0.650
    SCCOLVRB      0.000          0.000            0.590
    TCHCOLVR      0.000          0.000            0.463


            PSI

                HSGRADES        SLFCON          SUCCESS
    HSGRADES      1.000
    SLFCON        0.601          1.000                       (2a)
    SUCCESS       0.288          0.576            1.000


        CORRELATION MATRIX FOR ETA

                HSGRADES        SLFCON          SUCCESS
    HSGRADES      1.000
    SLFCON        0.601          1.000
    SUCCESS       0.288          0.576            1.000


    THE PROBLEM REQUIRED    1224  DOUBLE PRECISION WORDS,
    THE CPU-TIME WAS        0.55  SECONDS
```

FIGURE 16-7
LISREL output for hypothetical measurement model of college success.

```
DISSERTATION DATA/MEAS MODEL/REMOVAL
OF INDICATORS/ADD TE
```

LISREL ESTIMATES (MAXIMUM LIKELIHOOD)

LAMBDA Y

	HSGRADES	SLFCON	SUCCESS
HSMATH	1.000	0.000	0.000
HSVERBAL	0.917	0.000	0.000
HSANALYT	1.378	0.000	0.000
SCMATH	0.000	1.000	0.000
CSVERB	0.000	1.009	0.000
SCCOLMTH	0.000	0.000	1.000
TCHCOLMT	0.000	0.000	0.692
SCCOLVRB	0.000	0.000	0.629
TCHCOLVR	0.000	0.000	0.493

PSI

	HSGRADES	SLFCON	SUCCESS
HSGRADES	0.282		
SLFCON	0.233	0.531	
SUCCESS	0.144	0.394	0.882

THETA EPS

	HSMATH	HSVERBAL	HSANALYT	SCMATH	CSVERB
HSMATH	0.718				
HSVERBAL	0.000	0.763			
HSANALYT	0.000	0.000	0.465		
SCMATH	0.000	0.000	0.000	0.478	
CSVERB	0.000	0.000	0.000	0.000	0.450
SCCOLMTH	0.000	0.000	0.000	0.238	0.000
TCHCOLMT	0.000	0.000	0.000	0.092	0.000
SCCOLVRB	0.000	0.000	0.000	0.000	0.271
TCHCOLVR	0.000	0.000	0.000	0.000	0.146

	SCCOLMTH	TCHCOLMT	SCCOLVRB	TCHCOLVR	③a
HSMATH					
HSVERBAL					
HSANALYT					
SCMATH					
CSVERB					
SCCOLMTH	0.124				
TCHCOLMT	0.102	0.578			
SCCOLVRB	−0.095	0.000	0.656		
TCHCOLVR	0.000	0.326	0.420	0.812	

FIGURE 16-7 (CONTINUED)

W_A_R_N_I_N_G: THE MATRIX THETA EPS
IS NOT POSITIVE DEFINITE
SQUARED MULTIPLE CORRELATIONS FOR Y-VARIABLES

HSMATH	HSVERBAL	HSANALYT	SCMATH	CSVERB
0.282	0.237	0.535	0.522	0.550

SCCOLMTH	TCHCOLMT	SCCOLVRB	TCHCOLVR
0.876	0.422	0.344	0.188

SQUARED MULTIPLE CORRELATIONS FOR STRUCTURAL EQUATIONS

HSGRADES	SLFCON	SUCCESS
0.000	0.000	0.000

TOTAL COEFFICIENT OF DETERMINATION
FOR STRUCTURAL EQUATIONS IS 0.000

DISSERTATION DATA/MEAS MODEL/REMOVAL
OF INDICATORS/ADD TE

T-VALUES

LAMBDA Y

	HSGRADES	SLFCON	SUCCESS	
HSMATH	0.000	0.000	0.000	
HSVERBAL	3.227	0.000	0.000	
HSANALYT	3.488	0.000	0.000	
SCMATH	0.000	0.000	0.000	(1b)
CSVERB	0.000	3.752	0.000	
SCCOLMTH	0.000	0.000	0.000	
TCHCOLMT	0.000	0.000	4.139	
SCCOLVRB	0.000	0.000	2.307	
TCHCOLVR	0.000	0.000	1.976	

PSI

	HSGRADES	SLFCON	SUCCESS	
HSGRADES	2.259			
SLFCON	2.739	2.921		(2b)
SUCCESS	1.954	2.661	2.126	

FIGURE 16-7 (CONTINUED)

THETA EPS

	HSMATH	HSVERBAL	HSANALYT	SCMATH	CSVERB
HSMATH	5.643				
HSVERBAL	0.000	5.974			
HSANALYT	0.000	0.000	3.161		
SCMATH	0.000	0.000	0.000	3.216	
CSVERB	0.000	0.000	0.000	0.000	3.025
SCCOLMTH	0.000	0.000	0.000	1.880	0.000
TCHCOLMT	0.000	0.000	0.000	0.916	0.000
SCCOLVRB	0.000	0.000	0.000	0.000	2.508
TCHCOLVR	0.000	0.000	0.000	0.000	1.565 (3b)

	SCCOLMTH	TCHCOLMT	SCCOLVRB	TCHCOLVR
HSMATH				
HSVERBAL				
HSANALYT				
SCMATH				
CSVERB				
SCCOLMTH	0.307			
TCHCOLMT	0.381	2.522		
SCCOLVRB	−0.859	0.000	3.356	
TCHCOLVR	0.000	3.715	2.847	5.088

DISSERTATION DATA/MEAS MODEL/REMOVAL
OF INDICATORS/ADD TE

FITTED MOMENTS AND RESIDUALS

FITTED MOMENTS

	HSMATH	HSVERBAL	HSANALYT	SCMATH	CSVERB
HSMATH	1.000				
HSVERBAL	0.258	1.000			
HSANALYT	0.388	0.356	1.000		
SCMATH	0.233	0.213	0.321	1.009	
CSVERB	0.235	0.215	0.324	0.536	0.991
SCCOLMTH	0.144	0.132	0.198	0.632	0.398
TCHCOLMT	0.099	0.091	0.137	0.365	0.275
SCCOLVRB	0.090	0.083	0.124	0.248	0.521
TCHCOLVR	0.071	0.065	0.098	0.194	0.342

FIGURE 16-7 (CONTINUED)

	SCCOLMTH	TCHCOLMT	SCCOLVRB	TCHCOLVR
HSMATH				
HSVERBAL				
HSANALYT				
SCMATH				
CSVERB				
SCCOLMTH	1.006			
TCHCOLMT	0.712	1.000		
SCCOLVRB	0.459	0.383	1.005	
TCHCOLVR	0.434	0.627	0.693	1.026

FITTED RESIDUALS

	HSMATH	HSVERBAL	HSANALYT	SCMATH	CSVERB
HSMATH	0.000				
HSVERBAL	−0.057	0.000			
HSANALYT	0.035	−0.013	0.000		
SCMATH	−0.061	0.083	−0.038	−0.009	
CSVERB	0.025	0.107	−0.031	0.003	0.009
SCCOLMTH	0.049	0.017	−0.047	−0.010	0.001
TCHCOLMT	0.115	−0.021	0.125	0.005	−0.024
SCCOLVRB	0.112	0.134	0.003	0.000	0.010
TCHCOLVR	0.138	−0.061	0.037	−0.012	−0.027

	SCCOLMTH	TCHCOLMT	SCCOLVRB	TCHCOLVR
HSMATH				
HSVERBAL				
HSANALYT				
SCMATH				
CSVERB				
SCCOLMTH	−0.006			
TCHCOLMT	0.000	0.000		
SCCOLVRB	−0.005	−0.039	−0.005	
TCHCOLVR	−0.001	−0.021	−0.026	−0.026

NORMALIZED RESIDUALS

	HSMATH	HSVERBAL	HSANALYT	SCMATH	CSVERB
HSMATH	0.000				
HSVERBAL	−0.557	0.000			
HSANALYT	0.323	−0.124	0.000		
SCMATH	−0.589	0.804	−0.357	−0.062	
CSVERB	0.246	1.047	−0.292	0.025	0.065
SCCOLMTH	0.486	0.170	−0.460	−0.083	0.011
TCHCOLMT	1.140	−0.211	1.238	0.048	−0.235
SCCOLVRB	1.109	1.334	0.025	0.001	0.091
TCHCOLVR	1.361	−0.600	0.368	−0.118	−0.253

FIGURE 16-7 (CONTINUED)

	SCCOLMTH	TCHCOLMT	SCCOLVRB	TCHCOLVR
HSMATH				
HSVERBAL				
HSANALYT				
SCMATH				
CSVERB				
SCCOLMTH	−0.040			
TCHCOLMT	−0.003	0.001		
SCCOLVRB	−0.045	−0.368	−0.033	
TCHCOLVR	−0.013	−0.177	−0.214	−0.182

④a

MEASURES OF GOODNESS OF FIT FOR THE WHOLE MODEL:

CHI−SQUARE WITH 16 DEGREES OF FREEDOM
IS 21.33 (PROB. LEVEL = 0.166)

GOODNESS OF FIT INDEX IS 0.955

⑤a

ADJUSTED GOODNESS OF FIT INDEX IS 0.872

ROOT MEAN SQUARE RESIDUAL IS 0.052

FIGURE 16-7 (CONTINUED)

1. LISREL estimates individual parameters in a series of matrices. The standardized lambda matrix is the factor loading matrix, and as such, provides estimates of how well the the observed indicators load on their latent variables. On the LISREL printout in Figure 16-7 the latent variables are positioned at the top of each column of the lambda matrix (①a), while the observed indicators line up along the left side of the matrix.

When interpreting the lambda matrix on the printout, on the latent variable high-school grades, the standardized factor loading for high-school math is 0.531; for high-school verbal, 0.487; and for high-school analytic skills, 0.731. Similarly, the loadings on the latent variable academic self-confidence are 0.729 for the math self-confidence indicator and 0.736 for the verbal self-confidence indicator. The loadings for the indicators of the latent variable college success are 0.939 (college students' perceptions of math success), 0.650 (teacher's perception of student's math success), 0.590 (students' perceptions of verbal success), and 0.463 (teacher's perception of student's verbal success). These factor loadings are respectable and suggest the measures adequately measure their latent variables.

An additional benefit of LISREL is found in the lambda t-value matrix where the statistical significance of these loadings is recorded ①b. The t-values in this matrix are actually z-scores; therefore, scores greater than 1.96 are significant at $p \leq 0.05$. The loadings for all indicators are significant ($z \geq 1.96, p \leq 0.05$), suggesting that all observed indicators adequately measure their respective latent variable. (Note: z-scores are not available for one indicator on each latent variable in the lambda matrix [i.e., high-school math, math self-confidence, and students' perceptions of math success] because a "marker variable" strategy was used in this analysis. Each of these three indicators was the standardized "marker" on its respective latent variable, against which the other indicators were compared [Hayduk, 1987]).

In the measurement model the psi matrix (②ⓐ) is a correlation matrix, which reflects the correlation estimates between latent variables. Thus, the latent variable high-school grades correlates with academic self-confidence ($r = 0.601$), and its correlation with college success is 0.288. The relationship between academic self-confidence and college success is 0.576. When evaluating the statistical significance of the relationships between latent variables on the psi t-value matrix, two of the three latent variable intercorrelations are significant at $p \leq 0.05$. The correlation between high-school grades and college success is less than significant but was kept in the model because of theoretical support for the relationship and the hypothesized indirect effect of high-school grades on college success in the SEM.

The third matrix that is typically evaluated in measurement model estimation is the theta matrix (③ⓐ). This correlation matrix of observed indicators accounts for correlated method or measure variance between measures. Estimates of the correlated measurement error specified in the measurement model are presented in this matrix. For example the correlated measurement error between the verbal self-confidence measure and the student's perception of verbal success measure is $r = 0.271$. The associated theta t-value matrix (③ⓑ) shows this relationship is significant ($z = 2.505; p \leq 0.05$). Although not all specified correlated error is significant (e.g., correlated error between math self-confidence and teacher's perception of student's math success [$r = 0.092; z = 0.916; p \geq 0.05$]), the theoretical rationale for the original error specifications is judged to be strong enough to remain in the model.

In addition LISREL provides estimates of each observed indicator's standardized residuals, or systematic error. Standardized residual estimates $> +2$ standard deviation units indicate measures that do not fit the model well and may need to be deleted from the model. On examination of the standardized residual matrix (④ⓐ), all estimates are $< +2$, signifying they fit the model.

2. After estimating the individual parameters in the measurement model, LISREL provides a maximum likelihood X^2 goodness of fit measure for the model (⑤ⓐ). The measurement model of college success with three latent variables and nine observed indicators results in a $X^2(16, N = 101) = 21.33, p = 0.166$; GFI $= 0.955$; and RLR $<2:1$. These values suggested a model of good fit and substantiate subsequent examination of the SEM of college success.

Throughout all phases of the measurement and SEM processes, the LISREL printout also provides suggestions about specific modifications that can be made to the model to improve its fit. These suggestions, called *modification indices*, project a predicted decrease in X^2 for each parameter that is revised. The modification indices are driven solely by statistical merit and have no theoretical basis. For this reason the investigator must interpret the modification indices as statistical support for empirical evidence. These indices of model fit assist the investigator to respecify, test, and evaluate the model.

SEM

Specification

The theoretical SEM of college success specified causal relationships among three latent variables (see Fig. 16-5).

Identification

The SEM was theoretically and statistically identified. Applying the formula for determining the number of known parameters in the SEM:

$$\frac{N(N - 1)}{2},$$

where N equals the number of variables in the model, there were:

$$\frac{3(3 - 1)}{2} = 3$$

known parameters in the SEM of college success. The SEM hypothesized two causal paths, or unknown parameters. Thus, because there were more known parameters (three) than unknown parameters (two), the SEM met a basic condition of statistical identifiability.

Estimation and Model Fit

The SEM of college success was estimated using LISREL VI. The SEM's parameter estimates are shown in the LISREL printout in Figure 16-8. In this section the fit of individual parameter estimates is presented and then followed by a discussion of the model's overall fit.

1. LISREL estimates the causal parameters in the beta matrix (⑥ⓐ), in which the variables at the head of each column are cause variables and the variables to the left of each row are effect variables. The values in the beta matrix are Bs, which represent the expected amount of causal influence on the endogenous variable with a 1-unit change in the causal variable. In the standardized beta matrix the latent variable high-school grades demonstrated positive causal influence on academic self-confidence (B = 0.606), and academic self-confidence demonstrated positive causal influence on the latent variable college success (B = 0.580). When exploring the t value matrix (⑥ⓑ), both of these paths were significant ($p \leq 0.05$).

2. The SEM demonstrated a good fit (X^2 [17, $N = 101$] = 21.61; $p = 0.200$; GFI = 0.954; RLR < 2:1 [⑦ⓐ]). Also, the unexplained variance of the SEM's endogenous variables is determined by the formula, $\sqrt{1 - R^2}$. The squared multiple correlations (R^2) for the endogenous latent variables is found on the LISREL output (⑧ⓐ). Applying this formula, the amount of unexplained variance for the latent variable academic self-confidence is $\sqrt{1 - 0.368} = 0.788$, and $\sqrt{1 - 0.337} = 0.814$ for the latent endogenous variable college success (Fig. 16-9).

Thus, the hypothetical SEM of college success demonstrated that high-school grades had a direct causal influence on students' academic self-confidence (B = 0.606;

(*text continues on page 316*)

DISSERTATION DATA/STRUCT MODEL/REMOVAL
OF INDICATORS/ADD TE

STANDARDIZED SOLUTION

LAMBDA Y

	HSGRADES	SLFCON	SUCCESS
HSMATH	0.538	0.000	0.000
HSVERBAL	0.488	0.000	0.000
HSANALYT	0.723	0.000	0.000
SCMATH	0.000	0.722	0.000
CSVERB	0.000	0.741	0.000
SCCOLMTH	0.000	0.000	0.900
TCHCOLMT	0.000	0.000	0.651
SCCOLVRB	0.000	0.000	0.591
TCHCOLVR	0.000	0.000	0.475

BETA

	HSGRADES	SLFCON	SUCCESS	
HSGRADES	0.000	0.000	0.000	(6a)
SLFCON	0.606	0.000	0.000	
SUCCESS	0.000	0.580	0.000	

PSI

	HSGRADES	SLFCON	SUCCESS
HSGRADES	1.000		
SLFCON	0.000	0.632	
SUCCESS	0.000	0.000	0.663

CORRELATION MATRIX FOR ETA

	HSGRADES	SLFCON	SUCCESS
HSGRADES	1.000		
SLFCON	0.606	1.000	
SUCCESS	0.352	0.580	1.000

THE PROBLEM REQUIRED   1216 DOUBLE PRECISION WORDS,
THE CPU-TIME WAS   0.62 SECONDS

SQUARED MULTIPLE CORRELATIONS FOR STRUCTURAL EQUATIONS

HSGRADES	SLFCON	SUCCESS	
0.000	0.368	0.337	(8a)

TOTAL COEFFICIENT OF DETERMINATION
FOR STRUCTURAL EQUATIONS IS 0.000

FIGURE 16-8
LISREL output for hypothetical SEM of college success.

MEASURES OF GOODNESS OF FIT FOR THE WHOLE MODEL :

CHI–SQUARE WITH 17 DEGREES OF FREEDOM
IS 21.61 (PROB. LEVEL = 0.200)

GOODNESS OF FIT INDEX IS 0.954

ADJUSTED GOODNESS OF FIT INDEX IS 0.878

ROOT MEAN SQUARE RESIDUAL IS 0.048

DISSERTATION DATA/STRUCT MODEL/REMOVAL
OF INDICATORS/ADD TE

T–VALUES

LAMBDA Y

	HSGRADES	SLFCON	SUCCESS
HSMATH	0.000	0.000	0.000
HSVERBAL	3.236	0.000	0.000
HSANALYT	3.512	0.000	0.000
SCMATH	0.000	0.000	0.000
CSVERB	0.000	3.787	0.000
SCCOLMTH	0.000	0.000	0.000
TCHCOLMT	0.000	0.000	4.307
SCCOLVRB	0.000	0.000	2.473
TCHCOLVR	0.000	0.000	2.105

BETA

	HSGRADES	SLFCON	SUCCESS
HSGRADES	0.000	0.000	0.000
SLFCON	3.008	0.000	0.000
SUCCESS	0.000	5.224	0.000

6b

PSI

	HSGRADES	SLFCON	SUCCESS
HSGRADES	2.287		
SLFCON	0.000	2.493	
SUCCESS	0.000	0.000	1.817

THETA EPS

	HSMATH	HSVERBAL	HSANALYT	SCMATH	CSVERB
HSMATH	5.576				
HSVERBAL	0.000	5.962			
HSANALYT	0.000	0.000	3.292		
SCMATH	0.000	0.000	0.000	3.328	
CSVERB	0.000	0.000	0.000	0.000	2.988
SCCOLMTH	0.000	0.000	0.000	2.192	0.000
TCHCOLMT	0.000	0.000	0.000	1.058	0.000
SCCOLVRB	0.000	0.000	0.000	0.000	2.570
TCHCOLVR	0.000	0.000	0.000	0.000	1.589

FIGURE 16-8 (CONTINUED)

	SCCOLMTH	TCHCOLMT	SCCOLVRB	TCHCOLVR
HSMATH				
HSVERBAL				
HSANALYT				
SCMATH				
CSVERB				
SCCOLMTH	0.567			
TCHCOLMT	0.532	2.729		
SCCOLVRB	−0.793	0.000	3.524	
TCHCOLVR	0.000	3.661	2.943	5.111

FIGURE 16-8 (CONTINUED)

$p \leq 0.05$), and academic self-confidence had a strong causal effect on college success ($B = 0.580; p \leq 0.05$). In terms of variance the model accounted for 21% of the variance of the latent variable academic self-confidence and 17% on the latent variable college success. The nonsignificant chi-square demonstrates that the SEM of college success "held up" with this sample.

The following summary of the latent variable model process is provided to highlight the major points of this complex process:

1. The latent variable modeling process includes two sequential phases—measurement model testing, followed by SEM testing.
2. The measurement model underlies each SEM and hypothesizes and tests the adequacy of the model's latent variables and their observed indicators.

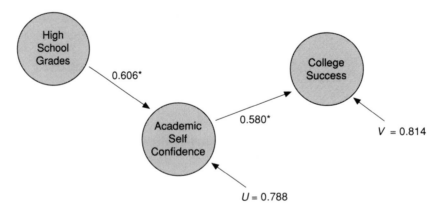

Chi-square (17, N = 101) = 21.61; p = 0.200; GFI = 0.954; RLR <2:1

Note: * = $p \leq 0.05$; U, V = disturbance or unexplained variance.

FIGURE 16-9
Hypothetical SEM of college success with parameter estimates.

3. Only after the measurement model demonstrates an adequate fit (i.e., nonsignificant chi-square) with the data of the study sample, suggesting that the model's latent variables and measures are adequate, can the SEM be tested.
4. The SEM estimates causal paths between latent variables.
5. A low, nonsignificant chi-square, suggesting that the SEM fits the data well, is sought.

EXAMPLE OF PUBLISHED LATENT VARIABLE MODEL

In a study by Dixon, Hickey, and Dixon (1992), a latent variable SEM was hypothesized with a sample of 243 professionally educated women for the purpose of understanding why some creatively productive people have an enhanced capacity for superior social adjustment and socioeconomic achievement, while others do not. Based on several theories a latent variable SEM with five latent variables and 13 observed indicators was specified (Fig. 16-10).

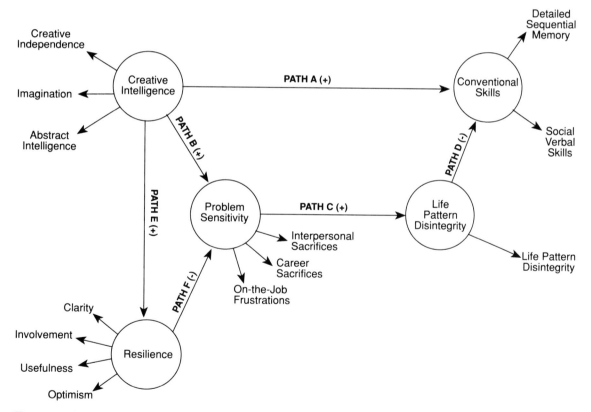

FIGURE 16-10

Originally specified SEM of social adjustment and socioeconomic achievement.
(Chi-square [55, $N = 243$] = 62.22; $p = 0.235$.)

Measurement Model Specification, Identification, Estimation, and Fit

The initial measurement model specified correlations between the five latent variables in the model, causal paths from the latent variables to their respective observed indicators, and no correlated error between observed measures. Because this measurement model was judged to be theoretically and empirically identified, its unknown parameters were estimated. The chi-square for the model was $X^2(56, N = 243) = 98.27$; $p \leq 0.0001$, suggesting the measurement model did not fit the data well.

The measurement model was respecified to include five correlations between

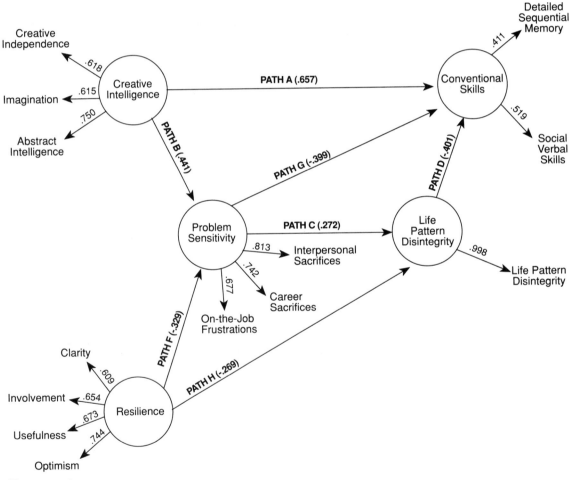

FIGURE 16-11

Respecified SEM of social adjustment and socioeconomic achievement.
(Chi-square [55, $N = 243$] = 51.55; $p = 0.607$.)

observed measures that were hypothesized to share common error variance between latent variables. The final measurement model resulted in a $X^2(51, N = 243) = 47.45$; $p = 0.615$, suggesting a model of good fit.

SEM Specification, Identification, Estimation, and Fit

After the measurement model demonstrated a fit consistent with the data, the causal paths in the SEM were specified. The SEM presented in Figure 16-10 was overidentified (i.e., 10 known parameters and six unknown parameters) and thus could be estimated. After estimation, the X^2 for the SEM was $(55, N = 243) = 62.22, p = 0.235$.

Although the chi-square indicated a good fit, the modification indices in the LISREL printout presented empirical information that was theoretically substantiated to support estimating a respecified SEM. The respecified SEM presented in Figure 16-11 had a $X^2(55, N = 243) = 51.55; p = 0.607$, suggesting a model that fit the data well.

Value and Limits of Structural Equation Modeling

SEM is valuable to the social and health sciences primarily when experimental designs are inappropriate. SEMs posit theoretically derived causal links between variables for the purpose of explaining their associations within the context of certain phenomena. In addition SEMs can be used to refine theory and state it more exactly (Kenny, 1979).

Although SEM has the potential to advance social and health sciences, it also has the potential to be misused. Models should be built from theory that is well grounded and should include variables that reflect the phenomenon under investigation. As Kenny (1979) suggests:

> There will be a temptation to dress up statistical analyses by calling them "causal analysis." Although the term causal modeling sounds impressive, remember it forces the researcher to make stronger assumptions in order to make stronger conclusions. (p. 8)

Bibliography

American Psychological Association. (1983). *Publication manual of the American Psychological Association* (3rd ed.). Washington, DC.

Aaronson, L. S. (1984). Health behavior in pregnancy: Testing a general model. *Dissertation Abstracts International, 44,* 11A, 3498.

Asher, A. B. (1983). *Causal modeling* (2nd ed.). Sage University Papers: Quantitative Applications in the Social Sciences Series, 3. Newbury Park, CA: Sage Publications, Inc.

Barnett, V., & Lewis, T. (1985). *Outliers in statistical data* (2nd ed.). New York: John Wiley & Sons.

Becker, P. T., Grunwald, P. C., Moorman, J., & Stuhr, S. (1991). Outcomes of developmentally supportive nursing care for very low birth weight infants. *Nursing Research, 40*(3), 150–155.

Bentler, P. M. (1989). *EQS structural equations program manual.* Los Angeles, CA:BMDP Statistical Software.

Berry, G. (1986). Statistical significance and confidence intervals. *Medical Journal of Australia, 144,* 618–619.

Blalock, H. M. (1961). Correlation and causality: The multivariate case. *Social Forces, 39,* 246–251.

Blalock, H. M. (1963). Making causal inferences for unmeasured variables from correlations among indicators. *American Journal of Sociology, 69,* 53–62.

Blalock, H. M. (1964). *Causal inferences in nonexperimental research.* Chapel Hill: The University of North Carolina Press.

Boudon, R. (1965). A method of linear causal analysis: Dependence analysis. *American Sociological Review, 30,* 365–373.

Braitman, L. E. (1988). Confidence intervals extract clinically useful information from data. *Annals of Internal Medicine, 108,* 296–298.

Braitman, L. E. (1991). Confidence intervals assess both clinical significance and statistical significance. *Annals of Internal Medicine, 114,* 515–517.

Bray, J. H., & Maxwell, S. E. (1985). *Multivariate analysis of variance.* Series: Quantitative Applications in the Social Sciences 54. Newbury Park, CA: Sage Publications, Inc.

Brooten, D. *Early hospital discharge and nurse specialist followup.* Program Grant, funded by the National Center for Nursing Research, PO1-NR1859.

Brown, J. S., Tanner, C. A., & Padrick, K. P. (1984). Nursing's search for scientific knowledge. *Nursing Research, 33,* 26–32.

Brown, M. S., & Tanner, C. (1990). Measurement of Type A behavior in preschoolers. *Nursing Research, 39,* 207–211.

Burns, N., & Grove, S. K. (1987). *The practice of nursing research: Conduct, critique and utilization*. Phildelphia: W.B. Saunders.

Burroughs, A. K., Asonye, U. O., Anderson-Shanklin, G. C., & Vidyasagar, D. (1978). The effect of nonnutritive sucking on transcutaneous oxygen tension in noncrying, preterm neonates. *Research in Nursing and Health, 1*, 69–75.

Campbell, D. T. (1988). *Methodology and epistemology for social science: Selected papers*. Chicago: University of Chicago Press.

Campbell, D. T., & Stanley, J. C. (1963). *Experimental and quasi-experimental designs for research*. Skokie, IL: Rand McNally.

Carmines, E. G., & McIver, J. P. (1981). Analyzing models with unobserved variables: Analysis of covariance structures. In G. W. Bohrnstedt & E. F. Borgatta (Eds.). *Social measurement: Current issues* (pp. 65–115). Newbury Park, CA: Sage Publications, Inc.

Carnap, R. (1953). What is probability? *Scientific American, 189*, 128–138.

Chatfield, C. (1988). *Problem solving: A statistician's guide*. London: Chapman and Hall.

Child, D. (1990). *The essentials of factor analysis* (2nd ed.). London: Holt, Rinehart, & Winston.

Cleveland, W. S. (1985). *The elements of graphing data*. Belmont, CA: Wadsworth.

Clinton, J. (1982). Ethnicity: The development of an empirical construct for cross-cultural health research. *Western Journal of Nursing Research, 4*(3), 281–300.

Cohen J. (1983). The cost of dichotomization. *Applied Psychological Measurement, 7*, 249–253.

Cohen, J. (1987). *Statistical power analysis for the behavioral sciences*. (Rev. ed.) Hillsdale, NJ: Lawrence Erlbaum Associates.

Cohen, J. (1990). Things I have learned (so far). *American Psychologist, 45*, 1304–1312.

Confidence Interval Analysis (CIA). IBM compatible microcomputer program available from Annals of Internal Medicine, Sixth Street at Race, Philadelphia, PA 19106-1657.

Cook, T. D., & Campbell, D. T. (1979). *Quasi-experimentation: Design and analysis issues for field settings*. Skokie, IL: Rand McNally.

Cox, C., & Roghmann, K. (1984). Empirical test of the interaction model of client health behavior. *Research in Nursing and Health, 7*, 275–285.

Daniel, W. W. (1987). *Biostatistics: A foundation for analysis in the health sciences* (4th ed.). New York: John Wiley & Sons.

Derdiarian, A. K., & Lewis, S. (1986). The D-L test of agreement: A stronger measure of interrater reliability. *Nursing Research, 35*, 375–378.

Dibble, S. L., Bostrom-Ezrati, J., & Rizzuto, C. (1991). Clinical predictors of intravenous site symptoms. *Research in Nursing and Health, 14*, 413–420.

Dixon, J. K., Dixon, J. P., Spinner, J., Sexton, D., & Perry, C. K. (1991). Psychometric and descriptive perspectives of illness impact over the lifespan. *Nursing Research, 40*, 51–56.

Dixon, J. P., Hickey, M., & Dixon, J. K. (1992). A causal model of the way emotions intervene between creative intelligence and conventional skills. *New Ideas in Psychology, 10*, 233–251.

Duncan, O. D. (1966). Path analysis: Sociological examples. *American Journal of Sociology, 72*, 1–16.

Ehrenberg, A. S. C. (1977). Rudiments of numeracy. *Journal of the Royal Statistical Society A, 140*(part 3), 277–297.

Ferketich, S., & Muller, M. (1990). Factor analysis revisited. *Nursing Research, 39*, 59–62.

Figueredo, A. J., Ferketich, S. L., & Knapp, T. R. (1991). More on MTMM: The role of confirmatory factor analysis. *Research in Nursing and Health, 14*, 387–391.

Finn, J. D., & Mattsson, I. (1978). *Multivariate analysis in educational research—Applications of the multivariance program*. Chicago: National Educational Resources.

Fisher, R. A. (1935). *The design of experiments*. London: Oliver & Boyd.

Fisher, R. A. (1970). *Statistical methods for research workers* (14th ed.). Darien, CT: Hafner Publishing Co.

Fletcher, R. H., & Fletcher, S. W. (1979). Clinical research in general medical journals: A 30-year perspective. *New England Journal of Medicine, 301,* 180–183.

Forrester, D. A. (1990). Aids-related risk factors, medical diagnosis, do-not-resuscitate orders and aggressiveness of nursing care. *Nursing Research, 39*(6), 350–354.

Freedman, D., Pisani, R., Purves, R., & Adhikari, A. (1991). *Statistics* (2nd ed.). New York: W. W. Norton.

Freund, J. E. (1988). *Modern elementary statistics* (7th ed.). Englewood Cliffs, NJ: Prentice-Hall.

Gable, R. (1986). *Instrument development in the affective domain.* Boston: Kluwer-Nijhoff.

Gardner, P. L. (1975). Scales and statistics. *Review of Educational Research, 45,* 43–57.

Glass, G. V., & Stanley, J. C. (1970). *Statistical methods in education and psychology.* Englewood Cliffs, NJ: Prentice-Hall.

Glymour, C., Scheines, R., Spirtes, P., & Kelly, K. (1987). *Discovering causal structure: Artificial intelligence, philosophy of science, and statistical modeling.* San Diego, CA: Academic.

Goodwin, L. D. (1984). Increasing efficiency and precision of data analysis: Multivariate vs univariate statistical techniques. Methodology Corner. *Nursing Research, 33*(4), 247–249.

Goodwin, L. D., & Goodwin, W. L. (1991). Estimating construct validity. *Research in Nursing and Health, 14,* 235–243.

Gould, S. J. (1985). The median isn't the message. *Discover, 6,* 40–42.

Gulick, E. E. (1987). Parsimony and model confirmation of the ADL self-care scale for multiple sclerosis persons. *Nursing Research, 36,* 278–283.

Gulick, E. E. (1989). Model confirmation of the MS-related symptom checklist. *Nursing Research, 38,* 147–153.

Gulick, E. E., & Bugg, A. (1992). Holistic health patterning in multiple sclerosis. *Research in Nursing and Health, 15*(3), 175–185.

Hackett, T. P., & Cassem, N. H. (1969). Factors contributing to delay in responding to the signs and symptoms of acute myocardial infarction. *American Journal of Cardiology, 24,* 651–658.

Hahn, G. J., & Meeker, W. Q. (1991). *Statistical intervals—A guide for practitioners.* New York: John Wiley & Sons.

Hald, A. (1952). *Statistical tables and formulas.* New York: John Wiley & Sons.

Hanley, J. A., & Lippman-Hand, A. (1983). If nothing goes wrong, is everything all right? Interpreting zero numerators. *Journal of the Amercian Medical Association, 249,* 1743–1745.

Hayduk, L. A. (1987). *Structural equation modeling with LISREL: Essentials and advances.* Baltimore, MD: The Johns Hopkins University Press.

Helwig, J. T., & Council, K. A. (Eds.). (1979). *SAS user's guide.* Cary, NC: SAS Institute, Inc.

Hildebrand, D. K. (1986). *Statistical thinking for behavioral scientists.* Boston: Duxbury Press.

Hinkle, D. E., Wiersma, W., & Jurs, S. G. (1988). *Applied statistics for the behavioral sciences* (2nd ed.). Boston: Houghton Mifflin.

Holm, K., & Christman, N. J. (1985). Post hoc tests following analysis of variance. *Research in Nursing and Health, 8,* 207–210.

Hosmer, D. W., & Lemeshow, S. (1989). *Applied logistic regression.* New York: John Wiley & Sons.

Jacobsen, B. S. (1981). Know thy data. *Nursing Research, 30,* 254–255.

Jacobsen, B. S., & Lowery, B. J. (1992). Further analysis of the psychometric properties of the Levine Denial of Illness Scale. *Psychosomatic Medicine, 54,* 372–381.

Jacobsen, B. S., & Meininger, J. C. (1985). The designs and methods of published nursing research: 1956–1983. *Nursing Research, 34,* 306–312.

Jacobsen, B. S., & Munro, B. H. (1991). Comparison of the new (revised) and original scoring systems for the multiple affect adjective checklist. [Summary] Symposia: Dorothy Brooten, Measurement of affect in pregnant and postpartal diabetic women, women following cesarean birth, and women post hysterectomy. *Proceedings of the Sigma Theta Tau International 31st Biennial convention scientific sessions,* Tampa, FL.

Jöreskog, K. G. (1973). A general method for estimating a linear structural equation system. In A. S. Goldberger & O. D. Duncan (Eds.). *Structural equation models in the social sciences.* New York: Academic Press.

Jöreskog, K. G., & Sörbom, D. (1986). *LISREL VI analysis of linear structural relationships by the method of maximum likelihood.* Mooresville, Indiana: Scientific Software, Inc.

Jöreskog, K. G., & Sörbom, D. (1989). *LISREL 7: A guide to the program and applications* (2nd ed.). Chicago: SPSS, Inc.

Kalisch, B. J., Kalisch, P. A., & McHugh, M. L. (1982). The nurse as a sex object in motion pictures, 1930–1980. *Research in Nursing and Health, 5*(3), 147–154.

Kenny, D. (1979). *Correlation and causality.* New York: John Wiley & Sons.

Kenny, D. (1987). *Statistics for the social and behavioral sciences.* Boston: Little, Brown, & Co.

Kerlinger, F. N. (1986). *Foundations of behavioral research* (3rd ed.). New York: Holt, Rinehart & Winston.

Kerlinger, F. N., & Pedhazur, E. S. (1973). *Multiple regression in behavioral research.* New York: Holt, Rinehart & Winston.

Ketterlinus, R. D., Henderson, S. H., & Lamb, M. E. (1990). Maternal age, sociodemographics, prenatal health and behavior: Influences on neonatal risk status. *Journal of Adolescent Health Care, 11*(5), 423–431.

Knapp, T. R. (1990). Treating ordinal scales as interval scales: An attempt to resolve the controversy. *Nursing Research, 39,* 121–123.

Koopmans, L. H. (1987). *Introduction to contemporary statistics* (2nd ed.). Boston: Duxbury Press.

Kotz, S., & Stroup, D. F. (1983). *Educated guessing: How to cope in an uncertain world.* New York: Marcel Dekker.

Last, J. M. (Ed.). (1983). *A dictionary of epidemiology.* New York: Oxford.

Lauter, E., Lauter, H., & Schmidtke, D. (1978). Properties and comparison of procedures of discriminant analysis. *Biometrika Journal, 20*(4), 407–424.

Lee, H. J. (1991). Relationship of hardiness and current life events to perceived health in rural adults. *Research in Nursing and Health, 14*(5), 351–359.

Lentner, C. (Ed.). (1982). *Geigy Scientific Tables,* Vol. 2. Basle: CIBA-Geigy: 89–102.

Lewis-Beck, M. S. (1980). Applied regression: An introduction. In *Quantitative Applications in the Social Sciences, 22.* Newbury Park, CA: Sage Publications, Inc.

Loehlin, J. C. (1987). *Latent variable models: An introduction to factor, path, and structural analysis.* New Jersey: Erlbaum Associates.

Lomax, R. G. (1982). A guide to LISREL—type structural equation modeling. *Behavior Research Methods & Instrumentation, 14,* 1–8.

Long, J. S. (1983). Confirmatory factor analysis. *Quantitative Applications in the Social Sciences, 33.* Newbury Park, CA: Sage Publications, Inc.

Lowery, B. J. (PI) (1992). *Attributions, control, and adjustment to breast cancer.* Grant funded by the National Center for Nursing Research, RO1-NR01897.

Lowery, B. J., Jacobsen, B. S., & Ducette, J. (1992). Causal attributions, control, and adjustment to breast cancer. *Psychosocial Oncology, 10*(4).

Lybrand, M., Medoff-Cooper, B., & Munro, B. H. (1990). Periodic comparisons of specific gravity using urine from a diaper and collecting bag. *The American Journal of Maternal/Child Nursing (MCN), 15*(4), 238–239.

Maikler, V. E. (1991). Effects of a skin refrigerant/anesthetic and age on the pain responses of infants receiving immunizations. *Research in Nursing and Health, 14,* 397–403.

Marascuilo, L. A., & Levin, J. R. (1983). *Multivariate statistics in the social sciences: A researcher's guide*. Monterey, CA: Brooks/Cole.

Meininger, J. C. (1985). The validity of Type A behavior scales for employed women. *Journal of Chronic Diseases, 38*, 375–383.

Moore, D. (1983). Prepared childbirth and marital satisfaction during the antepartum and postpartum periods. *Nursing Research, 32*(2), 73–79.

Moore, D. S. (1991). *Statistics: Concepts and controversies* (3rd ed.). New York: W. H. Freeman.

Muhlenkamp, A. F., & Sayles, J. A. (1986). Self-esteem, social support, and positive health practices. *Nursing Research, 35*(6), 334–338.

Munro, B. H. (1985). Predicting success in graduate clinical specialty programs. (Brief). *Nursing Research, 34*(1), 54–57.

Munro, B. H. (1989). Analyzing nominal data. *Clinical Nurse Specialist, 3*(4), 176–177.

Munro, B. H. (1990). Testing for interactions: The analysis of variance model. *Clinical Nurse Specialist, 4*(3), 128–129.

Munro, B. H., Brown, L., & Heitman, B. B. (1989). Pressure ulcers: One bed or another? *Geriatric Nursing, 10*(4), 190–192.

Munro, B. H., Jacobsen, B. S., & Brooten, D. A. (in preparation). Characteristics of the La Monica-Oberst patient satisfaction scale.

Murdaugh, C., & Verran, J. (1986). Theoretical modeling. *Nursing Research, 36*, 284–291.

Nie, N. H., Hull, C. H., Jenkins, J. G., Steinbrenner, K., & Bent, D. H. (1975). *Statistical package for the social sciences* (2nd ed.). New York: McGraw-Hill Book Co.

Norbeck, J. S., & Anderson, N. J. (1989). Life stress, social support, and anxiety in mid- and late-pregnancy among low income women. *Research in Nursing and Health, 12*(5), 281–287.

Norusis, M. J. (1990a). *The SPSS guide to data analysis for release 4*. Chicago, IL: SPSS Inc.

Norusis, M. J. (1990b). *SPSS/PC+ advanced statistics 4.0*. Chicago, IL: SPSS Inc.

Norusis, M. J. (1990c). *SPSS/PC+ 4.0 base manual*. Chicago, IL: SPSS Inc.

Norusis, M. J. (1990d). *SPSS/PC+ statistics 4.0*. Chicago, IL: SPSS Inc.

Nunnally, J. C. (1978). *Psychometric theory* (2nd ed.). New York: McGraw-Hill.

Olson, C. L. (1974). Comparative robustness of six tests of multivariate analysis of variance. *Journal of the American Statistical Association, 69*, 894–908.

Ott, L., & Mendenhall, W. (1990). *Understanding statistics* (5th ed.). Boston: PWS-Kent Publishing.

Pedhazur, E. J. (1982). *Multiple regression in behavioral research, explanation and prediction* (2nd ed.). New York: Holt, Rinehart & Winston.

Pender, N. J., Walker, S. N., Sechrist, K. R., & Frank-Stromberg, M. (1990). Predicting health-promoting lifestyles in the workplace. *Nursing Research, 39*(6), 326–332.

Pollock, S. E., Christian, B. J., & Sands, D. (1990). Responses to chronic illness: Analysis of psychological and physiological adaptation. *Nursing Research, 39*(5), 300–304.

Powell, R. W., McSweeney, M. B., & Wilson, C. E. (1983). X-ray calcifications as the only basis for breast biopsy. *Annals of Surgery, 197*, 555–559.

Remington, R. D., & Schork, M. A. (1970). *Statistics with application to the biological and health sciences*. Englewood Cliffs, NJ: Prentice-Hall.

Rice, V. H., & Johnson, J. E. (1984). Preadmission self-instruction booklets, post admission exercise performance, and teaching time. *Nursing Research, 33*(3), 147–151.

Riegelman, R. K. (1981). *Studying a study and testing a test: How to read the medical literature*. Boston: Little, Brown, & Co.

Rothert, M., Rovner, D., Holmes, M., Schmitt, N., Talarczyk, G. L., Kroll, J., & Gogate, J. (1990). Women's use of information regarding hormone replacement therapy. *Research in Nursing and Health, 13*, 355–366.

Rothman, K. J. (1986). *Modern epidemiology*. Boston: Little, Brown, & Company.

SAS Institute Inc. (1990). *SAS/STAT software: CALIS and LOGISTIC procedures, release 6.04* (SAS Technical Report, 6.04). North Carolina: SAS Institute Inc.

Schmid, C. F. (1983). *Statistical graphics: Design principles and practices.* New York: John Wiley & Son.

Schroeder, M. A. (1990). Diagnosing and dealing with multicollinearity. *Western Journal of Nursing Research, 12*(2), 175–187.

Skinner, B. F. (1972). *Cumulative record: A selection of papers* (3rd ed.). New York: Appleton-Century-Crofts, Meredith Corporation.

Snedecor, G. W. (1938). *Statistical methods.* Ames, Iowa: Collegiate Press.

Spearman, C. (1904). General intelligence, objectively determined and measured. *American Journal of Psychology, 15,* 201–293.

Spielberger, C. D. (1983). *Manual for the State-Trait anxiety inventory.* Palo Alto, CA: Consulting Psychologists Press.

Stevens, S. S. (1946). On the theory of scales of measurement. *Science, 102,* 677–680.

Stevens, S. S. (1968). Measurement, statistics, and the schemapiric view. *Science, 161,* 849–856.

Stuifbergen, A. K. (1990). Patterns of functioning in families with a chronically ill parent: An exploratory study. *Research in Nursing and Health, 13,* 35–44.

Tabachnick, B. G., & Fidell, L. S. (1983). *Using multivariate statistics.* New York: Harper & Row.

Teel, C., & Verran, J. A. (1991). Focus on psychometrics: Factor comparisons across studies. *Research in Nursing and Health, 14,* 67–72.

Thomas, S. P., & Williams, R. L. (1991). Perceived stress, trait anger, modes of anger expression, and health status of college men and women. *Nursing Research, 40* (5), 303–307.

Thorndike, R. M. (1988). Correlational procedures. In J. P. Keeves (Ed.). *Educational research, methodology, and measurement: An international handbook.* New York: Pergamon Press.

Thurstone, L. L. (1947). *Multiple-factor analysis.* Chicago: University of Chicago Press.

Tufte, E. R. (1983). *The visual display of quantitative information.* Cheshire, CT: Graphics Press.

Tukey, J. W. (1977). *Exploratory data analysis.* Reading, MA: Addison-Wesley.

Tulman, L. R., & Jacobsen, B. S. (1989). Goldilocks and variability. *Nursing Research, 38,* 377–379.

Valanis, B. G., & Yeaworth, R. (1982). Ratings of physical and mental health in the older bereaved. *Research in Nursing and Health, 5*(3), 137–146.

Verran, J. A., & Ferketich, S. L. (1987). Testing linear model assumptions: Residual analysis. *Nursing Research, 36*(2), 127–129.

Visintainer, M. A., & Wolfer, J. A. (1975). Psychological preparation for surgical pediatric patients: The effect on children's and parents' stress responses and adjustment. *Pediatrics, 56,* 187–202.

Wainer, H., & Thissen, D. (1981). Graphical data analysis. *Annual Review of Psychology, 32,* 191–241.

Walker, S. N., Sechrist, K. R., & Pender, N. J. (1987). The health promoting lifestyle profile: Development and psychometric characteristics. *Nursing Research, 36,* 76–81.

Weisberg, H. F. (1992). *Central tendency and variability,* Series: Quantitative Applications in the Social Sciences, No. 83. Newbury Park, CA: Sage Publications.

Wikoff, R. L., & Miller, P. (1991). Canonical analysis in nursing research. Methodology Corner. *Nursing Research, 40*(6), 367–370.

Wiley, D. E. (1973). The identification problem for structural equation models with unmeasured variables. In A. S. Goldberger & O. D. Duncan (Eds.). *Structural equation models in the social sciences* (pp. 69–83). New York: Academic Press.

Winer, B. J. (1971). *Statistical principles in experimental design* (2nd ed.). New York: McGraw-Hill.

Wolfer, J. A., & Visintainer, M. A. (1975). Pediatric surgical patients' and mothers' distress and coping behavior as a function of psychological preparation and stress-point nursing care. *Nursing Research, 24,* 244–255.

Wonnacott, R. J., & Wonnacott, T. H. (1985). *Introductory statistics* (4th ed.). New York: John Wiley & Son.

Wright, S. (1918). On the nature of size factors. *Genetics, 3,* 367–374.

Wright, S. (1921). Correlation and causation. *Journal of Agricultural Research, 20,* 557–585.

Wu, Y. B., & Slakter, M. J. (1990). Increasing the precision of data analysis: Planned comparisons versus omnibus tests. Methodology Corner. *Nursing Research, 39*(4), 251–253.

Youngblut, J. M., Loveland-Cherry, C. J., & Horan, M. (1991). Maternal employment effects on family and preterm infants at three months. *Nursing Research, 40*(5), 272–275.

APPENDICES

APPENDIX A

Percent of Total Area of Normal Curve Between a z-Score and the Mean

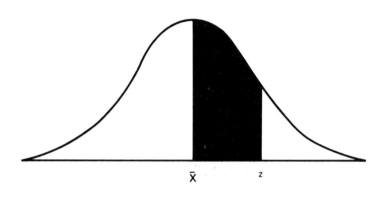

z	0.00	0.01	0.02	0.03	0.04	0.05	0.06	0.07	0.08	0.09
0.0	00.00	00.40	00.80	01.20	01.60	01.99	02.39	02.79	03.19	03.59
0.1	03.98	04.38	04.78	05.17	05.57	05.96	06.36	06.75	07.14	07.53
0.2	07.93	08.32	08.71	09.10	09.48	09.87	10.26	10.64	11.03	11.41
0.3	11.79	12.17	12.55	12.93	13.31	13.68	14.06	14.43	14.80	15.17
0.4	15.54	15.91	16.28	16.64	17.00	17.36	17.72	18.08	18.44	18.79
0.5	19.15	19.50	19.85	20.19	20.54	20.88	21.23	21.57	21.90	22.24
0.6	22.57	22.91	23.24	23.57	23.89	24.22	24.54	24.86	25.17	25.49
0.7	25.80	26.11	26.42	26.73	27.04	27.34	27.64	27.94	28.23	28.52
0.8	28.81	29.10	29.39	29.67	29.95	30.23	30.51	30.78	31.06	31.33
0.9	31.59	31.86	32.12	32.38	32.64	32.90	33.15	33.40	33.65	33.89
1.0	34.13	34.38	34.61	34.85	35.08	35.31	35.54	35.77	35.99	36.21
1.1	36.43	36.65	36.86	37.08	37.29	37.49	37.70	37.90	38.10	38.30
1.2	38.49	38.69	38.88	39.07	39.25	39.44	39.62	39.80	39.97	40.15
1.3	40.32	40.49	40.66	40.82	40.99	41.15	41.31	41.47	41.62	41.77
1.4	41.92	42.07	42.22	42.36	42.51	42.65	42.79	42.92	43.06	43.19
1.5	43.32	43.45	43.57	43.70	43.83	43.94	44.06	44.18	44.29	44.41
1.6	44.52	44.63	44.74	44.84	44.95	45.05	45.15	45.25	45.35	45.45
1.7	45.54	45.64	45.73	45.82	45.91	45.99	46.08	46.16	46.25	46.33

(continued)

z	0.00	0.01	0.02	0.03	0.04	0.05	0.06	0.07	0.08	0.09
1.8	46.41	46.49	46.56	46.64	46.71	46.78	46.86	46.93	46.99	47.06
1.9	47.13	47.19	47.26	47.32	47.38	47.44	47.50	47.56	47.61	47.67
2.0	47.72	47.78	47.83	47.88	47.93	47.98	48.03	48.08	48.12	48.17
2.1	48.21	48.26	48.30	48.34	48.38	48.42	48.46	48.50	48.54	48.57
2.2	48.61	48.64	48.68	48.71	48.75	48.78	48.81	48.84	48.87	48.90
2.3	48.93	48.96	48.98	49.01	49.04	49.06	49.09	49.11	49.13	49.16
2.4	49.18	49.20	49.22	49.25	49.27	49.29	49.31	49.32	49.34	49.36
2.5	49.38	49.40	49.41	49.43	49.45	49.46	49.48	49.49	49.51	49.52
2.6	49.53	49.55	49.56	49.57	49.59	49.60	49.61	49.62	49.63	49.64
2.7	49.65	49.66	49.67	49.68	49.69	49.70	49.71	49.72	49.73	49.74
2.8	49.74	49.75	49.76	49.77	49.77	49.78	49.79	49.79	49.80	49.81
2.9	49.81	49.82	49.82	49.83	49.84	49.84	49.85	49.85	49.86	49.86
3.0	49.87									
3.5	49.98									
4.0	49.997									
5.0	49.99997									

(From Hald, A. [1952]. Statistical tables and formulas. New York: John Wiley & Sons. [Table 1].)

APPENDIX B
Distribution of χ^2 Probability

df	0.20	0.10	0.05	0.02	0.01	0.001
1	1.642	2.706	3.841	5.412	6.635	10.827
2	3.219	4.605	5.991	7.842	9.210	13.815
3	4.642	6.251	7.815	9.837	11.345	16.266
4	5.989	7.779	9.488	11.668	13.277	18.467
5	7.289	9.236	11.070	13.388	15.086	20.515
6	8.558	10.645	12.592	15.033	16.812	22.457
7	9.803	12.017	14.067	16.622	18.475	24.322
8	11.030	13.362	15.507	18.168	20.090	26.125
9	12.242	14.684	16.919	19.679	21.666	27.877
10	13.442	15.987	18.307	21.161	23.209	29.588
11	14.631	17.275	19.675	22.618	24.725	31.264
12	15.812	18.549	21.026	24.054	26.217	32.909
13	16.985	19.812	22.362	25.472	27.688	34.528
14	18.151	21.064	23.685	26.873	29.141	36.123
15	19.311	22.307	24.996	28.259	30.578	37.697
16	20.465	23.542	26.296	29.633	32.000	39.252
17	21.615	24.769	27.587	30.995	33.409	40.790
18	22.760	25.989	28.869	32.346	34.805	42.312
19	23.900	27.204	30.144	33.687	36.191	43.820
20	25.038	28.412	31.410	35.020	37.566	45.315
21	26.171	29.615	32.671	36.343	38.932	46.797
22	27.301	30.813	33.924	37.659	40.289	48.268
23	28.429	32.007	35.172	38.968	41.638	49.728
24	29.553	33.196	36.415	40.270	42.980	51.179
25	30.675	34.382	37.652	41.566	44.314	52.620
26	31.795	35.563	38.885	42.856	45.642	54.052
27	32.912	36.741	40.113	44.140	46.963	55.476
28	34.027	37.916	41.337	45.419	48.278	56.893
29	35.139	39.087	42.557	46.693	49.588	58.302
30	36.250	40.256	43.773	47.962	50.892	59.703

(From Fisher, R. A. [1970]. Statistical methods for research workers [14th ed.]. Darien, CT: Hafner Publishing. [Taken from Table III, pp. 112–113].)

APPENDIX C
Distribution of t

	Level of Significance for One-Tailed Test					
	0.10	0.05	0.025	0.01	0.005	0.0005
	Level of Significance for Two-Tailed Test					
df	0.20	0.10	0.05	0.02	0.01	0.001
1	3.078	6.314	12.706	31.821	63.657	636.619
2	1.886	2.920	4.303	6.965	9.925	31.598
3	1.638	2.353	3.182	4.541	5.841	12.941
4	1.533	2.132	2.776	3.747	4.604	8.610
5	1.476	2.015	2.571	3.365	4.032	6.859
6	1.440	1.943	2.447	3.143	3.707	5.959
7	1.415	1.895	2.365	2.998	3.499	5.405
8	1.397	1.860	2.306	2.896	3.355	5.041
9	1.383	1.833	2.262	2.821	3.250	4.781
10	1.372	1.812	2.228	2.764	3.169	4.587
11	1.363	1.796	2.201	2.718	3.106	4.437
12	1.356	1.782	2.179	2.681	3.055	4.318
13	1.350	1.771	2.160	2.650	3.012	4.221
14	1.345	1.761	2.145	2.624	2.977	4.140
15	1.341	1.753	2.131	2.602	2.947	4.073
16	1.337	1.746	2.120	2.583	2.921	4.015
17	1.333	1.740	2.110	2.567	2.898	3.965
18	1.330	1.734	2.101	2.552	2.878	3.922
19	1.328	1.729	2.093	2.539	2.861	3.883
20	1.325	1.725	2.086	2.528	2.845	3.850
21	1.323	1.721	2.080	2.518	2.831	3.819
22	1.321	1.717	2.074	2.508	2.819	3.792
23	1.319	1.714	2.069	2.500	2.807	3.767
24	1.318	1.711	2.064	2.492	2.797	3.745
25	1.316	1.708	2.060	2.485	2.787	3.725
26	1.315	1.706	2.056	2.479	2.779	3.707
27	1.314	1.703	2.052	2.473	2.771	3.690
28	1.313	1.701	2.048	2.467	2.763	3.674

(continued)

df	Level of Significance for One-Tailed Test					
	0.10	0.05	0.025	0.01	0.005	0.0005
	Level of Significance for Two-Tailed Test					
	0.20	0.10	0.05	0.02	0.01	0.001
29	1.311	1.699	2.045	2.462	2.756	3.659
30	1.310	1.697	2.042	2.457	2.750	3.646
40	1.303	1.684	2.021	2.423	2.704	3.551
60	1.296	1.671	2.000	2.390	2.660	3.460
120	1.289	1.658	1.980	2.358	2.617	3.373
∞	1.282	1.645	1.960	2.326	2.576	3.291

(From Fisher, R. A. [1970]. Statistical methods for research workers (14th ed.). Darien, CT: Hafner Publishing [Table IV, p. 176].)

APPENDIX D

The 5% and 1% Points for the Distribution of F

n_1 Degrees of Freedom (For Greater Mean Square)*

n_2^+	1	2	3	4	5	6	7	8	9	10	11	12	14	16	20	24	30	40	50	75	100	200	500	∞
1	161 / 4,052	200 / 4,999	216 / 5,403	225 / 5,625	230 / 5,764	234 / 5,859	237 / 5,928	239 / 5,981	241 / 6,022	242 / 6,056	243 / 6,082	244 / 6,106	245 / 6,142	246 / 6,169	248 / 6,208	249 / 6,234	250 / 6,258	251 / 6,286	252 / 6,302	253 / 6,323	253 / 6,334	254 / 6,352	254 / 6,361	254 / 6,366
2	18.51 / 98.49	19.00 / 99.00	19.16 / 99.17	19.25 / 99.25	19.30 / 99.30	19.33 / 99.33	19.36 / 99.34	19.37 / 99.36	19.38 / 99.38	19.39 / 99.40	19.40 / 99.41	19.41 / 99.42	19.42 / 99.43	19.43 / 99.44	19.44 / 99.45	19.45 / 99.46	19.46 / 99.47	19.47 / 99.48	19.47 / 99.48	19.48 / 99.49	19.49 / 99.49	19.49 / 99.49	19.50 / 99.50	19.50 / 99.50
3	10.13 / 34.12	9.55 / 30.82	9.38 / 29.46	9.12 / 28.71	9.01 / 28.47	8.94 / 27.91	8.88 / 27.67	8.84 / 27.49	8.81 / 27.34	8.78 / 27.23	8.76 / 27.13	8.74 / 27.05	8.71 / 26.92	8.69 / 26.83	8.66 / 26.69	8.64 / 26.60	8.62 / 26.50	8.60 / 26.41	8.58 / 26.35	8.57 / 26.27	8.56 / 26.23	8.54 / 26.18	8.54 / 26.14	8.53 / 26.12
4	7.71 / 21.20	6.94 / 18.00	6.59 / 16.69	6.39 / 15.98	6.26 / 15.52	6.16 / 15.21	6.09 / 14.98	6.04 / 14.80	6.00 / 14.66	5.96 / 14.54	5.93 / 14.45	5.91 / 14.37	5.87 / 14.24	5.84 / 14.15	5.80 / 14.02	5.77 / 13.93	5.74 / 13.83	5.71 / 13.74	5.70 / 13.69	5.68 / 13.61	5.66 / 13.57	5.65 / 13.52	5.64 / 13.48	5.63 / 13.46
5	6.61 / 16.26	5.79 / 13.27	5.41 / 12.06	5.19 / 11.39	5.05 / 10.97	4.95 / 10.67	4.88 / 10.45	4.82 / 10.27	4.78 / 10.15	4.74 / 10.05	4.70 / 9.96	4.68 / 9.89	4.64 / 9.77	4.60 / 9.68	4.56 / 9.55	4.53 / 9.47	4.50 / 9.38	4.46 / 9.29	4.44 / 9.24	4.42 / 9.17	4.40 / 9.13	4.38 / 9.07	4.37 / 9.04	4.36 / 9.02
6	5.99 / 13.74	5.14 / 10.92	4.76 / 9.78	4.53 / 9.15	4.39 / 8.75	4.28 / 8.47	4.21 / 8.26	4.15 / 8.10	4.10 / 7.98	4.06 / 7.87	4.03 / 7.79	4.00 / 7.72	3.96 / 7.60	3.92 / 7.52	3.87 / 7.39	3.84 / 7.31	3.81 / 7.23	3.77 / 7.14	3.75 / 7.09	3.72 / 7.02	3.71 / 6.99	3.69 / 6.94	3.68 / 6.90	3.67 / 6.88
7	5.59 / 12.25	4.74 / 9.55	4.35 / 8.45	4.12 / 7.85	3.97 / 7.46	3.87 / 7.19	3.79 / 7.00	3.73 / 6.84	3.68 / 6.71	3.63 / 6.62	3.60 / 6.54	3.57 / 6.47	3.52 / 6.35	3.49 / 6.27	3.44 / 6.15	3.41 / 6.07	3.38 / 5.98	3.34 / 5.90	3.32 / 5.85	3.29 / 5.78	3.28 / 5.75	3.25 / 5.70	3.24 / 5.67	3.23 / 5.65
8	5.32 / 11.26	4.46 / 8.65	4.07 / 7.59	3.84 / 7.01	3.69 / 6.63	3.58 / 6.37	3.50 / 6.19	3.44 / 6.03	3.39 / 5.91	3.34 / 5.82	3.31 / 5.74	3.28 / 5.67	3.23 / 5.56	3.20 / 5.48	3.15 / 5.36	3.12 / 5.28	3.08 / 5.20	3.05 / 5.11	3.03 / 5.06	3.00 / 5.00	2.98 / 4.96	2.96 / 4.91	2.94 / 4.88	2.93 / 4.86
9	5.12 / 10.56	4.26 / 8.02	3.86 / 6.99	3.63 / 6.42	3.48 / 6.06	3.37 / 5.80	3.29 / 5.62	3.23 / 5.47	3.18 / 5.35	3.13 / 5.26	3.10 / 5.18	3.07 / 5.11	3.02 / 5.00	2.98 / 4.92	2.93 / 4.80	2.90 / 4.73	2.86 / 4.64	2.82 / 4.56	2.80 / 4.51	2.77 / 4.45	2.76 / 4.41	2.73 / 4.36	2.72 / 4.33	2.71 / 4.31
10	4.96 / 10.04	4.10 / 7.56	3.71 / 6.55	3.48 / 5.99	3.33 / 5.64	3.22 / 5.39	3.14 / 5.21	3.07 / 5.06	3.02 / 4.95	2.97 / 4.85	2.94 / 4.78	2.91 / 4.71	2.86 / 4.60	2.82 / 4.52	2.77 / 4.41	2.74 / 4.33	2.70 / 4.25	2.67 / 4.17	2.64 / 4.12	2.61 / 4.05	2.59 / 4.01	2.56 / 3.96	2.55 / 3.93	2.54 / 3.91
11	4.84 / 9.65	3.98 / 7.20	3.59 / 6.22	3.36 / 5.67	3.20 / 5.32	3.09 / 5.07	3.01 / 4.88	2.95 / 4.74	2.90 / 4.63	2.86 / 4.54	2.82 / 4.46	2.79 / 4.40	2.74 / 4.29	2.70 / 4.21	2.65 / 4.10	2.61 / 4.02	2.57 / 3.94	2.53 / 3.86	2.50 / 3.80	2.47 / 3.74	2.45 / 3.70	2.42 / 3.66	2.41 / 3.62	2.40 / 3.60
12	4.75 / 9.33	3.88 / 6.93	3.49 / 5.95	3.26 / 5.41	3.11 / 5.06	3.00 / 4.82	2.92 / 4.65	2.85 / 4.50	2.80 / 4.39	2.76 / 4.30	2.72 / 4.22	2.69 / 4.16	2.64 / 4.05	2.60 / 3.98	2.54 / 3.86	2.50 / 3.78	2.46 / 3.70	2.42 / 3.61	2.40 / 3.56	2.36 / 3.49	2.35 / 3.46	2.32 / 3.41	2.31 / 3.38	2.30 / 3.36
13	4.67 / 9.07	3.80 / 6.70	3.41 / 5.74	3.18 / 5.20	3.02 / 4.86	2.92 / 4.62	2.84 / 4.44	2.77 / 4.30	2.72 / 4.19	2.67 / 4.10	2.63 / 4.02	2.60 / 3.96	2.55 / 3.85	2.51 / 3.78	2.46 / 3.67	2.42 / 3.59	2.38 / 3.51	2.34 / 3.42	2.32 / 3.37	2.28 / 3.30	2.26 / 3.27	2.24 / 3.21	2.22 / 3.18	2.21 / 3.16
14	4.60 / 8.86	3.74 / 6.51	3.34 / 5.56	3.11 / 5.03	2.96 / 4.69	2.85 / 4.46	2.77 / 4.28	2.70 / 4.14	2.65 / 4.03	2.60 / 3.94	2.56 / 3.86	2.53 / 3.80	2.48 / 3.70	2.44 / 3.62	2.39 / 3.51	2.35 / 3.43	2.31 / 3.34	2.27 / 3.26	2.24 / 3.21	2.21 / 3.14	2.19 / 3.11	2.16 / 3.06	2.14 / 3.02	2.13 / 3.00
15	4.54 / 8.68	3.68 / 6.36	3.29 / 5.42	3.06 / 4.89	2.90 / 4.56	2.79 / 4.32	2.70 / 4.14	2.64 / 4.00	2.59 / 3.89	2.55 / 3.80	2.51 / 3.73	2.48 / 3.67	2.43 / 3.56	2.39 / 3.48	2.33 / 3.36	2.29 / 3.29	2.25 / 3.20	2.21 / 3.12	2.18 / 3.07	2.15 / 3.00	2.12 / 2.97	2.10 / 2.92	2.08 / 2.89	2.07 / 2.87
16	4.49 / 8.53	3.63 / 6.23	3.24 / 5.29	3.01 / 4.77	2.85 / 4.44	2.74 / 4.20	2.66 / 4.03	2.59 / 3.89	2.54 / 3.78	2.49 / 3.69	2.45 / 3.61	2.42 / 3.55	2.37 / 3.45	2.33 / 3.37	2.28 / 3.25	2.24 / 3.18	2.20 / 3.10	2.16 / 3.01	2.13 / 2.96	2.09 / 2.89	2.07 / 2.86	2.04 / 2.80	2.02 / 2.77	2.01 / 2.75
17	4.45 / 8.40	3.59 / 6.11	3.20 / 5.18	2.96 / 4.67	2.81 / 4.34	2.70 / 4.10	2.62 / 3.93	2.55 / 3.79	2.50 / 3.68	2.45 / 3.59	2.41 / 3.52	2.38 / 3.45	2.33 / 3.35	2.29 / 3.27	2.23 / 3.16	2.19 / 3.08	2.15 / 3.00	2.11 / 2.92	2.08 / 2.86	2.04 / 2.79	2.02 / 2.76	1.99 / 2.70	1.97 / 2.67	1.96 / 2.65

Critical values table (F-distribution), continued. Each denominator df (left column) has two rows of values: the upper (roman) and lower (bold) entries. Values are listed from df1 = 1 (largest) to higher df1 (smallest).

df																								
18	4.41	3.55	3.16	2.93	2.77	2.66	2.58	2.51	2.46	2.41	2.37	2.34	2.29	2.25	2.19	2.15	2.11	2.07	2.04	2.00	1.98	1.95	1.93	1.92
	8.28	**6.01**	**5.09**	**4.58**	**4.25**	**4.01**	**3.85**	**3.71**	**3.60**	**3.51**	**3.44**	**3.37**	**3.27**	**3.19**	**3.07**	**3.00**	**2.91**	**2.83**	**2.78**	**2.71**	**2.68**	**2.62**	**2.59**	**2.57**
19	4.38	3.52	3.13	2.90	2.74	2.63	2.55	2.48	2.43	2.38	2.34	2.31	2.26	2.21	2.15	2.11	2.07	2.02	2.00	1.96	1.94	1.91	1.90	1.88
	8.18	**5.93**	**5.01**	**4.50**	**4.17**	**3.94**	**3.77**	**3.63**	**3.52**	**3.43**	**3.36**	**3.30**	**3.19**	**3.12**	**3.00**	**2.92**	**2.84**	**2.76**	**2.70**	**2.63**	**2.60**	**2.54**	**2.51**	**2.49**
20	4.35	3.49	3.10	2.87	2.71	2.60	2.52	2.45	2.40	2.35	2.31	2.28	2.23	2.18	2.12	2.08	2.04	1.99	1.96	1.92	1.90	1.87	1.85	1.84
	8.10	**5.85**	**4.94**	**4.43**	**4.10**	**3.87**	**3.71**	**3.56**	**3.45**	**3.37**	**3.30**	**3.23**	**3.13**	**3.05**	**2.94**	**2.86**	**2.77**	**2.69**	**2.63**	**2.56**	**2.53**	**2.47**	**2.44**	**2.42**
21	4.32	3.47	3.07	2.84	2.68	2.57	2.49	2.42	2.37	2.32	2.28	2.25	2.20	2.15	2.09	2.05	2.00	1.96	1.93	1.89	1.87	1.84	1.82	1.81
	8.02	**5.78**	**4.87**	**4.37**	**4.04**	**3.81**	**3.65**	**3.51**	**3.40**	**3.31**	**3.24**	**3.17**	**3.07**	**2.99**	**2.88**	**2.80**	**2.72**	**2.63**	**2.58**	**2.51**	**2.47**	**2.42**	**2.38**	**2.36**
22	4.30	3.44	3.05	2.82	2.66	2.55	2.47	2.40	2.35	2.30	2.26	2.23	2.18	2.13	2.07	2.03	1.98	1.93	1.91	1.87	1.84	1.81	1.80	1.78
	7.94	**5.72**	**4.82**	**4.31**	**3.99**	**3.76**	**3.59**	**3.45**	**3.35**	**3.26**	**3.18**	**3.12**	**3.02**	**2.94**	**2.83**	**2.75**	**2.67**	**2.58**	**2.53**	**2.46**	**2.42**	**2.37**	**2.33**	**2.31**
23	4.28	3.42	3.03	2.80	2.64	2.53	2.45	2.38	2.32	2.28	2.24	2.20	2.14	2.10	2.04	2.00	1.96	1.91	1.88	1.84	1.82	1.79	1.77	1.76
	7.88	**5.66**	**4.76**	**4.26**	**3.94**	**3.71**	**3.54**	**3.41**	**3.30**	**3.21**	**3.14**	**3.07**	**2.97**	**2.89**	**2.78**	**2.70**	**2.62**	**2.53**	**2.48**	**2.41**	**2.37**	**2.32**	**2.28**	**2.26**
24	4.26	3.40	3.01	2.78	2.62	2.51	2.43	2.36	2.30	2.26	2.22	2.18	2.13	2.09	2.02	1.98	1.94	1.89	1.86	1.82	1.80	1.76	1.74	1.73
	7.82	**5.61**	**4.72**	**4.22**	**3.90**	**3.67**	**3.50**	**3.36**	**3.25**	**3.17**	**3.09**	**3.03**	**2.93**	**2.85**	**2.74**	**2.66**	**2.58**	**2.49**	**2.44**	**2.36**	**2.33**	**2.27**	**2.23**	**2.21**
25	4.24	3.38	2.99	2.76	2.60	2.49	2.41	2.34	2.28	2.24	2.20	2.16	2.11	2.06	2.00	1.96	1.92	1.87	1.84	1.80	1.77	1.74	1.72	1.71
	7.77	**5.57**	**4.68**	**4.18**	**3.86**	**3.63**	**3.46**	**3.32**	**3.21**	**3.13**	**3.05**	**2.99**	**2.89**	**2.81**	**2.70**	**2.62**	**2.54**	**2.45**	**2.40**	**2.32**	**2.29**	**2.23**	**2.19**	**2.17**
26	4.22	3.37	2.98	2.74	2.59	2.47	2.39	2.32	2.27	2.22	2.18	2.15	2.10	2.05	1.99	1.95	1.90	1.85	1.82	1.78	1.76	1.72	1.70	1.69
	7.72	**5.53**	**4.64**	**4.14**	**3.82**	**3.59**	**3.42**	**3.29**	**3.17**	**3.09**	**3.02**	**2.96**	**2.86**	**2.77**	**2.66**	**2.58**	**2.50**	**2.41**	**2.36**	**2.28**	**2.25**	**2.19**	**2.15**	**2.13**
27	4.21	3.35	2.96	2.73	2.57	2.46	2.37	2.30	2.25	2.20	2.16	2.13	2.08	2.03	1.97	1.93	1.88	1.84	1.80	1.76	1.74	1.71	1.68	1.67
	7.68	**5.49**	**4.60**	**4.11**	**3.79**	**3.56**	**3.39**	**3.26**	**3.14**	**3.06**	**3.00**	**2.93**	**2.83**	**2.74**	**2.63**	**2.55**	**2.47**	**2.38**	**2.33**	**2.25**	**2.21**	**2.16**	**2.12**	**2.10**
28	4.20	3.34	2.95	2.71	2.56	2.44	2.36	2.29	2.24	2.19	2.15	2.12	2.06	2.02	1.96	1.91	1.87	1.81	1.78	1.75	1.72	1.69	1.67	1.65
	7.64	**5.45**	**4.57**	**4.07**	**3.76**	**3.53**	**3.36**	**3.23**	**3.11**	**3.03**	**2.95**	**2.90**	**2.80**	**2.71**	**2.60**	**2.52**	**2.44**	**2.35**	**2.30**	**2.22**	**2.18**	**2.13**	**2.09**	**2.06**
29	4.18	3.33	2.93	2.70	2.54	2.43	2.35	2.28	2.22	2.18	2.14	2.10	2.05	2.00	1.94	1.90	1.85	1.80	1.77	1.73	1.71	1.68	1.65	1.64
	7.60	**5.42**	**4.54**	**4.04**	**3.73**	**3.50**	**3.33**	**3.20**	**3.08**	**3.00**	**2.92**	**2.87**	**2.77**	**2.68**	**2.57**	**2.49**	**2.41**	**2.32**	**2.27**	**2.19**	**2.15**	**2.10**	**2.06**	**2.03**
30	4.17	3.32	2.92	2.69	2.53	2.42	2.34	2.27	2.21	2.16	2.12	2.09	2.04	1.99	1.93	1.89	1.84	1.79	1.76	1.72	1.69	1.66	1.64	1.62
	7.56	**5.39**	**4.51**	**4.02**	**3.70**	**3.47**	**3.30**	**3.17**	**3.06**	**2.98**	**2.90**	**2.84**	**2.74**	**2.66**	**2.55**	**2.47**	**2.38**	**2.29**	**2.24**	**2.16**	**2.13**	**2.07**	**2.03**	**2.01**
32	4.15	3.30	2.90	2.67	2.51	2.40	2.32	2.25	2.19	2.14	2.10	2.07	2.02	1.97	1.91	1.86	1.82	1.76	1.74	1.69	1.67	1.64	1.61	1.59
	7.50	**5.34**	**4.46**	**3.97**	**3.66**	**3.42**	**3.25**	**3.12**	**3.01**	**2.94**	**2.86**	**2.80**	**2.70**	**2.62**	**2.51**	**2.42**	**2.34**	**2.25**	**2.20**	**2.12**	**2.08**	**2.02**	**1.98**	**1.96**
34	4.13	3.28	2.88	2.65	2.49	2.38	2.30	2.23	2.17	2.12	2.08	2.05	2.00	1.95	1.89	1.84	1.80	1.74	1.71	1.67	1.64	1.61	1.59	1.57
	7.44	**5.29**	**4.42**	**3.93**	**3.61**	**3.38**	**3.21**	**3.08**	**2.97**	**2.89**	**2.82**	**2.76**	**2.66**	**2.58**	**2.47**	**2.38**	**2.30**	**2.21**	**2.15**	**2.08**	**2.04**	**1.98**	**1.94**	**1.91**
36	4.11	3.26	2.86	2.63	2.48	2.36	2.28	2.21	2.15	2.10	2.06	2.03	1.98	1.93	1.87	1.82	1.78	1.71	1.69	1.65	1.62	1.59	1.56	1.55
	7.39	**5.25**	**4.38**	**3.89**	**3.58**	**3.35**	**3.18**	**3.04**	**2.94**	**2.86**	**2.78**	**2.72**	**2.62**	**2.54**	**2.43**	**2.35**	**2.26**	**2.17**	**2.12**	**2.04**	**2.00**	**1.94**	**1.90**	**1.87**
38	4.10	3.25	2.85	2.62	2.46	2.35	2.26	2.19	2.14	2.09	2.05	2.02	1.96	1.92	1.85	1.80	1.76	1.69	1.67	1.63	1.60	1.57	1.54	1.53
	7.35	**5.21**	**4.34**	**3.86**	**3.54**	**3.32**	**3.15**	**3.02**	**2.91**	**2.82**	**2.75**	**2.69**	**2.59**	**2.51**	**2.40**	**2.32**	**2.22**	**2.14**	**2.08**	**2.00**	**1.97**	**1.90**	**1.86**	**1.84**
40	4.08	3.23	2.84	2.61	2.45	2.34	2.25	2.18	2.12	2.07	2.04	2.00	1.95	1.90	1.84	1.79	1.74	1.69	1.66	1.61	1.59	1.55	1.53	1.51
	7.31	**5.18**	**4.31**	**3.83**	**3.51**	**3.29**	**3.12**	**2.99**	**2.88**	**2.80**	**2.73**	**2.66**	**2.56**	**2.49**	**2.37**	**2.29**	**2.20**	**2.11**	**2.05**	**1.97**	**1.94**	**1.88**	**1.84**	**1.81**
42	4.07	3.22	2.83	2.59	2.44	2.32	2.24	2.17	2.11	2.06	2.02	1.99	1.94	1.89	1.82	1.78	1.73	1.68	1.64	1.60	1.57	1.54	1.51	1.49
	7.27	**5.15**	**4.29**	**3.80**	**3.49**	**3.26**	**3.10**	**2.96**	**2.86**	**2.77**	**2.70**	**2.64**	**2.54**	**2.46**	**2.35**	**2.26**	**2.17**	**2.08**	**2.02**	**1.94**	**1.91**	**1.85**	**1.80**	**1.78**
44	4.06	3.21	2.82	2.58	2.43	2.31	2.23	2.16	2.10	2.05	2.01	1.98	1.92	1.88	1.81	1.76	1.72	1.66	1.63	1.58	1.56	1.52	1.50	1.48
	7.24	**5.12**	**4.26**	**3.78**	**3.46**	**3.24**	**3.07**	**2.94**	**2.84**	**2.75**	**2.68**	**2.62**	**2.52**	**2.44**	**2.32**	**2.24**	**2.15**	**2.06**	**2.00**	**1.92**	**1.88**	**1.82**	**1.78**	**1.75**

(continued)

n_1 Degrees of Freedom (For Greater Mean Square)*

$n_2^†$	1	2	3	4	5	6	7	8	9	10	11	12	14	16	20	24	30	40	50	75	100	200	500	∞
46	4.05	3.20	2.81	2.57	2.42	2.30	2.22	2.14	2.09	2.04	2.00	1.97	1.91	1.87	1.80	1.75	1.71	1.65	1.62	1.57	1.54	1.51	1.48	1.46
	7.21	**5.10**	**4.24**	**3.76**	**3.44**	**3.22**	**3.05**	**2.92**	**2.82**	**2.73**	**2.66**	**2.60**	**2.50**	**2.42**	**2.30**	**2.22**	**2.13**	**2.04**	**1.98**	**1.90**	**1.86**	**1.80**	**1.76**	**1.72**
48	4.04	3.19	2.80	2.56	2.41	2.30	2.21	2.14	2.08	2.03	1.99	1.96	1.90	1.86	1.79	1.74	1.70	1.64	1.61	1.56	1.53	1.50	1.47	1.45
	7.19	**5.08**	**4.22**	**3.74**	**3.42**	**3.20**	**3.04**	**2.90**	**2.80**	**2.71**	**2.64**	**2.58**	**2.48**	**2.40**	**2.28**	**2.20**	**2.11**	**2.02**	**1.96**	**1.88**	**1.84**	**1.78**	**1.73**	**1.70**
50	4.03	3.18	2.79	2.56	2.40	2.29	2.20	2.13	2.07	2.02	1.98	1.95	1.90	1.85	1.78	1.74	1.69	1.63	1.60	1.55	1.52	1.48	1.46	1.44
	7.17	**5.06**	**4.20**	**3.72**	**3.41**	**3.18**	**3.02**	**2.88**	**2.78**	**2.70**	**2.62**	**2.56**	**2.46**	**2.39**	**2.26**	**2.18**	**2.10**	**2.00**	**1.94**	**1.86**	**1.82**	**1.76**	**1.71**	**1.68**
55	4.02	3.17	2.78	2.54	2.38	2.27	2.18	2.11	2.05	2.00	1.97	1.93	1.88	1.83	1.76	1.72	1.67	1.61	1.58	1.52	1.50	1.46	1.43	1.41
	7.12	**5.01**	**4.16**	**3.68**	**3.37**	**3.15**	**2.98**	**2.85**	**2.75**	**2.66**	**2.59**	**2.53**	**2.43**	**2.35**	**2.23**	**2.15**	**2.06**	**1.96**	**1.90**	**1.82**	**1.78**	**1.71**	**1.66**	**1.64**
60	4.00	3.15	2.76	2.52	2.37	2.25	2.17	2.10	2.04	1.99	1.95	1.92	1.86	1.81	1.75	1.70	1.65	1.59	1.56	1.50	1.48	1.44	1.41	1.39
	7.08	**4.98**	**4.13**	**3.65**	**3.34**	**3.12**	**2.95**	**2.82**	**2.72**	**2.63**	**2.56**	**2.50**	**2.40**	**2.32**	**2.20**	**2.12**	**2.03**	**1.93**	**1.87**	**1.79**	**1.74**	**1.68**	**1.63**	**1.60**
65	3.99	3.14	2.75	2.51	2.36	2.24	2.15	2.08	2.02	1.98	1.94	1.90	1.85	1.80	1.73	1.68	1.63	1.57	1.54	1.49	1.46	1.42	1.39	1.37
	7.04	**4.95**	**4.10**	**3.62**	**3.31**	**3.09**	**2.93**	**2.79**	**2.70**	**2.61**	**2.54**	**2.47**	**2.37**	**2.30**	**2.18**	**2.09**	**2.00**	**1.90**	**1.84**	**1.76**	**1.71**	**1.64**	**1.60**	**1.56**
70	3.98	3.13	2.74	2.50	2.35	2.23	2.14	2.07	2.01	1.97	1.93	1.89	1.84	1.79	1.72	1.67	1.62	1.56	1.53	1.47	1.45	1.40	1.37	1.35
	7.01	**4.92**	**4.08**	**3.60**	**3.29**	**3.07**	**2.91**	**2.77**	**2.67**	**2.59**	**2.51**	**2.45**	**2.35**	**2.28**	**2.15**	**2.07**	**1.98**	**1.88**	**1.82**	**1.74**	**1.69**	**1.62**	**1.56**	**1.53**
80	3.96	3.11	2.72	2.48	2.33	2.21	2.12	2.05	1.99	1.95	1.91	1.88	1.82	1.77	1.70	1.65	1.60	1.54	1.51	1.45	1.42	1.38	1.35	1.32
	6.96	**4.88**	**4.04**	**3.56**	**3.25**	**3.04**	**2.87**	**2.74**	**2.64**	**2.55**	**2.48**	**2.41**	**2.32**	**2.24**	**2.11**	**2.03**	**1.94**	**1.84**	**1.78**	**1.70**	**1.65**	**1.57**	**1.52**	**1.49**
100	3.94	3.09	2.70	2.46	2.30	2.19	2.10	2.03	1.97	1.92	1.88	1.85	1.79	1.75	1.68	1.63	1.57	1.51	1.48	1.42	1.39	1.34	1.30	1.28
	6.90	**4.82**	**3.98**	**3.51**	**3.20**	**2.99**	**2.82**	**2.69**	**2.59**	**2.51**	**2.43**	**2.36**	**2.26**	**2.19**	**2.06**	**1.98**	**1.89**	**1.79**	**1.73**	**1.64**	**1.59**	**1.51**	**1.46**	**1.43**
125	3.92	3.07	2.68	2.44	2.29	2.17	2.08	2.01	1.95	1.90	1.86	1.83	1.77	1.72	1.65	1.60	1.55	1.49	1.45	1.39	1.36	1.31	1.27	1.25
	6.84	**4.78**	**3.94**	**3.47**	**3.17**	**2.95**	**2.79**	**2.65**	**2.56**	**2.47**	**2.40**	**2.33**	**2.23**	**2.15**	**2.03**	**1.94**	**1.85**	**1.75**	**1.68**	**1.59**	**1.54**	**1.46**	**1.40**	**1.37**
150	3.91	3.06	2.67	2.43	2.27	2.16	2.07	2.00	1.94	1.89	1.85	1.82	1.76	1.71	1.64	1.59	1.54	1.47	1.44	1.37	1.34	1.29	1.25	1.22
	6.81	**4.75**	**3.91**	**3.44**	**3.14**	**2.92**	**2.76**	**2.62**	**2.53**	**2.44**	**2.37**	**2.30**	**2.20**	**2.12**	**2.00**	**1.91**	**1.83**	**1.72**	**1.66**	**1.56**	**1.51**	**1.43**	**1.37**	**1.33**
200	3.89	3.04	2.65	2.41	2.26	2.14	2.05	1.98	1.92	1.87	1.83	1.80	1.74	1.69	1.62	1.57	1.52	1.45	1.42	1.35	1.32	1.26	1.22	1.19
	6.76	**4.71**	**3.88**	**3.41**	**3.11**	**2.90**	**2.73**	**2.60**	**2.50**	**2.41**	**2.34**	**2.28**	**2.17**	**2.09**	**1.97**	**1.88**	**1.79**	**1.69**	**1.62**	**1.53**	**1.48**	**1.39**	**1.33**	**1.28**
400	3.86	3.02	2.62	2.39	2.23	2.12	2.03	1.96	1.90	1.85	1.81	1.78	1.72	1.67	1.60	1.54	1.49	1.42	1.38	1.32	1.28	1.22	1.16	1.13
	6.70	**4.66**	**3.83**	**3.36**	**3.06**	**2.85**	**2.69**	**2.55**	**2.46**	**2.37**	**2.29**	**2.23**	**2.12**	**2.04**	**1.92**	**1.84**	**1.74**	**1.64**	**1.57**	**1.47**	**1.42**	**1.32**	**1.24**	**1.19**
1000	3.85	3.00	2.61	2.38	2.22	2.10	2.02	1.95	1.89	1.84	1.80	1.76	1.70	1.65	1.58	1.53	1.47	1.41	1.36	1.30	1.26	1.19	1.13	1.08
	6.66	**4.62**	**3.80**	**3.34**	**3.04**	**2.82**	**2.66**	**2.53**	**2.43**	**2.34**	**2.26**	**2.20**	**2.09**	**2.01**	**1.89**	**1.81**	**1.71**	**1.61**	**1.54**	**1.44**	**1.38**	**1.28**	**1.19**	**1.11**
∞	3.84	2.99	2.60	2.37	2.21	2.09	2.01	1.94	1.88	1.83	1.79	1.75	1.69	1.64	1.57	1.52	1.46	1.40	1.35	1.28	1.24	1.17	1.11	1.00
	6.64	**4.60**	**3.78**	**3.32**	**3.02**	**2.80**	**2.64**	**2.51**	**2.41**	**2.32**	**2.24**	**2.18**	**2.07**	**1.99**	**1.87**	**1.79**	**1.69**	**1.59**	**1.52**	**1.41**	**1.36**	**1.25**	**1.15**	**1.00**

5% = roman type; 1% = boldface type

* numerator.

† denominator.

(From Snedecor, G. W. [1938]. Statistical methods. Ames, Iowa: Collegiate Press. [Table 10-3, pp. 184–187].)

APPENDIX E

Critical Values of the Correlation Coefficient

	Level of Significance for One-Tailed Test			
	.05	.025	.01	.005
	Level of Significance for Two-Tailed Test			
df	.10	.05	.02	.01
1	.988	.997	.9995	.9999
2	.900	.950	.980	.990
3	.805	.878	.934	.959
4	.729	.811	.882	.917
5	.669	.754	.833	.874
6	.622	.707	.789	.834
7	.582	.666	.750	.798
8	.549	.632	.716	.765
9	.521	.602	.685	.735
10	.497	.576	.658	.708
11	.476	.553	.634	.684
12	.458	.532	.612	.661
13	.441	.514	.592	.641
14	.426	.497	.574	.623
15	.412	.482	.558	.606
16	.400	.468	.542	.590
17	.389	.456	.528	.575
18	.378	.444	.516	.561
19	.369	.433	.503	.549
20	.360	.423	.492	.537
21	.352	.413	.482	.526
22	.344	.404	.472	.515
23	.337	.396	.462	.505
24	.330	.388	.453	.496
25	.323	.381	.445	.487

(continued)

	Level of Significance for One-Tailed Test			
	.05	.025	.01	.005
	Level of Significance for Two-Tailed Test			
df	.10	.05	.02	.01
26	.317	.374	.437	.479
27	.311	.367	.430	.471
28	.306	.361	.423	.463
29	.301	.355	.416	.456
30	.296	.349	.409	.449
35	.275	.325	.381	.418
40	.257	.304	.358	.393
45	.243	.288	.338	.372
50	.231	.273	.322	.354
60	.211	.250	.295	.325
70	.195	.232	.274	.303
80	.183	.217	.256	.283
90	.173	.205	.242	.267
100	.164	.195	.230	.254
125		.174		.228
150		.159		.208
200		.138		.181
300		.113		.148
400		.098		.128
500		.088		.115
1000		.062		.081

(From Fisher, R. A. [1970]. Statistical methods for research workers [14th ed.]. Darien, CT: Hafner Publishing Co. [Table V.A., p. 211].)

APPENDIX F
Transformation of r to z_r

r	z_r	r	z_r	r	z_r	r	z_r	r	z_r
.000	.000	.200	.203	.400	.424	.600	.693	.800	1.099
.005	.005	.205	.208	.405	.430	.605	.701	.805	1.113
.010	.010	.210	.213	.410	.436	.610	.709	.810	1.127
.015	.015	.215	.218	.415	.442	.615	.717	.815	1.142
.020	.020	.220	.224	.420	.448	.620	.725	.820	1.157
.025	.025	.225	.229	.425	.454	.625	.733	.825	1.172
.030	.030	.230	.234	.430	.460	.630	.741	.830	1.188
.035	.035	.235	.239	.435	.466	.635	.750	.835	1.204
.040	.040	.240	.245	.440	.472	.640	.758	.840	1.221
.045	.045	.245	.250	.445	.478	.645	.767	.845	1.238
.050	.050	.250	.255	.450	.485	.650	.775	.850	1.256
.055	.055	.255	.261	.455	.491	.655	.784	.855	1.274
.060	.060	.260	.266	.460	.497	.660	.793	.860	1.293
.065	.065	.265	.271	.465	.504	.665	.802	.865	1.313
.070	.070	.270	.277	.470	.510	.670	.811	.870	1.333
.075	.075	.275	.282	.475	.517	.675	.820	.875	1.354
.080	.080	.280	.288	.480	.523	.680	.829	.880	1.376
.085	.085	.285	.293	.485	.530	.685	.838	.885	1.398
.090	.090	.290	.299	.490	.536	.690	.848	.890	1.422
.095	.095	.295	.304	.495	.543	.695	.858	.895	1.447
.100	.100	.300	.310	.500	.549	.700	.867	.900	1.472
.105	.105	.305	.315	.505	.556	.705	.877	.905	1.499
.110	.110	.310	.321	.510	.563	.710	.887	.910	1.528
.115	.116	.315	.326	.515	.570	.715	.897	.915	1.557
.120	.121	.320	.332	.520	.576	.720	.908	.920	1.589
.125	.126	.325	.337	.525	.583	.725	.918	.925	1.623
.130	.131	.330	.343	.530	.590	.730	.929	.930	1.658
.135	.136	.335	.348	.535	.597	.735	.940	.935	1.697
.140	.141	.340	.354	.540	.604	.740	.950	.940	1.738
.145	.146	.345	.360	.545	.611	.745	.962	.945	1.783

(continued)

r	z_r	r	z_r	r	z_r	r	z_r	r	z_r
.150	.151	.350	.365	.550	.618	.750	.973	.950	1.832
.155	.156	.355	.371	.555	.626	.755	.984	.955	1.886
.160	.161	.360	.377	.560	.633	.760	.996	.960	1.946
.165	.167	.365	.383	.565	.640	.765	1.008	.965	2.014
.170	.172	.370	.388	.570	.648	.770	1.020	.970	2.092
.175	.177	.375	.394	.575	.655	.775	1.033	.975	2.185
.180	.182	.380	.400	.580	.662	.780	1.045	.980	2.298
.185	.187	.385	.406	.585	.670	.785	1.058	.985	2.443
.190	.192	.390	.412	.590	.678	.790	1.071	.990	2.647
.195	.198	.395	.418	.595	.685	.795	1.085	.995	2.994

(From Hinkle, D. E., Wiersma, W., & Jurs, S. G. [1981]. Applied statistics for the behavioral sciences [2nd ed.]. [Appendix C.6, p. 658]. Boston: Houghton Mifflin. Copyright ©1988 by Houghton Mifflin Company. Used by permission.)

APPENDIX G
Exercises

Following the advice of the reviewers of the first edition, all the exercises have been designed to be carried out on a computer. Given the ready access to personal computers, it is more important to develop some skill in entering and analyzing data than to practice hand calculations. We have decided, therefore, to restrict these exercises to ones that you can manage yourself. The exercises are fairly simple, aimed at helping you to learn to enter data and grasp the concepts of data analysis without overwhelming you with numbers. If you want to attempt some of the more sophisticated topics in the book, you will need access to larger data sets than we are able to provide in these exercises.

Since not everyone has access to a personal computer with statistical software, we have included an introductory program (MYSTAT) with this book. If you do have access to more sophisticated software, you will probably want to use that. The exercises in this book provide many examples of the use of the SPSS/PC+ package.

What Is MYSTAT?

Software for statistics range in power and cost. One very large and powerful package is called SYSTAT, which can perform most statistics in common use. The SYSTAT company has also produced a smaller set of procedures called MYSTAT, which they supply as a way of introducing their product. Although it will not handle such sophisticated techniques as factor analysis and logistic regression, it can be used with up to 32,000 cases and 50 variables.

What Do You Need to Use MYSTAT?

You need access to an IBM-compatible personal computer with a 3½ inch disk drive.

CHAPTER 1

Your tasks are to:

1. Enter data.
2. Run frequencies to produce output like that in Table 1-2.
3. Group the data and run frequencies on the grouped data, as in Table 1-3. Use five intervals (30–39, 40–49, 50–59, 60–69, 70–79).
4. Create a histogram of your data.

Rather than ask you to enter all 113 hysterectomy patients, we have taken a subset of cases. They are in Table G-1. Enter the data into a data file. If you are using MYSTAT, here is how to do it.

Creating a Data Base in MYSTAT

1. Turn on your computer.
2. Put MYSTAT disk into the 3½ inch drive, probably designated A or B.
3. At the prompt, type the letter of the drive with the MYSTAT disk, followed by a colon. For example for the A drive, you type **A:**. Press the "Enter" (sometimes called "Return") key.

TABLE G-1
Ages of Hysterectomy Patients

Subject	Age
1	39
2	44
3	48
4	30
5	47
6	78
7	42
8	45
9	75
10	60
11	49
12	58
13	44
14	40
15	71
16	63
17	56
18	53
19	46
20	42
21	37
22	42
23	32
24	45
25	69
26	41
27	50
28	47
29	43
30	35

4. At the prompt for the drive with the MYSTAT disk, type **MYSTAT** and then press the Enter key.
5. You will see the MYSTAT logo. Follow the directions, "Press Enter or Return."
6. To view the demonstration, type **DEMO**, then use the Enter key. NOTE: Do not type any commands. Simply proceed through the demonstration by pressing the Enter key. You must proceed to the end of **DEMO** before moving on to Step 7.
7. Now let's try to create a data set. If you have just viewed the demo, you will first have to type **NEW** at the MYSTAT prompt (>), then type **EDIT**, and then press the Enter key [ENTER].
8. You will see a spreadsheet with cases (subjects) down the left side of the screen. The cursor is at the top left corner of the spreadsheet above Case 1.
9. Since the subject numbers are already on the screen, you just have to add the ages of the hysterectomy patients.
10. First, name your variable. Variable names must be surrounded by single or double quotation marks, and be no longer than 8 characters.
11. Type **'AGE'** [ENTER].
12. Press the Home key and the cursor will be in position to enter the age for Subject 1.
13. Now type the age for Subject 1 (39) and press [ENTER]. Continue to enter the rest of the ages:

   44 [ENTER]
   48 [ENTER]
   30 [ENTER]
   etc.

   If you make a mistake, use the cursor keys to move up and down and just type over the mistake.
14. After checking for any errors, press the Escape key. The cursor will move below the spreadsheet.
15. MYSTAT added 3 zeros after the decimal point. To get rid of them, type **FORMAT = 0** (zero) [ENTER]. Try it.
16. Press the Escape key again. Note that it moves back into the spreadsheet. You can move in and out of the spreadsheet by pressing the Escape key.
17. Move back to the bottom prompt (press Escape) and type **SAVE HYSTER**. That will save the data set you created under the name of HYSTER.SYS (MYSTAT adds the SYS). Filenames can be up to 8 characters long and must begin with a letter.

   Congratulations! You have created your first MYSTAT data file.

Running Frequencies With MYSTAT

You have entered ages for 30 subjects. Now you want to describe the sample in relation to age by creating a frequency distribution like the one in Table 1-2.

1. Starting after you saved HYSTER, still in EDIT, with the data sheet on your screen, type **QUIT** [ENTER]. The main menu will appear.
2. Enter the following commands, being sure to check them before pressing Enter, as they will disappear from view.

USE HYSTER [ENTER] (This tells the program which data file you are using.)

OUTPUT @ [ENTER] (The @ character stands for the printer. It says that you want the output printed. If your printer is not on, you will get an error message.)

FORMAT = 0 (zero) (This takes the 3 decimal places out.)

NOTE 'FREQUENCY DISTRIBUTION OF AGE OF HYSTERECTOMY PATIENTS' [ENTER] (NOTE tells the system that it is to copy as a header what is included between the quotes. This creates a title for your output.)

TABULATE AGE/LIST [ENTER] (TABULATE is a MYSTAT keyword from the main menu, AGE is the variable you want to tabulate, and LIST is an option for the way the table will appear.)

On your screen you will see a listing of the frequencies for each age. If the printout does not appear, take the printer off line and push the form feed button.

The format is different from Table 1-2, in which the ages are listed down the left side of the table. Here the ages are on the far right. The first age listed is 30, and the last 78. Fifteen of the ages or 50% of the distribution are between 30 and 45. Take some time to familiarize yourself with this form. Your output should look like that in Figure G-1.

If you want to stop for a while before completing the last two tasks in this assignment, type **QUIT** at the main menu. Always be sure that you have saved your work before leaving MYSTAT. After typing **QUIT**, you should see the DOS prompt.

Frequencies on Grouped Data

In Table 1-3, Barbara Jacobsen demonstrates a frequency distribution of the ages of the hysterectomy patients. She used 11 classes, each with an interval of 5 years. Because there are only 30 subjects in your data set, use 5 intervals of 10 years each (30–39, 40–49, 50–59, 60–69, 70–79).

1. If you are not in MYSTAT, reenter it.
2. At the main menu type **EDIT HYSTER** [ENTER]. This will move you back to the spreadsheet with your scores. We need to create a new variable for these groupings. We can call it AGEGRP.
3. At the lower prompt, type **FORMAT = 0** (zero) to get rid of the decimals. Then, to create the new variable with ages grouped into 10-year periods, type the following commands. You will see the numbers being added to your file.

    LET AGEGRP = 0 (zero). (This creates your new variable and gives all subjects a zero for the value.) Now, to create your groups you want to give all subjects in a given group a common number. One way is:

Ages 30–39 = 1
Ages 40–49 = 2
Ages 50–59 = 3
Ages 60–69 = 4
Ages 70–79 = 5

FREQUENCY DISTRIBUTION OF AGE OF HYSTERECTOMY PATIENTS

COUNT	CUM COUNT	PCT	CUM PCT	AGE
1	1	3.3	3.3	30
1	2	3.3	6.7	32
1	3	3.3	10.0	35
1	4	3.3	13.3	37
1	5	3.3	16.7	39
1	6	3.3	20.0	40
1	7	3.3	23.3	41
3	10	10.0	33.3	42
1	11	3.3	36.7	43
2	13	6.7	43.3	44
2	15	6.7	50.0	45
1	16	3.3	53.3	46
2	18	6.7	60.0	47
1	19	3.3	63.3	48
1	20	3.3	66.7	49
1	21	3.3	70.0	50
1	22	3.3	73.3	53
1	23	3.3	76.7	56
1	24	3.3	80.0	58
1	25	3.3	83.3	60
1	26	3.3	86.7	63
1	27	3.3	90.0	69
1	28	3.3	93.3	71
1	29	3.3	96.7	75
1	30	3.3	100.0	78

FIGURE G-1

Frequency Distribution of Age of Hysterectomy Patients.

MYSTAT will do this with some rather tedious commands using IF statements. The general format of these statements is:

IF <expression> THEN LET <variable> = <expression>

One way to create our categories is to type the following:

IF AGE <40 THEN LET AGEGRP = 1 [ENTER] (30–39)
IF AGE <50 AND AGE >39 THEN LET AGEGRP = 2 [ENTER] (40–49)
IF AGE <60 AND AGE >49 THEN LET AGEGRP = 3 [ENTER] (50–59)
IF AGE <70 AND AGE >59 THEN LET AGEGRP = 4 [ENTER] (60–69)
IF AGE >69 THEN LET AGEGRP = 5 [ENTER] (70–79)

As you can see on your screen, MYSTAT has created a new variable with ages grouped into decades.

4. **SAVE HYSTER**. This will save your file with your new variable, AGEGRP. You will be warned:

WARNINGTHE FILE YOU HAVE NAMED ALREADY EXISTS.
DO YOU WANT TO WRITE OVER IT? (Y OR N)

This is to protect you from destroying perfectly good data sets by using the same name for some new data. But in this case, you have added on and want to save the new file, so press **Y** [ENTER]. You will see the message that "30 CASES ARE SAVED INTO HYSTER."

5. Now move to the main menu to execute the TABULATE command. (Type **QUIT**.)
6. To produce the frequencies of the grouped data, type the following:

USE HYSTER
OUTPUT @
FORMAT = 0
NOTE 'GROUPED FREQUENCY DATA'
TABULATE AGEGRP/LIST

Your output should look like Figure G-2. The largest age group is 2 (40–49 year olds) with 15 subjects or 50% of the total. Again, **congratulations!** You have completed three of your four assigned tasks.

GROUPED FREQUENCY DATA

COUNT	CUM COUNT	PCT	CUM PCT	AGEGRP	
5	5	16.7	16.7		1
15	20	50.0	66.7		2
4	24	13.3	80.0		3
3	27	10.0	90.0		4
3	30	10.0	100.0		5

FIGURE G-2
Grouped Frequency Data.

Creating a Histogram

1. At the main menu the following commands will create a histogram.

USE HYSTER
OUTPUT @
NOTE 'HISTOGRAM OF AGES'
HISTOGRAM AGE

In this initial session, you have learned how to create a data file and run some procedures using MYSTAT or some other computer software. In the exercises for Chapter 2 we will look at other ways to describe our data.

CHAPTER 2

Your tasks are to:

1. Produce measures of central tendency and dispersion, as in Tables 2-3 and 2-4.
2. Create a box-and-whisker plot or some other graph of your data. Use the same data set you used for Chapter 1 exercises (i.e., the ages of the hysterectomy patients).

MYSTAT Users

1. Enter the program by typing **MYSTAT** at the appropriate prompt.
2. At the MYSTAT prompt (>) type the following:

USE HYSTER [ENTER] (This brings this file into the active mode.)
OUTPUT @ [ENTER] (This causes output to go to the printer. Remember that you may have to use the form feed button to activate the printing.)
NOTE 'put an appropriate title in here' [ENTER]
STATS [ENTER] (This gives descriptive statistics.)

You will get the following statistics for all the variables in your data set: N of cases, minimum, maximum, mean, and standard deviation. See Figure G-3. The mean age is 49 with a standard deviation of 12 years.

DESCRIPTIVE STATISTICS FOR AGES OF HYSTERECTOMY PATIENTS

TOTAL OBSERVATIONS: 30

	AGE	AGEGRP
N OF CASES	30	30
MINIMUM	30	1
MAXIMUM	78	5
MEAN	49	2
STANDARD DEV	12	1

FIGURE G-3
Descriptive Statistics for Ages of Hysterectomy Patients.

You can ask for additional statistics and control which variables are included. The general format for this procedure is:

STATS <name of variable/s>/ <names of statistics>

Statistics available include:

MEAN SD SKEWNESS KURTOSIS MINIMUM MAXIMUM RANGE SUM SEM (standard error of measurement)

Try the following:

STATS AGE / MEAN SD SKEWNESS KURTOSIS

2. For a box-and-whiskers plot type:

BOX AGE

Compare your box-and-whiskers plot with Figure 2-10.

CHAPTERS 3 AND 4

There are no computer exercises for these chapters.

CHAPTER 5

Chi-Square

Let's use a fairly simple example, so you can get some more practice entering data. This example is based on one in an editorial in *Clinical Nurse Specialist* (Munro, 1989). We want to know whether the sex of the student is related to his or her choice of clinical specialty. The null hypothesis is that there is no difference between men and women in relation to specialty choice. The data are contained in Table G-2. There are 60 subjects.

TABLE G-2
Specialty Choice and Sex of Student

Subject Number	SEX (1 = M; 2 = F)	SPECIAL (1 = M/S; 2 = PSYCH)
1	1	1
2	2	1
3	2	2
4	2	1
5	2	2
6	1	1
7	2	1
8	2	2
9	1	2
10	2	1
11	2	1
12	1	1
13	2	2
14	2	1
15	2	2
16	1	1
17	2	2
18	1	1
19	1	2
20	2	2
21	2	1
22	2	2
23	1	1
24	2	1
25	1	1
26	1	1
27	2	1
28	1	1
29	2	2

(continued)

TABLE G-2 (CONTINUED)
Specialty Choice and Sex of Student

Subject Number	SEX (1 = M; 2 = F)	SPECIAL (1 = M/S; 2 = PSYCH)
30	2	1
31	1	2
32	2	1
33	2	1
34	2	2
35	2	1
36	1	1
37	2	2
38	2	1
39	2	1
40	1	1
41	2	2
42	2	1
43	2	2
44	1	1
45	2	2
46	2	1
47	2	1
48	1	2
49	2	1
50	2	1
51	1	2
52	2	1
53	2	1
54	1	1
55	2	1
56	1	1
57	2	2
58	2	1
59	2	2
60	1	1

Sex is coded as follows: 1 = male, 2 = female. Specialty is coded as follows: 1 = Medical-Surgical Nursing, 2 = Psychiatric Nursing.

Your tasks for chi-square are to:

1. Enter the data.
2. Run a chi-square analysis.
   For those of you using SPSS, the commands are listed in Figure 5-3.

MYSTAT Users

1. At the main menu in MYSTAT, type **EDIT**.
2. On the spreadsheet, enter your variable names as:

   'SEX' [ENTER]
   'SPECIAL' [ENTER]

3. Press the Home key.
4. Press the Escape key. (You should be at the system prompt below the spreadsheet.)
5. Type **FORMAT = 0**.
6. Press the Escape key. (You should be ready to enter data for the first subject.)
7. Enter the data for the first two subjects as follows:

   1 [ENTER] **1** [ENTER]
   2 [ENTER] **2** [ENTER]

   Enter all data and check your work.

8. You are now ready to save your file. Press the Escape key to get the lower prompt and then type **SAVE CHOICE**. You have saved a file called CHOICE.
9. Move to the main menu by typing **QUIT**.
10. At the main menu prompt type:

    USE CHOICE
    OUTPUT @
    NOTE 'CHI-SQUARE ANALYSIS'
    TABULATE SPECIAL * SEX

    Your output should look like Figure G-4. In the table, the columns describe the sex of the respondent, and the rows are the specialty choice. There were 20 men (1) and 40 women (2). Among the men 15 (75%) chose Medical-Surgical Nursing (1), and 5 (25%) chose Psychiatric Nursing (2). Among the women, 24 (60%) chose Medical-Surgical Nursing. Although a higher percent of men (75%) than women (60%) chose Medical-Surgical Nursing, this difference was not statistically significant (Chi-square = 1.319, $df = 1, p = .251$). The null hypothesis of no difference between the genders in relation to specialty choice was upheld.

Friedman and Wilcoxon Tests

In addition to the chi-square, you should try to use the computer to perform other nonparametric tests. Figures 5-8 and 5-9 provide examples of Wilcoxon and Friedman tests. Friedman was used to compare subjects under three different conditions, walking, group meeting, and control. This is a repeated measures design in which the subjects were exposed to each of the treatments. The Wilcoxon test was used to make paired comparisons. The data used in these examples are contained in Table G-3.

Enter the data and run the analysis. SPSS users can follow the commands in the Figures 5-5 and 5-6.

```
CHI-SQUARE ANALYSIS
TABLE OF   SPECIAL      (ROWS) BY      SEX     (COLUMNS)
FREQUENCIES
                  1         2      TOTAL

           1     15        24       39

           2      5        16       21

TOTAL            20        40       60
```

TEST STATISTIC	VALUE	DF	PROB
PEARSON CHI-SQUARE	1.319	1	.251
LIKELIHOOD RATIO CHI-SQUARE	1.359	1	.244
MCNEMAR SYMMETRY CHI-SQUARE	12.448	1	.000
YATES CORRECTED CHI-SQUARE	.742	1	.389
FISHER EXACT TEST (TWO-TAIL)			.390

COEFFICIENT	VALUE	ASYMPTOTIC STD ERROR
PHI	.1482	
CONTINGENCY	.1466	
GOODMAN-KRUSKAL GAMMA	.3333	.27065
KENDALL TAU-B	.1482	.12224
STUART TAU-C	.1333	.11089
YULE Q	.3333	.27065
YULE Y	.1716	.14776
COHEN KAPPA	.1212	.10184
SPEARMAN RHO	.1482	.12224
SOMERS D (COLUMN DEPENDENT)	.1465	.12127
LAMBDA (COLUMN DEPENDENT)	.0000	.00000
UNCERTAINTY (COLUMN DEPENDENT)	.0178	.02986

FIGURE G-4
Chi-Square Analysis.

MYSTAT Users

1. Enter MYSTAT, move to the spread sheet.
2. Enter your variable names: WALKING, GROUPMTG, AND CONTROL. (Remember to use single quotes around the names.)
3. Press Home, then Escape, and type **FORMAT = 0** at prompt. Push Escape again to move into position to enter data.
4. For subject 1, enter data as:

   2 [ENTER] **1** [ENTER] **1** [ENTER]

5. Enter all data, check your results. Use Escape key to get prompt and save your data set as **NONPAR**.
6. Type **QUIT** to move to main menu.

TABLE G-3
Data Used for Figures 5-8 and 5-9 in Text

Subjects	WALKING	GROUPMTG	CONTROL
1	2	1	1
2	3	2	1
3	2	1	1
4	3	2	1
5	4	3	2
6	3	2	2
7	4	1	2
8	3	2	2
9	4	3	3
10	3	4	3
11	4	2	3
12	4	3	3
13	4	3	4
14	3	4	4
15	4	4	4

7. At the main menu, type the following:

USE NONPAR
OUTPUT @
FRIEDMAN WALKING GROUPMTG CONTROL

After getting that output, type:

WILCOXON WALKING GROUPMTG CONTROL

```
FRIEDMAN TWO-WAY ANALYSIS OF VARIANCE RESULTS FOR   15 CASES


    VARIABLE      RANK SUM


    WALKING        40.000
    GROUPMTG       25.500
    CONTROL        24.500


FRIEDMAN TEST STATISTIC = 10.033
KENDALL COEFFICIENT OF CONCORDANCE =    .334


PROBABILITY IS   .007 ASSUMING CHI-SQUARE DISTRIBUTION WITH   2 DF
```

FIGURE G-5
Friedman Two-Way Analysis of Variance.

WILCOXON SIGNED RANKS TEST RESULTS

COUNTS OF DIFFERENCES (ROW VARIABLE GREATER THAN COLUMN)

	WALKING	GROUPMTG	CONTROL
WALKING	0	12	11
GROUPMTG	2	0	4
CONTROL	1	3	0

Z = (SUM OF SIGNED RANKS)/SQUARE ROOT(SUM OF SQUARED RANKS)

	WALKING	GROUPMTG	CONTROL
WALKING	.000		
GROUPMTG	−2.675	.000	
CONTROL	−2.810	−.378	.000

TWO-SIDED PROBABILITIES USING NORMAL APPROXIMATION

	WALKING	GROUPMTG	CONTROL
WALKING	1.000		
GROUPMTG	.007	1.000	
CONTROL	.005	.705	1.000

FIGURE G-6
Wilcoxon Signed Ranks Test.

8. You should now have output that is similar to that in Figures 5-8 and 5-9. Let's look at it. Figures G-5 and G-6 contain the output.

In the MYSTAT version, rank sums are given, rather than mean ranks, but we see that the Friedman test statistic of 10.033 is the same as the chi-square listed on the SPSS printout. The p value has been rounded to .007.

The Wilcoxon printout looks very different from the SPSS printout, but contains the same information. In the SPSS printout (Fig. 5-9), when comparing WALKING with GROUPMTG, we saw that GROUPMTG had 12 cases with lower ranks than WALKING, that there were 2 cases where GROUPMTG was greater than WALKING and there was 1 tie. Now look at the MYSTAT printout. All the differences are contained in the first table. It is set up so that the row variable is greater than the column. Let's look at WALKING and GROUPMTG again. We see that WALKING was greater than GROUPMTG 12 times, GROUPMTG was greater 2 times. Although ties aren't listed, because there were 15 cases, we know that 1 must have been a tie. In the same manner, you could compare WALKING and GROUPMTG with the CONTROL group.

The Z scores are slightly different in the two versions. In the SPSS version the Z for the WALKING/GROUPMTG comparison is -2.4794. In the MYSTAT version it is -2.675 (second table in Fig. G-6). The probabilities are given next. The probability for the WALKING/CONTROL comparison is .005.

CHAPTER 6

Independent t Test

The data are contained in Table G-4. Enter them into the computer and run a *t* test to compare the mean scores of the two groups.

TABLE G-4
Data for Independent t Test

Subject	GROUP (1 = Experimental; 2 = Control)	SCORE
1	1	21
2	1	18
3	1	14
4	1	20
5	1	11
6	1	19
7	1	8
8	1	12
9	1	13
10	1	15
11	2	12
12	2	14
13	2	10
14	2	8
15	2	16
16	2	5
17	2	3
18	2	9
19	2	11

Correlated or Paired t Test

The data for this analysis are in Table G-5. Enter them into the computer and run a paired *t* test to determine if the group's scores varied at the two time periods.

MYSTAT Users

1. Enter the data set for the independent *t* test.
2. Save it as IT.
3. The following commands issued at the main menu will result in a *t* test. You may, of course, add a **NOTE**, if you wish.

   USE IT
   OUTPUT @
   TTEST SCORE * GROUP

4. Enter the data set for the paired *t* test.
5. Save it as CT.
6. The following commands issued at the main menu will result in a paired *t* test.

   USE CT
   OUTPUT @
   TTEST PRETEST POSTTEST

Your printouts should look like those in Figures G-7 and G-8. In the independent t-test the means of the two groups were significantly different ($p = .014$). MYSTAT does not provide a test of the assumption of homogeneity of variance. The formula for the F test is the larger variance over the smaller variance. Squaring the standard deviations (SDs) results in the following variances:

Group 1 18.3184
Group 1 16.9415

TABLE G-5
Data for Correlated (Paired or Dependent) t Test

Subject	PRETEST	POSTTEST
1	20	25
2	11	18
3	9	5
4	8	20
5	22	28
6	18	20
7	15	22
8	10	12
9	12	18
10	14	19

```
INDEPENDENT SAMPLES T-TEST ON      SCORE      GROUPED BY      GROUP

              GROUP        N       MEAN          SD
              1.000        10      15.100        4.280
              2.000         9       9.778        4.116


    SEPARATE VARIANCES T =        2.761 DF =     16.9 PROB = .014
        POOLED VARIANCES T =      2.755 DF =       17 PROB = .014
```

FIGURE G-7
Independent Samples *t* Test.

```
  PAIRED SAMPLES T-TEST ON    PRETEST    VS POSTTEST    WITH        10
CASES


  MEAN DIFFERENCE =        -4.800
  SD DIFFERENCE =         4.185
  T =        3.627 DF =       9 PROB = .006
```

FIGURE G-8
Paired Samples *t* Test.

18.3184/16.9415 = 1.08 with 9,8 *df*s. In Appendix D we see that with 9 and 8 degrees of freedom, the critical value for the .05 level is 3.39. Thus, the assumption of homogeneity of variance has been met, and the pooled *t* test is the appropriate formula to use. The mean for group 1 of 15.1 is significantly higher than the mean of 9.778 for group 2.

On the paired *t* test we see that the groups scored significantly higher ($p = .006$) on the posttest than on the pretest.

CHAPTER 7

One-Way Analysis of Variance

Add a third group to the data contained in Table G-4, and then run a one-way analysis of variance to determine whether the means of the three groups differ. Table G-6 contains the data for the additional subjects. For SPSS users, follow the example in Figure 7-4. Use the Scheffe post-hoc test.

MYSTAT Users

1. Reenter the data set for the independent *t* test by typing:

   EDIT IT

   at the MYSTAT prompt.
2. Enter the additional subjects (20 thru 30). Save the new data set.

TABLE G-6
Additional Data for One-Way Analysis of Variance

Subject	Group	Score
20	3	19
21	3	10
22	3	21
23	3	17
24	3	15
25	3	10
26	3	11
27	3	18
28	3	16
29	3	14
30	3	22

3. The following commands issued at the main menu will result in a one-way analysis of variance. (Add an appropriate NOTE.)

USE IT
OUTPUT @
CATEGORY GROUP = 3 (number of groups included in analysis)
ANOVA SCORE (dependent variable is score)
ESTIMATE (tells it to begin)

4. Your output should look like that in Figure G-9. You can see that the groups differed significantly, but since MYSTAT does not do post-hoc tests, we cannot tell where the paired differences lie.

```
DEP VAR:   SCORE      N:   30   MULTIPLE R:   .547   SQUARED MULTIPLE R:   .299



                      ANALYSIS OF VARIANCE

   SOURCE   SUM-OF-SQUARES   DF   MEAN-SQUARE   F-RATIO      P

    GROUP         203.229     2      101.615     5.756    0.008

    ERROR         476.637    27       17.653
```

FIGURE G-9
One-Way Analysis of Variance.

CHAPTER 8

Two-Way Analysis of Variance

The data from Table 8-3 in the text are presented here in Table G-7 in the way they should be entered into the computer. Create a new data set for the 20 subjects. Then run a two-way analysis of variance where SEX and RX are the independent variables and X is the dependent variable. SPSS users should follow the example in Figure 8-1.

MYSTAT Users

1. Create a new data set with variables named SEX, RX, and X. Save it as TWOWAY.
2. The following commands issued at the main menu will result in a two-way analysis of variance.

   USE TWOWAY
   OUTPUT @
   CATEGORY SEX = 2 RX = 2
   ANOVA X
   ESTIMATE

3. The output should look like Figure G-10. Compare it to Figure 8-1 in the text.

TABLE G-7
Data from Table 8-3 for Two-Way Analysis of Variance

Subject	Sex	RX	X
1	1	1	1
2	1	1	3
3	1	1	4
4	1	1	2
5	1	1	2
6	1	2	8
7	1	2	9
8	1	2	10
9	1	2	6
10	1	2	7
11	2	1	10
12	2	1	9
13	2	1	9
14	2	1	7
15	2	1	8
16	2	2	4
17	2	2	2
18	2	2	3
19	2	2	4
20	2	2	1

```
DEP VAR:        X      N:   20    MULTIPLE R:   .926    SQUARED MULTIPLE R:   .858
```

ANALYSIS OF VARIANCE

SOURCE	SUM-OF-SQUARES	DF	MEAN-SQUARE	F-RATIO	P
SEX	1.250	1	1.250	0.735	0.404
RX	0.050	1	0.050	0.029	0.866
SEX* RX	162.450	1	162.450	95.559	0.000
ERROR	27.200	16	1.700		

FIGURE G-10
Two-Way Analysis of Variance.

CHAPTER 9

Analysis of Covariance

Add a covariate to the data used for the two-way analysis of variance (Table G-7). The scores for the covariate are in Table G-8. Add the additional variable and run an analysis of covariance. For SPSS users, Figure 9-3 contains an example.

MYSTAT Users

1. **EDIT TWOWAY**
2. Add the variable **COV**.
3. Give the 20 subjects their scores on **COV**.
4. Save the new data.
5. The following commands issued at the main menu will result in an analysis of covariance.

> **USE TWOWAY**
> **OUTPUT** @
> **CATEGORY SEX = 2 RX = 2**
> **COVARIATE COV**
> **ANOVA X**
> **ESTIMATE**

Your output should look like Figure G-11. You cannot check the homogeneity of regression assumption with MYSTAT. The results indicate no significant main effects, but there is a significant interaction between SEX and RX ($p = 0.015$). The covariate is making a significant contribution to the amount of variance accounted for in the dependent variable ($p = 0.012$).

TABLE G-8
Covariate

Subject	COV
1	2
2	2
3	3
4	1
5	1
6	6
7	10
8	8
9	8
10	8
11	12
12	10
13	10
14	6
15	6
16	5
17	1
18	2
19	3
20	2

```
DEP VAR:      X     N:   20   MULTIPLE R:   .953    SQUARED MULTIPLE R:   .908
```

ANALYSIS OF VARIANCE

SOURCE	SUM-OF-SQUARES	DF	MEAN-SQUARE	F-RATIO	P
SEX	0.100	1	0.100	0.085	0.775
RX	0.050	1	0.050	0.043	0.839
SEX* RX	8.845	1	8.845	7.522	0.015
COV	9.561	1	9.561	8.130	0.012
ERROR	17.639	15	1.176		

FIGURE G-11
Analysis of Covariance.

CHAPTER *10*

Repeated Measures Analysis of Variance

There are no exercises for this chapter.

CHAPTER *11*

Correlation

Use the data in Table 12-1 in the text. Create a data set with 20 subjects and their scores on ANGER and STRESS. SPSS users see Figure 11-3 for commands.

MYSTAT Users

1. Create a new data file. Name it CORR.
2. The following commands issued at the main menu will result in a Pearson Correlation Matrix.

   USE CORR
   OUTPUT @
   PEARSON ANGER STRESS

3. Your output should look like Figure G-12.

```
               PEARSON CORRELATION MATRIX

                                    ANGER        STRESS

                       ANGER        1.000
                       STRESS       0.840        1.000
```

FIGURE G-12
Pearson Correlation Matrix.   NUMBER OF OBSERVATIONS: 20

CHAPTER *12*

Regression

Use the same data set you created for Chapter 11. Run a regression with STRESS as the dependent variable, and ANGER as the independent variable. SPSS users note Figure 12-5.

```
DEP VAR: STRESS      N:  20    MULTIPLE R: .840    SQUARED MULTIPLE R: .705
ADJUSTED SQUARED MULTIPLE R:  .688      STANDARD ERROR OF ESTIMATE:     2.911


    VARIABLE     COEFFICIENT   STD ERROR   STD COEF TOLERANCE    T    P(2 TAIL)
    CONSTANT        0.361        1.552       0.000    .        0.233   0.819
      ANGER         1.257        0.192       0.840  .100E+01   6.557   0.000



                        ANALYSIS OF VARIANCE


    SOURCE      SUM-OF-SQUARES    DF   MEAN-SQUARE     F-RATIO      P


  REGRESSION       364.277       1      364.277       42.990     0.000
   RESIDUAL        152.523      18        8.474
```

FIGURE G-13
Regression Analysis.

MYSTAT Users

1. The following commands issued at the main menu will result in a regression analysis.

    USE CORR
    OUTPUT @
    MODEL STRESS = CONSTANT + ANGER
    ESTIMATE

2. Your output should look like Figure G-13.

CHAPTERS 13, 14, 15, & 16

There are no exercises for these chapters, because MYSTAT cannot run such analyses. For those of you with access to more sophisticated software, you may want to try some of the examples in the book. Since the techniques in these chapters require fairly large numbers of subjects, it is most helpful to have access to data sets with appropriate variables and requisite numbers of subjects.

Appendix H

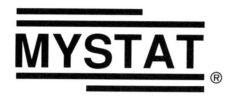

An instructional version of SYSTAT
for IBM-PC/compatibles

MYSTAT Version 2.1

An instructional version of SYSTAT

SYSTAT, Inc.
1800 Sherman Avenue
Evanston, IL 60201
Tel. 708.**864.5670**
FAX 708.**492.3567**

Introduction

This is a real statistics program—it is not just a demonstration. You can use MYSTAT to enter, transform, and save data, and to perform a wide range of statistical evaluations. Please use MYSTAT to solve *real* problems.

MYSTAT is a fully operational subset of SYSTAT, our premier statistics package. We've geared MYSTAT especially for teaching, with descriptive statistics, cross-tabulation, Pearson and Spearman correlation coefficients, regression, ANOVA, nonparametric tests, and graphics all in a single, easy-to-use package.

An instructional business version of MYSTAT is also available. MYSTAT has special forecasting and time series routines in addition to most of the regular MYSTAT features.

Both versions of MYSTAT are available in Macintosh, IBM-PC/compatible, and VAX/VMS versions. Copies are available at a nominal cost.

For more information about SYSTAT, SYGRAPH, and our other top-rated professional statistics and graphics packages, please call or write.

Installation   MYSTAT requires 256K of RAM and a floppy or hard disk drive. It can handle up to 50 variables and up to 32,000 cases.

Your MYSTAT disk contains three files: MYSTAT.EXE (the program), MYSTAT.HLP (a file with information for on-line help), and DEMO.CMD (a demonstration that creates a data file and demonstrates some of MYSTAT's features).

Hard disk   ### Set up the CONFIG.SYS file
The CONFIG.SYS file in your root directory must have a line that says FILES=20. You can modify your existing CONFIG.SYS file, or create one if you don't have one, by typing the following lines from the DOS prompt (>).

```
COPY CONFIG.SYS + CON: CONFIG.SYS
FILES=20
```

To finish, press the F6 key and then press Enter or Return.

Set up the AUTOEXEC.BAT file
You may find it convenient to install MYSTAT in its own directory and add that directory to the PATH statement in your AUTOEXEC.BAT file. This file should be located in the root directory (\) of your boot disk (the hard disk). *If you do not already have an AUTOEXEC.BAT file, or if your AUTOEXEC.BAT file does not have a PATH statement already,* please do the following:

```
COPY AUTOEXEC.BAT + CON: AUTOEXEC.BAT
PATH=C:\;C:\MYSTAT
[F6, ENTER]
```

If you already have an AUTOEXEC.BAT file that has a PATH statement, use a text editor to add the MYSTAT directory to the existing PATH statement.

Reboot your machine

Copy the files on the MYSTAT disk into a \SYSTAT directory
Now, make a \SYSTAT directory, insert the MYSTAT disk in drive A, and copy the MYSTAT files into the directory. (You must have the help file in the same directory as MYSTAT.EXE. If you put MYSTAT.EXE in a directory other than \SYSTAT, the help file MYSTATB.HLP must be either in that directory or the \SYSTAT directory.)

```
>MD \SYSTAT
>CD \SYSTAT
>COPY A:*.*
```

You are now ready to begin using MYSTAT. From now on, all you need to do to get ready to use MYSTAT is boot and move (CD) into the \SYSTAT directory. Save your MYSTAT master disk as a back up copy.

Floppy disk   ***Boot your machine***

Insert a "boot disk" into drive A. Close the door of the disk drive and turn on the machine.

Set up a CONFIG.SYS file on your boot disk

The boot disk must contain a file named CONFIG.SYS with a line FILES=20. You can modify your existing CONFIG.SYS file, or create one if you don't have one, by typing the following lines from the DOS prompt (>).

```
COPY CONFIG.SYS + CON: CONFIG.SYS
FILES=20
```

To finish, press the F6 key and then press Enter or Return.

Set up an AUTOEXEC.BAT file on your boot disk

You must be sure that you have a file called AUTOEXEC.BAT containing the line PATH=A:\;B:\ on your boot disk. If you do not, type the following lines from the DOS prompt (>)

```
COPY CON AUTOEXEC.BAT + CON: AUTOEXEC.BAT
PATH=A:\;B:\
[F6, Enter]
```

Reboot your machine

Make a copy of the MYSTAT disk

When you get a DOS prompt (>), remove the boot disk. Put the MYSTAT disk in drive A and a blank, formatted disk in drive B and type the COPY command at the prompt:

```
>COPY A:*.* B:
```

Remove the master disk from drive A and store it. If anything happens to your working copy, use the master to make a new copy.

Use MYSTAT

Now, switch your working copy into drive A. If necessary, make drive A the "logged" drive (the drive your machine reads from) by issuing the command A: at the DOS prompt (>).

MYSTAT reads and writes its temporary work files to the currently logged drive. Since there is limited room on the MYSTAT disk, you should read and write all your data, output, and command files from a data disk in drive B.

From now on, all you need to do to use MYSTAT is boot, insert your working copy, and log the A drive.

Getting started

To start, type MYSTAT and press Enter.

>MYSTAT

When you see the MYSTAT logo, press Enter. You'll see a command menu listing all the commands you can use in MYSTAT.

Command menu

The command menu shows a list of all the commands that are available for MYSTAT. The commands are divided into six groups: information, file handling, miscellaneous, graphics, statistics, and forecasting.

```
MYSTAT --- An Instructional Version of SYSTAT

DEMO        EDIT        MENU        PLOT        STATS       MODEL
HELP                    NAMES       BOX         TABULATE    CATEGORY
SYSTAT      USE         LIST        HISTOGRAM   TTEST       ANOVA
            SAVE        FORMAT      STEM        PEARSON     COVARIATE
            PUT         NOTE        TPLOT                   ESTIMATE
            SUBMIT

QUIT        OUTPUT      SORT        CHARSET     SIGN
                        RANK                    WILCOXON
                        WEIGHT                  FRIEDMAN
```

As you become more experienced with MYSTAT, you might want to turn the menu off. You can use the MENU command to turn it on and off.

>MENU

Data Editor

MYSTAT has a built-in Data Editor with its own set of commands. To enter the Editor, use the EDIT command.

>EDIT

Inside the Editor, you can enter, view, edit, and transform data. When you are done with the Editor, type QUIT to get out of the Editor and back to MYSTAT, where you can do statistical and graphical analyses. To quit MYSTAT itself, type QUIT again.

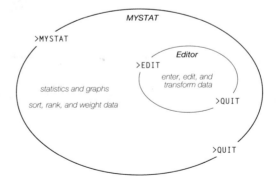

The Data Editor is an independent program inside MYSTAT and has its own commands. Five commands—USE, SAVE, HELP, QUIT, and FORMAT—appear both inside *and* outside the Editor.

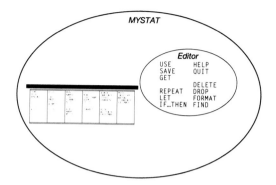

Demo

To see an on-line demonstration of MYSTAT, use the DEMO command. (Remember to press Enter after you type the command.)

>DEMO

When the demonstration is finished, MYSTAT returns you to the command menu. After you've seen the demo, you might want to remove the DEMO.CMD file and the CITIES.SYS data file that it creates to save disk space.

Help

The HELP command provides instructions for any command—inside *or* outside the Editor. HELP lists all the commands with brief descriptions.

>HELP

You can get help for any specific command . For example:

>HELP EDIT
EDIT starts the MYSTAT full screen editor.

EDIT [filename]

EDIT (edit a new file)
EDIT CITIES (edit CITIES.SYS)

For further information, type EDIT [Enter], [ESC], and then type HELP
[Enter] inside the data editor.

The second line shows *a* summary of the command. You see that any EDIT command must begin with the command word EDIT. The brackets indicate that specifying a file is optional. Anything in lower-case, like "filename," is just a placeholder—you should type a real file name (or a real variable name, or whatever).

Customizing DEMO and HELP
All help information is stored in the text file MYSTATB.HLP. You can use a text editor to customize your help information. Similarly, teachers can design special demonstrations by editing the file DEMO.CMD.

Information about SYSTAT
For information about SYSTAT and how to order it, use the SYSTAT command.

Data Editor

The MYSTAT Data Editor lets you enter and edit data, view data, and transform variables. First, we enter data; later, we show you how to use commands.

To use the Editor to create a new file, type EDIT and press Enter. If you already have a MYSTAT data file that you want to edit, specify a filename with the EDIT command.

```
>EDIT [<filename>]
```

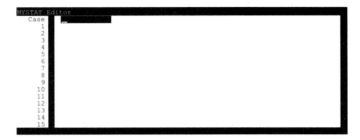

If you do not specify a filename, you get an empty Editor like the one above. MYSTAT stores data in a rectangular worksheet. *Variables* fill vertical columns and each horizontal row represents a *case*.

Entering data

First enter variable names in the top row. Variable names *must* be surrounded by single or double quotation marks, must begin with a letter, and can be no longer than 8 characters.

Character variables (those whose values are words and letters) must have names ending with a dollar sign ($). The quotation marks and dollar sign do not count toward the eight character limit.

Numeric variables (those whose values are numbers) can be named with subscripts; e.g., ITEM(3). Subscripts are useful because they allow you to specify a range of variables for analyses. For example, STATS ITEM(1-3) does descriptive statistics on the first three ITEM(*i*) variables.

The cursor is already positioned in the first cell in the top row of the worksheet. Type 'CITY$' or "CITY$" and then press Enter.

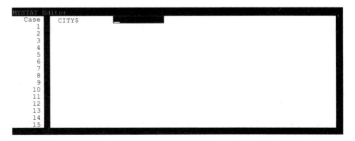

MYSTAT enters variable names in upper-case whether you enter them in lower- or upper-case.

The cursor automatically moves to the second column. You are now ready to name the rest of the variables, pressing Enter to store each name in the worksheet.

```
'STATE$'
"POP"
'RAINFALL'
```

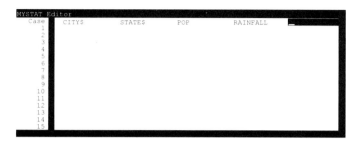

Now you can enter values. Move the cursor to the first blank cell under CITY$ by pressing Home. (On most machines, Home is the 7 key on the numeric keypad. If pressing the 7 key types a 7 rather than moving the cursor, press the NumLock key and try again.)

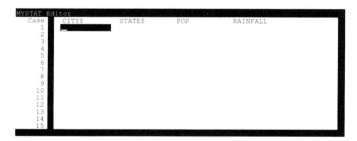

When the cell under CITY$ is selected, enter the first data value:

```
'New York'
```

When you press Enter, MYSTAT accepts the value and moves the cursor to the right. You can also use the cursor arrow keys to move the cursor.

Character values can be no longer than twelve characters. Like variable names, character values must be surrounded by single or double quotation marks. Unlike variable names, character values are case sensitive—upper-case is not the same as lower-case (for example, 'TREE' is not the same as 'tree' or 'Tree'). Enter a blank space surrounded by quotation marks for missing character values. To use single or double quotation marks as part of a value, surround the whole value with the opposite marks.

Numeric values can be up to 10^{35} in absolute magnitude. Scientific notation is used for long numbers; e.g., .000000000015 is equivalent to 1.5E–11. Enter a decimal (.) for missing numeric values.

Enter the first few cases: type a value, press Enter, and type the next value. The cursor automatically moves to the beginning of the next case when a row is filled.

```
    "New York"      "NY"    7164742      57.03
 "Los Angeles"      "CA"    3096721       7.81
      "Chicago"     "IL"    2992472         34
```
(etc.)

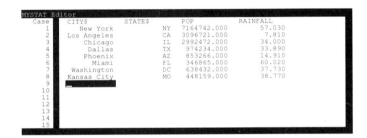

Moving around

Use the cursor keys on the numeric keypad to move around in the Editor.

Esc		toggle between Editor and command prompt (>)
Home	7	move to first cell in worksheet
↑	8	move upward one cell
PgUp	9	scroll screen up
←	4	move left one cell
→	6	move right one cell
End	1	move to last case in worksheet
↓	2	move down one cell
PgDn	3	scroll screen down

If these keys type numbers rather than move the cursor, press the NumLock key which toggles the keypad back and forth between typing numbers and performing the special functions. (If your computer does not have a NumLock key or something similar, consult the manual that came with your machine.)

Editing data

To change a value or variable name move to the cell you want, type the new value, and press Enter. Remember to enclose character values and variable names in quotation marks.

Data Editor commands

When you have entered your data, press the Esc key to move the cursor to the prompt (>) below the worksheet. You can enter editor commands at this prompt. Commands can be typed in upper- or lower-case. Items in <angle brackets> are placeholders; for instance, you should type a specific filename in place of <filename>.

DELETE and DROP	DELETE lets you remove an entire case (row) from the dataset in the Editor. You can specify a range or list of cases to be deleted. The following are valid DELETE commands.

```
DELETE 3                Deletes third case from dataset.
DELETE 3-10             Deletes cases 3 through 10.
DELETE 3, 5-8, 10       Deletes cases 3, 5, 6, 7, 8, and 10.
```

DROP removes variables from the dataset in the Editor. You can specify several variables or a range of subscripted variables.

```
DROP RAINFALL           Drops RAINFALL from dataset.
DROP X(1-3)             Drops subscripted variables X(1-3).
DROP X(1-3), GROUP$     Drops X(1-3) and GROUP$.
```

Saving files

The SAVE command saves the data in the Editor to a MYSTAT data file. You must save data in a data file before you can analyze them with statistical and graphic commands.

```
SAVE <filename>         Saves data in a MYSTAT file.
 /DOUBLE | SINGLE       Choose single or double precision.
```

MYSTAT filenames can be up to 8 characters long and must begin with a letter. MYSTAT adds a ".SYS" extension that labels the file as a MYSTAT data file. To specify a path name for a file, enclose the entire file name, including the file extension, in single or double quotation marks.

MYSTAT stores data in double-precision by default. You can choose single precision with the SINGLE option if you prefer: add /SINGLE to the end of the command. Always type a slash before command options.

```
SAVE CITIES/SINGLE      Saves CITIES.SYS in single precision
```

Single precision requires approximately half as much disk space as double precision and is accurate to about 9 decimal places. The storage option (single or double precision) does not affect computations, which always use double precision arithmetic (accurate to about 15 places).

```
SAVE CITIES             Creates data file CITIES.SYS.
SAVE b:new              Creates file NEW.SYS on B drive.
SAVE 'C:\DATA\FIL.SYS'  Creates FIL.SYS in \DATA directory of C.
```

You can save data in text files for exporting to other programs with the PUT command. PUT is not an Editor command, though. First QUIT the Editor, USE the data file, and PUT the data to a text file.

Reading files

USE reads a MYSTAT data file into the Editor.

```
USE [<filename>]        Reads data from MYSTAT data file.
```

Starting new data files

Use the NEW command to clear the worksheet and start editing a new data file.

Importing data from other programs

You can import data from other programs through plain text (ASCII) file. ASCII files contain only plain text and numbers—they have no special characters or formatting commands.

Start the program and save your data in a plain ASCII file according to the instructions given by that program's manual. The ASCII file must have a ".DAT" extension, data values must be separated by blanks or commas, and each case must begin on a new line.

Then, start MYSTAT. Use EDIT to get an empty worksheet, and enter variable names in the worksheet for each variable in the ASCII file. Next, use GET to read the text file. Finally, SAVE the data in a MYSTAT file.

```
GET [<filename>]              Reads data from ASCII text file.
```

Finding a case

FIND searches through the Editor starting from the current cursor position, and moves the cursor to the first value that meets the condition you specify. Try this:

```
>FIND POP<1000000
```

This moves the cursor to case 4. After MYSTAT finds a value, use the FIND command without an argument (that is, "FIND" is the entire command) to find the next case meeting the same condition. All functions, relations, and operators listed above are available.

Some valid FIND commands:

```
>FIND AGE>45 AND SEX$='MALE'
>FIND INCOME<10000 AND STATE$='NY'
>FIND (TEST1+TEST2+TEST3)>90
```

Decimal places in the Editor

The FORMAT command specifies the number (0–9) of decimal places to be shown in the Editor. The default is 3. Numbers are stored the way you enter them regardless of the FORMAT setting; FORMAT affects the Editor display only.

```
FORMAT=<#>                    Sets number of decimal places to <#>.
    /UNDERFLOW                Displays tiny numbers in scientific notation.
```

For example, to set a two-place display with scientific notation for tiny numbers use the command:

```
>FORMAT=2/UNDERFLOW
```

Transforming variables

Use LET and IF...THEN to transform variables or create new ones.

```
LET <var>=<exprn>             Transforms <var> according to <exprn>.
IF <exprn> THEN LET           Transforms <var> conditionally according to
    <var>=<exprn>                 <exprn>.
```

For example, we can use LET to create a variable LOGPOP from POP:

```
>LET LOGPOP=LOG(POP)
```

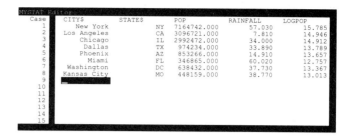

LET labels the last column of the worksheet LOGPOP and sets the values to the natural logs of the POP values. (If LOGPOP had already existed, its values would have been replaced.)

Use IF...THEN for *conditional* transformations. For example:

```
>IF POP>1000000 THEN LET SIZE$='BIG'
```

creates a new character variable, SIZE$, and assigns the value BIG for every city that has population greater than one million.

For both LET and IF...THEN, character values must be enclosed in quotation marks and are case sensitive (i.e., "MALE" is not the same as "male"). Use a period to indicate missing values.

Some valid LET and IF-THEN commands:

```
>LET ALPHA$='abcdef'
>LET LOGIT1=1/(1+EXP(A+B*X))
>LET TRENDY=INCOME>40000 AND CAR$='BMW'
>IF SEX$='Male' THEN LET GROUP=1
>IF group>2 THEN LET NEWGROUP=2
>IF A=-9 AND B<10 OR B>20 THEN LET C=LOG(D)*SQR(E)
```

Functions, relations, and operators for FIND, LET, and IF...THEN			
+	addition	SQR	square root
-	subtraction	ABS	absolute value
*	multiplication	CASE	current case number
/	division	INT	integer truncation
^	exponentiation		
<	less than	URN	uniform random number
<=	less than or equal to	ZRN	normal random number
=	equal to	ZCF	standard normal CDF
<>	not equal to	ZIF	inverse normal CDF
>=	greater than or equal		
>	greater than	SIN	sine (argument in radians)
		COS	cosine
AND	logical and	TAN	tangent
OR	logical or	ASN	arcsine
		ACS	arccosine
LOG	natural log	ATN	arctangent
EXP	exponential function	ATH	hyperbolic arctangent

Logical expressions

Logical expressions evaluate to one if true and to zero if false. For example, for LET CHILD=AGE<12, a variable AGE would be filled with ones for those cases where AGE is less than 12 and zeros whenever AGE is 12 or greater.

Random data

You can generate random numbers using the REPEAT, LET, and SAVE commands in the Editor. First, enter variable names. Press Esc to move the cursor to the command line. Then, use REPEAT to fill cases with missing values and LET to redefine the values.

REPEAT 20	Fills 20 cases with missing values.
LET A=URN	Fills A with uniform random data.
LET B=ZRN	Fills B with normal random data.
SAVE RANDOM	Saves data in file RANDOM.SYS.

Leaving the Data Editor

Use the QUIT command to leave the Editor and return to the main MYSTAT menu.

    >QUIT

**General
MYSTAT
commands**

Once your data are in a MYSTAT data file, you can use MYSTAT's statistical and graphics routines to examine them.

Open a data file
First, you must open the file containing the data you want to analyze:

```
USE <filename>              reads the data in <filename>
```

To analyze the data we entered earlier, type:

```
>USE CITIES
```

MYSTAT responds by listing the variables in the file.

```
VARIABLES IN MYSTAT FILE ARE:
     CITY$     STATE$     POP     RAINFALL   LOGPOP
```

See variable names and data values
The NAMES command shows the variable names in the current file.

```
>NAMES
VARIABLES IN MYSTAT FILE ARE:
     CITY$     STATE$     POP     RAINFALL   LOGPOP
```

The LIST command displays the values of variables you specify. If you specify no variables, all variables are shown.

```
>LIST CITY$
                          CITY$

CASE     1          New York
CASE     2       Los Angeles
CASE     3           Chicago
CASE     4            Dallas
CASE     5           Phoenix
CASE     6             Miami
CASE     7        Washington
CASE     8       Kansas City

  8 CASES AND    5 VARIABLES PROCESSED
```

Decimal places
Use the FORMAT command to specify the number of digits to be displayed after the decimal in statistical output. This FORMAT command has the same syntax and works the same as in the Editor:

```
FORMAT=<#>                  Sets number of decimal places to <#>.
   /UNDERFLOW               Uses scientific notation for tiny numbers.
```

Sorting and ranking data

SORT reorders the cases in a file in ascending order according to the variables you specify. You can specify up to ten numeric or character variables for nested sorts. Use a SAVE command after the USE command to save the sorted data into a MYSTAT file. Then, USE the sorted file to do analysis.

```
>USE MYDATA
>SAVE SORTED
>SORT CITY$ POP
>USE SORTED
```

RANK replaces each value of a variable with its rank order within that variable. Specify an output file before ranking.

```
>USE MYDATA
>SAVE RANKED
>RANK RAINFALL
>USE RANKED
```

Weighting data

WEIGHT replicates cases according to the integer parts of the values of the weighting variable you specify.

    WEIGHT <variable>   Weights according to variable specified.

To turn weighting off, use WEIGHT without an argument.

```
>WEIGHT
```

Quitting

When you are done with your analyses, you can end your session with the QUIT command. Remember that the Data Editor also has a QUIT. To quit MYSTAT from the Editor, enter QUIT twice.

```
>QUIT
```

Notation used in command summaries

Any item in angled brackets (< >) is representative—insert an actual value or variable in its place. Replace <var> with a variable name, replace <#> with a number, <var$> with a character variable, and <gvar> with a numeric or character grouping variable.

Some commands have *options* you can use to change the type of output you get. Place a slash / before listing any options for your command. You only need one slash before the option list, no matter how many options you use.

A vertical line (|) means "or." Items in brackets ([ ]) are optional. Commas and spaces are interchangeable, except that *you must use a comma at the end of the line when a command continues to a second line.*

You can abbreviate commands and options to the first two or three characters. You may use upper- and lower-case interchangeably.

Most commands allow you to specify particular variables. If you don't specify variables, MYSTAT uses its defaults (usually the first numeric variable or all numeric variables, depending on the command).

Statistics

Descriptive
statistics

STATS produces basic descriptive statistics. Here we use STATS with
the POP, RAINFALL, and LOGPOP variables of the dataset we
entered earlier.

```
>STATS
TOTAL OBSERVATIONS:  8

                        POP      RAINFALL  LOGPOP

N OF CASES             8           8         8
MINIMUM          346865.000      7.810    12.757
MAXIMUM         7164742.000     60.020    15.785
MEAN            2064361.375     35.520    14.028
STANDARD DEV    2335788.226     18.032     1.068
```

Here is a summary of the STATS command. The box on the facing
page describes the notation we use for command summaries in this
manual.

```
STATS <var1> <var2>…          Statistics for the variables specified.
   MEAN SD SKEWNESS, KURTOSIS  Choose which statistics you want.
      MINIMUM, MAXIMUM RANGE SUM,
      SEM
   /BY <gvar>                  Statistics for each group defined by the group-
                               ing variable <gvar>. The data must first be
                               SORTed on the grouping variable.
```

For example, you can get the mean, standard deviation, and range for
RAINFALL with the following command.

```
>STATS RAINFALL / MEAN SD RANGE
TOTAL OBSERVATIONS:  8

                   RAINFALL

N OF CASES        8
MEAN             35.520
STANDARD DEV     18.032
RANGE            52.210
```

Tabulation

TABULATE provides one-way and multi-way frequency tables. For
two-way tables, MYSTAT provides the Pearson chi-square statistic.
You can produce a table of frequencies, percents, row percents, or
column percents. You can tell MYSTAT to ignore missing data with
the MISS option.

```
TAB <var1>*<var2>…            Tabulates the variables you specify
   /LIST                      Special list format table.
   FREQUENCY PERCENT ROWPCT   Different types of tables
      COLPCT MISS
TABULATE                      Frequency tables of all numeric variables.
TABULATE AGE/LIST             Frequency table of AGE in list format.
TAB AGE*SEX                   Two-way table with chi-square.
TAB AGE*SEX$*STATE$/ROWPCT    Three-way row percent table.
TAB A,AGE*SEX/FREQ, PERC      Two two-way frequency and cell percent
                                tables (A*SEX and AGE*SEX).
TAB AGE*SEX/MISS              Two-way table excluding missing values.
```

One-way frequency tables show the number of times a distinct value appears in a variable. Two-way and multi-way tables count the appearances of each unique combination of values. Multi-way tables count the appearances of a value in each subgroup. Percent tables convert the frequencies to percentages of the total count; row percent tables show percentages of the total for each row; and column percent tables show percentages of the total for each column.

T-tests

TTEST does dependent and independent *t*-tests. A dependent (paired samples) *t*-test tests whether the means of two continuous variables differ. An independent test tests whether the means of two groups of a single variable differ.

To request an independent (two-sample) *t*-test, specify one or more continuous variables and one grouping variable. Separate the continuous variable(s) from the grouping variable with an asterisk. The grouping variable must have only two values.

To request a dependent (paired) *t*-test, specify two or more continuous variables. MYSTAT does separate dependent *t*-tests for each possible pairing of the variables.

TTEST <var1>…[*<gvar>]	Does *t*-tests of the variables you specify.
TTEST A B	Dependent (paired) t-test of A and B.
TTEST A B C	Paired tests of A and B, A and C, B and C.
TTEST A*SEX$	Independent test.
TTEST A B C*SEX	Three independent tests.

You can also do a one-sample test by adding a variable to your data file that has a constant value corresponding to the population mean of your null hypothesis. Then do a dependent *t*-test on this variable and your data variable.

Correlation

PEARSON computes Pearson product moment correlation coefficients for the variables you specify (or all numerical variables). You can select pairwise or listwise deletion of missing data; pairwise is the default. RANK the variables before correlating to compute Spearman rank-order correlations.

PEARSON <var1> ...	Pearson correlation matrix.
/PAIRWISE | LISTWISE	Pairwise or listwise deletion of missing values.
PEARSON	Correlation matrix of all numeric variables.
CORR HEIGHT IQ AGE	Matrix of three variables.
PEARSON /LISTWISE	Listwise deletion rather than pairwise.

Correlation measures the strength of linear association between two variables. A value of 1 or –1 indicates a perfect linear relationship; a value of 0 indicates that neither variable can be linearly predicted from the other.

Regression
and ANOVA

MYSTAT computes simple and multiple regression and balanced or unbalanced ANOVA designs. For unbalanced designs, MYSTAT uses the method of weighted squares of means.

The MODEL and ESTIMATE commands provide linear regression. MODEL specifies the regression equation and ESTIMATE tells MYSTAT to start working. Your MODEL should almost always include a CONSTANT term.

```
>MODEL Y=CONSTANT+X
>ESTIMATE
```
Simple linear regression.

```
>MODEL Y=CONSTANT+X+Z
>ESTIMATE
```
Multiple linear regression.

Use CATEGORY and ANOVA commands for fully factorial ANOVA. CATEGORY specifies the number of categories (levels) for one or more variables used as categorical predictors (factors). ANOVA specifies the dependent variable and produces a fully-factorial design from the factors given by CATEGORY.

All CATEGORY variables must have integer values from 1 to k, where k is the number of categories.

```
>CATEGORY SEX=2
>ANOVA SALARY
>ESTIMATE
```
One-way design with independent variable SALARY and one factor (SEX) with 2 levels

```
>CATEGORY A=2,B=3
>ANOVA Y
>ESTIMATE
```
Two-by-three ANOVA

Use COVARIATE to specify covariates in a fully factorial design.

```
>CATEGORY A=2 B=3
>COVARIATE X
>ANOVA Y
>ESTIMATE
```
This ANOCOVA includes factor (A,B) by covariate (X) interactions, which test the assumption of homogeneity of regression slopes.

Saving residuals

Use a SAVE command before MODEL or ANOVA to save residuals in a file. MYSTAT saves model variables, estimated values, residuals, and standard error of prediction as the variables ESTIMATE, RESIDUAL, and SEPRED. When you use SAVE with a linear model, MYSTAT lists cases with extreme studentized residuals or leverage values and prints the Durbin-Watson and autocorrelation statistics.

```
>SAVE RESIDS
>MODEL Y=CONSTANT+X+Z
>ESTIMATE
```

```
>SAVE RESID2
>CATEGORY SEX=2
>ANOVA SALARY
>ESTIMATE
```

You can USE the residuals file to analyze your residuals with MYSTAT's statistical and graphic routines.

Non-parametric tests

SIGN computes a sign test on all pairs of specified variables, omitting zero differences.

SIGN <varlist>	Sign tests on each pairing of the variables specified.
SIGN	Sign tests on all pairs of numeric variables in the file.
SIGN A B C	Sign tests on A and B, A and C, and B and C.

WILCOXON calculates a Wilcoxon signed-rank test on all pairs of specified variables, omitting zero differences and averaging ties.

WILCOXON <varlist>	Wilcoxon signed-rank tests on each pairing of the variables specified.
SIGN	Wilcoxon signed-rank tests on all pairs of numeric variables in the file.
SIGN A B C	Wilcoxon signed-rank tests on A and B, A and C, and B and C.

FRIEDMAN computes a two-way Friedman nonparametric analysis of variance, averaging tied ranks.

FRIEDMAN <varlist>	Friedman tests on each pairing of the variables specified.
SIGN	Friedman tests on all pairs of numeric variables in the file.
SIGN A B C	Friedman tests on A and B, A and C, and B and C.

Graphics

Use the CHARSET command to choose the type of graphic characters to be used for printing and screen display. If you have IBM screen or printer graphic characters, use GRAPHICS; if not, use GENERIC. The GENERIC setting uses characters like +, −, and |.

```
CHARSET GRAPHICS        For IBM graphic characters.
CHARSET GENERIC         For any screen or printer.
```

Scatterplots

PLOT draws a two-way scatterplot of one or more Y variables on a vertical scale against an X variable on a horizontal scale. Use different plotting symbols to distinguish Y variables.

```
PLOT <yvar1>…*<xvar>        Plots <yvar(s)> against <xvar>.
  /SYMBOL=<var$> | '<char>'  Use character variable values or character
                               string as plotting symbol.
  YMAX=<#> YMIN=<#> XMAX=<#>  Specify range of X and Y values.
    XMIN=<#>
  LINES=<#>                  Specify number of screen lines for graph.
PLOT A*B/SYMBOL='*'         Uses asterisk as plotting symbol.
PLOT A*B/SYMBOL=SEX$        Uses SEX$ values for plotting symbol.
PL Y1 Y2*X/SY='1','2'       Plot Y1 points as 1 and Y2 points as 2.
PLOT A*B/LINES=40           Limits graph size to 40 lines on screen.
```

For example, we can plot LOGPOP against RAINFALL using the first letter of the values of CITY$ for plotting symbols.

```
>PLOT LOGPOP*RAINFALL/SYMBOL=CITY$
```

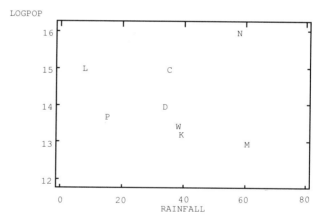

The SYMBOL option is powerful. If you are plotting several Y variables, you can label each variable by specifying its own plotting symbol.

```
>PLOT Y1 Y2*X/SYMBOL='1','2'
```

Or, you can name a character variable to plot each point with the first letter of the variable's value for the corresponding case:

```
>PLOT WEIGHT*AGE/SYMBOL=SEX$
```

Box-and-whisker plots

BOX produces box-and-whisker plots. Include an asterisk and a grouping variable for grouped box plots.

BOX <var1>...[*<gvar>]	[Grouped] box plots of the variables.
/GROUPS=<#>,	Show only the first <#> groups.
MIN=<#> MAX=<#>	Specify scale limits.
BOX	Box plots of every numeric variable.
BOX SALARY	Box plot of SALARY only.
BOX SALARY*RANK	Grouped box plots of SALARY by RANK
BOX INCOME*STATE$/GR=10	Box plots of first 10 groups only

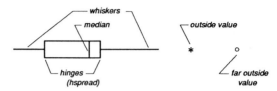

The center line of the box marks the *median*. The edges of the box show the upper and lower *hinges*. The median splits the ordered batch of numbers in half and the hinges split these halves in half again. The distance between the hinges is called the *Hspread*. The *whiskers* show the range of points within 1.5 Hspreads of the hinges. Points outside this range are marked by asterisks and those more than 3 Hspreads from the hinges are marked with circles.

Histograms

HISTOGRAM displays histograms for one or more variables.

HISTOGRAM <var1> ...	Histograms of variables specified
/BARS=<#>	Limits the number of bars used.
SCALE,	Forces round cutpoints between bars.
MIN=<#> MAX=<#>	Specifies scale limits.
HISTOGRAM	Histograms of every numeric variable.
HISTOGRAM A B/BARS=18	Forces 18 bars for histograms of A and B.
HIST A/MIN=0 MAX=10	Histogram of A with scale from 0 to 20.

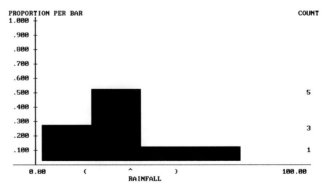

A histogram shows the *distribution* of a variable. The data are divided into equal-sized intervals along the horizontal axis. The number of values in each interval is represented by a vertical bar. The height of each bar is measured two ways: the right axis shows the number of cases, and the left axis shows the proportion of the sample in each bar.

Stem-and-leaf
diagrams

STEM plots a stem-and-leaf diagram.

```
STEM <var1>..                    Diagrams of variables specified.
   /LINES=<#>                    Specify number of lines in diagram.
STEM                             Stem-and-leaf of every numeric variable.
STEM TAX                         Stem-and-leaf of TAX.
STEM TAX/LINES=20                Stem-and-leaf with 20 lines.
```

The numbers on the left side are *stems* (the most significant digits in which variation occurs) . The *leaves* (the subsequent digits) are printed on the right. For example, in the following plot, the stems are 10's digits and the leaves are 1's digits.

```
         STEM AND LEAF PLOT OF VARIABLE: RAINFALL, N =    48

MINIMUM IS:         7.000
LOWER HINGE IS:        26.500
MEDIAN IS:       36.000
UPPER HINGE IS:        43.000
MAXIMUM IS:        60.000

                        0   78
                        1   0114
                        1   55556
                        2
                        2 H 588
                        3   00113333
                        3 M 5557999
                        4 H 001123333
                        4   55567999
                        5   0
                        5   9
                        6   0
```

(We added 40 more cases to the dataset for this plot. You will get a different plot if you try this example with the CITIES.SYS data file.)

Hinges are defined under "Box-and-whisker plots," above.

Time series
plots

TPLOT produces time series plots, which plot a variable against Case (time). TPLOT's STANDARDIZE option removes the series mean from each value and divides each by the standard deviation. MYSTAT uses the first fifteen cases unless you specify otherwise with the LAG option.

```
TPLOT <var>                      Case plot of variable specified.
   /LAG=<#>                      Plots first <#> cases.
   STANDARDIZE,                  Standardizes before plotting.
   MIN=<#>,MAX=<#>               Sets scale limits.
TPLOT                            Case plot of first numeric variable.
TPLOT PRICE/LAG=10               First 10 cases of PRICE.
TPLOT PRICE/STAN                 Standardizes before plotting.
```

Submitting files of commands

You can operate MYSTAT in batch mode, where MYSTAT executes a series of commands from a file and you sit back and watch. (You've already seen a command file in action: the DEMO demonstration uses a file of commands, DEMO.CMD.)

The SUBMIT command reads commands from a file and executes the commands as though they were typed from the keyboard. Command files must have a ".CMD" file extension.

Use a word processor to create a file of commands—one command per line, with no extraneous characters. Save the file as a text (ASCII) file. (Use the command "COPY CON BATCH.CMD" and [F6] to type commands into a file if you have no word processor.)

```
SUBMIT <filename>        Submits file of commands.
SUBMIT COMMANDS          Reads commands from COMMANDS.CMD.
SUBMIT B:NEWJOB          Reads commands from file on drive B.
```

Redirecting output

Ordinarily, MYSTAT sends its results to the screen. OUTPUT routes *subsequent* output to an ASCII file or a printer.

```
OUTPUT *                 Sends output to the screen only
OUTPUT @                 Sends output to the screen and the printer.
OUTPUT <filename>        Sends output to the screen and a text file.
```

MYSTAT adds a .DAT suffix to ASCII files produced by OUTPUT. You must use OUTPUT *or QUIT the program to stop redirecting.

Printing and saving analysis results

To print analysis results, use OUTPUT @ before doing the analysis or analyses. Use OUTPUT <filename> to save analysis results in a file. Use OUTPUT * to turn saving or printing off when you are finished.

Printing data or variable names

You can print your data by using OUTPUT @ and then using the LIST command. Use LIST <var1>... to print only certain variables. Don't forget to turn printing off when you are done.

You can print your variable names by using OUTPUT @ and then NAMES. Don't forget to turn printing off when you are done.

**Putting
comments in
output**

NOTE allows you to write comments in your output. Surround each line with quotation marks, and issue another NOTE command for additional lines:

```
>NOTE 'Following are descriptive statistics for the POP'
>NOTE "and RAINFALL variables of the CITIES dataset."
>STATS POP RAINFALL
TOTAL OBSERVATIONS:  8

                            POP      RAINFALL

N OF CASES              8         8
MINIMUM         346865.000     7.810
MAXIMUM        7164742.000    60.020
MEAN           2064361.375    35.520
STANDARD DEV   2335788.226    18.032
>NOTE "Note that the average annual rainfall for these"
>NOTE 'cities is 35.52 inches.'
```

**Saving data
in text files**

You can save datasets to ASCII text files with the PUT command. PUT saves the current dataset in a plain text file suitable for use with most other programs. Text files have a .DAT extension.

```
USE <filename>                 Opens the dataset to be exported
PUT <filename>                 Saves the dataset as a text file
```

Note that the PUT command is *not* an Editor command. To save a newly created dataset in a plain text file, you must QUIT from the Editor, USE the datafile, and finally PUT the data in an ASCII file.

```
>EDIT
[editing session here]
>SAVE A:NEWSTUFF
>QUIT
>USE A:NEWSTUFF
>PUT A:NEWTEXT
```

The above commands would create a plain ASCII file called NEWTEXT.DAT on the A disk.

Index of commands

This index lists all of MYSTAT's commands and the Editor commands

Editor commands

DELETE	delete a row (case)
DROP	drop a column (variable)
Esc key	toggle between command line and worksheet
FIND	find a particular data value
FORMAT	set number of decimal places in Editor
GET	read data from an ASCII file
HELP	get help for Editor commands
IF...THEN	conditionally transform or create a variable
LET	transform or create a variable
NEW	create a new data file
QUIT	quit the Editor and return to MYSTAT
REPEAT	fill cases with missing values
SAVE	save data in a data file
USE	read a data file into Editor

MYSTAT commands

ANOVA	analysis of variance
BOX	box-and-whisker plot
CATEGORY	specify factors for ANOVA
CHARSET	choose type of characters for graphs
COVARIATE	specify covariate term for ANOCOVA
DEMO	demonstration of MYSTAT
EDIT	edit a new or existing data file
ESTIMATE	start computations for regression
FORMAT	set number of decimal places in output
FRIEDMAN	Friedman nonparametric analysis of variance
HELP	get help for MYSTAT commands
HISTOGRAM	draw histogram
LIST	display data values
MENU	turn the command menu on/off
MODEL	specify a regression model
NAMES	display variable names
NOTE	put comment in output
OUTPUT	redirect output to printer or text file
PEARSON	Pearson correlation matrix
PLOT	scatterplot (X-Y plot)
PUT	save data in text file
QUIT	quit the MYSTAT program
RANK	rank data
SAVE	save results in a file
SIGN	sign test
SORT	sort data
STATS	descriptive statistics
STEM	stem-and-leaf diagram
SUBMIT	submit a batch file of commands
SYSTAT	get information about SYSTAT
TABULATE	one-way or multi-way tables
TPLOT	case plot
TTEST	independent and dependent t-tests
USE	read a data file for analysis
WEIGHT	weight data
WILCOXON	Wilcoxon signed-rank test

Index

Numbers followed by *f* indicate a figure; *t* following a page number indicates tabular material.